...edg...
...essi...

Recent Advances

Cardio...

15

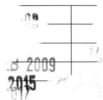

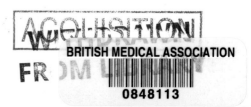

Recent Advances in Cardiology 14
Edited by Derek J Rowlands and Bernard Clarke

ISBN   978–1–85315–715–8

Recent Advances in

Cardiology
15

Edited by

Derek J Rowlands BSc MD FRCP FACC FESC

Honorary Consultant Cardiologist, Manchester Heart Centre,
Manchester Royal Infirmary, Manchester, UK.
Consultant Cardiologist, Alexandra Hospital,
The Beeches Consulting Centre, Cheadle, Cheshire, UK

Bernard Clarke BSc MD FRCP(Lond.) FRCP(Edin.) FESC FACC

Consultant Cardiologist, Manchester Heart Centre, Manchester
Royal Infirmary, Central Manchester and Manchester Children's
University Hospitals NHS Trust, Manchester, UK.
Honorary Lecturer in Medicine, University of
Manchester, UK

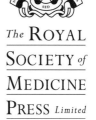

The ROYAL
SOCIETY *of*
MEDICINE
PRESS *Limited*

Published by the Royal Society of Medicine Press Ltd
1 Wimpole Street, London W1G 0AE, UK
Tel: +44 (0)20 7290 2921
Fax: +44 (0)20 7290 2929
Email: publishing@rsm.ac.uk
Website: www.rsmpress.co.uk

British Library Cataloguing in Publication Data
A catalogue record for this book is available from the British Library
ISBN 978–1–85315–729–5

Distribution in Europe and Rest of World:

Marston Book Services Ltd
PO Box 269, Abingdon
Oxon OX14 4YN, UK
Tel: +44 (0)1235 465500
Fax: +44 (0)1235 465555
Email: direct.order@marston.co.uk

Distribution in the USA and Canada:

Royal Society of Medicine Press Ltd
c/o BookMasters Inc
30 Amberwood Parkway
Ashland, OH 44805, USA
Tel: +1 800 247 6553/+1 800 266 5564
Fax: +1 419 281 6883
Email: order@bookmasters.com

Distribution in Australia and New Zealand:

Elsevier Australia
30–52 Smidmore Street
Marrickville NSW 2204, Australia
Tel: +61 2 9517 8999
Fax: +61 2 9517 2249
Email: service@elsevier.com.au

Editorial services and typesetting by BA & GM Haddock, Ford, Midlothian, UK
Printed in Great Britain by Bell & Bain, Glasgow, UK

Contents

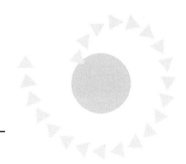

Contributors

Yvonne Alexander BSc PhD
Lecturer and Postgrduate Tutor in Cardiovascular Medicine, Cardiovascular
Research Group, School of Clinical and Laboratory Sciences, University of
Manchester, Manchester, UK

Emma J. Birks MRCP PhD
Consultant Cardiologist in Transplantation and Mechanical Circulatory Support,
Royal Brompton and Harefield NHS Trust, Harefield, Middlesex, UK

Isabelle Boutron MD PhD
INSERM U738, Paris, France; Université Paris 7 Denis Diderot, UFR de Médecine,
Paris, France; AP-HP, Hôpital Bichat, Département d'Epidémiologie,
Biostatistique et Recherche Clinique, Paris, France

Hee Cheol Cho PhD
Program Manager, Excigen, Inc., Baltimore, Maryland, USA

Jeremy P.R. Dick MA MB BChir PhD FRCP
Clinical Director of Greater Manchester Neuroscience Centre; Movement Disorder
Neurologist and Lead Neurologist at South Manchester University Hospital
Foundation Trust.

Kim A. Eagle MD FACC
Cardiovascular Center, University of Michigan Health Services, Ann Arbor,
Michigan, USA

Finn G. Farquharson MBBS MSc FRCR
Consultant Vascular Radiologist, Manchester Royal Infirmary, Manchester, UK

Richard Grocott-Mason MD FRCP
Consultant Cardiologist, Hillingdon Hospital, Uxbridge, Middlesex, UK

Anthony Heagerty MD FRCP FMedSci
Professor of Medicine, Cardiovascular Research Group, School of Clinical and
Laboratory Sciences, University of Manchester, Manchester, UK

Charles Ilsley FRCP FRACP
Director of Cardiology, Harefield Hospital, Harfield, Middlesex, UK

Petra Jenkins MB ChB MRCP
Specialist Registrar in Cardiology, Manchester Heart Centre, Manchester Royal Infirmary, Manchester, UK

Daniel Keenan BSc MB BCh FRCS
Consultant Cardiothoracic Surgeon, Manchester Royal Infirmary, Manchester, UK

Niall G. Keenan BM BCh MRCP
Research Fellow, Cardiovascular Magnetic Resonance Unit, Royal Brompton Hospital, London, UK

Wei C. Lau MD
Cardiovascular Center, University of Michigan Health Services, Ann Arbor, Michigan, USA

Vaikom S. Mahadevan MD MRCP
Consultant Cardiologist and Interventionist in Adult Congenital Heart Disease, Manchester Heart Centre, Manchester Royal Infirmary, Manchester, UK

Eduardo Marbán MD PhD
Heart Institute, Cedars-Sinai Medical Center, Los Angeles, California, USA

K. Edward McLaughlin MD FRCS
Consultant Cardiothoracic Surgeon, Manchester Heart Centre, Manchester Royal Infirmary, Manchester, UK

James B. Meigs MD MPH
Associate Professor of Medicine, Harvard Medical School; Associate Physician, General Medicine Division, Department of Medicine, Massachusetts General Hospital Boston, Massachusetts, USA

Gregory J. Mishkel MD
Prairie Education & Research Cooperative, Prairie Heart Institute of St John's Hospital, Springfield, Illinois, USA

Anna L. Moore MPH
Prairie Education & Research Cooperative, Prairie Heart Institute of St John's Hospital, Springfield, Illinois, USA

Philip R. Moore MRCP PhD
SpR in Cardiology, Harefield Hospital, Royal Brompton and Harefield NHS Trust, Harefield, Middlesex, UK

Dudley J. Pennell MD FRCP FESC FACC
Director Cardiovascular Magnetic Resonance Unit, Royal Brompton Hospital, London, UK and Professor, Imperial College, London UK

Amanda M. Pfeiffer BS
Prairie Education & Research Cooperative, Prairie Heart Institute of St John's Hospital, Springfield, Illinois, USA

Derek J. Rowlands BSc MD FRCP FACC FESC
Honorary Consultant Cardioloist, Manchester Heart Centre, Manchester Royal Infirmary, Manchester, UK. Consultant Cardiologist, Alexandra Hospital, The Beeches Consulting Centre, Cheadle, Cheshire, UK

Martin K. Rutter MD FRCP
Consultant Physician and Honorary Senior Lecturer, Cardiovascular Research
Group, Division of Cardiovascular and Endocrine Sciences, University of
Manchester and Manchester Diabetes Centre, Manchester Royal Infirmary,
Manchester, UK

Marc E. Shelton MD
Prairie Cardiovascular Consultants Ltd, Springfield, Illinois, USA

Philippe Gabriel Steg MD FESC FACC FCCP
Professor, INSERM U-698 et Université Paris VII – Denis Diderot, Hôpital Bichat-
Claude Bernard; Assistance Publique, Hôpitaux de Paris, Paris, France

Jane E. Wainwright MD MRCP
Clinical Governance Lead for the Greater Manchester Neuroscience Centre
Neurologists and Consultant Neurologist, Hope Hospital, Salford, UK

John G. Webb MD
McLeod Professor of Heart Valve Interventions, University of British Columbia;
Director Cardiac Catheterization, Division of Cardiology, St Paul's Hospital,
Vancouver, British Columbia, Canada

Peter W.F. Wilson MD
Professor of Medicine and Public Health Emory University; Director of
Epidemiology and Genomic Medicine, Altanta VA Medical Centre, GA, USA

Eduardo Marbán Hee Cheol Cho

1

Gene and cell therapy for cardiac arrhythmias

Cardiac rhythm disorders are caused by malfunctions of impulse generation and/or conduction. Present therapies span a wide array of approaches but remain largely palliative. Progress in understanding the underlying biology opens up new prospects for better alternatives to the present routine. Here, we review the current state of the art in gene- and cell-based approaches to correct cardiac rhythm disturbances. These include gene therapy for atrial fibrillation, genetic suppression of an ionic current, stem-cell therapies, an adult somatic cell-fusion approach, novel synthetic pacemaker channels, and creating a self-contained pacemaker in non-excitable cells. We then conclude by discussing advantages and disadvantages of the new possibilities.

The heart requires a steady rhythm and rate in order to fulfil its physiological role as the pump for the circulation. An excessively rapid heart rate (tachycardia) allows insufficient time for the mechanical events of ventricular emptying and filling. Cardiac output drops, the lungs become congested and, in the extreme, the circulation collapses. An equally morbid chain of events ensues if the heart beats too slowly (bradycardia). Serious disturbances of cardiac rhythm, known as arrhythmias, afflict more than 3 million Americans and account for > 479,000 deaths annually.[1] In 2001, $2.7 billion ($6634 per discharge) was paid to Medicare beneficiaries for cardiac arrhythmia-related diseases.[1]

Current therapy has serious limitations: anti-arrhythmic drugs can sometimes be effective, but their utility is limited by their propensity to create new arrhythmias while suppressing others.[2–5] Ablation of targeted tissue can readily cure simple wiring errors, but is less effective in treating more complex

Eduardo Marbán MD PhD
Heart Institute, 8700 Beverly Blvd, Cedars-Sinai Medical Center, Los Angeles, CA 90048, USA
E-mail: eduardo.marban@csmc.edu

Hee Cheol Cho PhD
Program Manager, Excigen, Inc., 6200 Seaforth Street, Baltimore, MD 21224, USA.
E-mail: heecheol@exigen.com

and common arrhythmias, such as atrial fibrillation or ventricular tachycardia.[6,7] Implantable devices can serve as surrogate pacemakers to sustain heart rate, or as defibrillators to treat excessively rapid rhythms. Such devices are expensive, and implantation involves a number of acute and chronic risks (pulmonary collapse, bacterial infection, lead or generator failure[8]). In short, arrhythmias are a serious threat of public health proportions, and current treatment is inadequate. Given these limitations, we have begun to develop biological therapies as alternatives to conventional treatment.

The most obvious application of gene therapy is to correct monogenic deficiency disorders such as haemophilia or severe combined immuno-deficiency syndrome. Indeed, the latter is the only disease to have been cured (in a few infants) by gene therapy.[9] Gene therapy for cardiovascular disorders, as it is most commonly being developed today, focuses not on correcting deficiency disorders but rather on attempts to foster angiogenesis in ischaemic myocardium,[10,11] or to suppress vascular stenosis in a variety of iatrogenic settings.[12,13] The concept of gene or cell therapy for cardiac arrhythmias differs conceptually from conventional applications. We seek to achieve functional re-engineering of cardiac tissue, so as to alter a specific electrical property of the tissue in a salutary manner. For example, genes or cells are introduced to alter the velocity of electrical conduction in a defined region of the heart, or to create a spontaneously-active biological pacemaker from normally-quiescent myocardium. A relevant analogy is the use of off-the-shelf or customised parts to improve the performance of a lacklustre automobile engine. Our 'parts' are wild-type (or mutant) genes and engineered cells; our engine is the heart.

Here we will review our progress in two areas: the treatment of atrial fibrillation, and the creation of biological pacemakers. The reader is referred to the original articles describing the work for more details. We then conclude by considering future directions of this type of gene therapy.

ATRIAL FIBRILLATION

Atrial fibrillation affects more than 2 million people in the US, including 5–10% of people over the age of 65 years and 10–35% of the 5 million patients with congestive heart failure.[14] Accepted therapy for atrial fibrillation includes either anti-arrhythmic drugs to maintain sinus rhythm, or drugs which suppress conduction in the atrioventricular node to control the ventricular rate. Although appealing, the maintenance of sinus rhythm is often unsuccessful. Within 1 year of conversion to sinus rhythm, 25–50% of patients revert to atrial fibrillation in spite of anti-arrhythmic drug treatment.[15] The usual long-term clinical scenario, then, is to accept the inevitability of chronic atrial fibrillation and focus on ventricular rate control. The equivalence of rate and rhythm control strategies in asymptomatic patients was recently confirmed in AFFIRM and RACE, two multicentre clinical trials.[16]

Medical therapies to control heart rate during atrial fibrillation have targeted the conduction properties of the atrioventricular node by suppressing the calcium current (calcium channel blockers) or by affecting the balance of adrenergic and cholinergic tone (β-blockers and digoxin). For patients with normal ventricular function, atrioventricular nodal suppressing drugs reduce the heart rate by 15–30%,[15] but the frequent side-effects of these drugs include

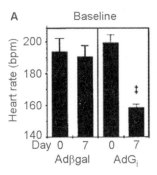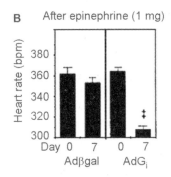

Fig. 1 Ventricular rate after induction of atrial fibrillation in a porcine model. The heart rate was measured during acutely induced atrial fibrillation at baseline and 7 days after atrioventricular nodal gene transfer of β-galactosidase (control) or $G\alpha_{i2}$. (A) Drug-free state; (B) after 1 mg epinephrine intravenously.

bronchospasm, hypotension, depression, fatigue, and constipation.[17] When atrioventricular nodal blocking drugs are not tolerated or not effective, the only remaining option is radiofrequency ablation of the atrioventricular node and implantation of a pacemaker. We evaluated the possibility of gene transfer-mediated control of the ventricular rate during atrial fibrillation.[18] In a porcine model of acute atrial fibrillation, we delivered recombinant adenoviruses containing a gene for the a subunit of the inhibitory G protein ($G\alpha_{i2}$) into the atrioventricular nodal artery. This transgene was chosen following the premise that overexpression of $G\alpha_{i2}$ would suppress basal adenylate cyclase activity and, thereby, indirectly suppress calcium channel activity in the atrioventricular node. The efficiency of gene transfer was optimised by pretreatment with nitroglycerin, vascular endothelial growth factor, and sildenafil.[19,20] Slightly less than half of all cells in the atrioventricular node showed evidence of gene transfer, and Western blot analysis documented a 6-fold overexpression of $G\alpha_{i2}$. Gene transfer occurred rarely (< 1% of cells) throughout the rest of the heart and the body. The transgene had obvious phenotypic consequences which were evident by measuring various indices of cardiac conduction. During sinus rhythm, the treatment group had evidence of conduction slowing and increased refractoriness in the atrioventricular node. In atrial fibrillation, the heart rate was reduced by 20% when compared to controls (Fig. 1). The relative decrease in heart rate persisted after the application of a β-adrenergic agonist. Since these results were obtained using clinically-available catheters and equipment, translation to human therapy would be relatively straightforward. Major steps between the current state of development and clinical applicability include the use of longer-lasting, non-inflammatory vectors (such as adeno-associated virus), and tests of safety and efficacy in animal models of chronic atrial fibrillation.

BIOLOGICAL PACEMAKERS

BIOLOGICAL PACEMAKER BY I_{K1} KNOCKOUT

The pacemaker of the heart is normally encompassed within a small region known as the sino-atrial node. The sino-atrial node initiates the heartbeat, sustains the circulation and sets the rate and rhythm of cardiac contraction.[21] The working muscle of the heart (myocardium), comprising the pumping chambers known as the atria and the ventricles, is normally excited by pacemaker activity originating in the sino-atrial node. However, in the absence of such activity, the myocardium lacks spontaneous activity. Therefore, loss of specialised pacemaker cells in the sino-atrial node, as occurs in a variety of common diseases, results in circulatory collapse, necessitating the implantation of an electronic pacemaker.[22] Such devices are effective, but have a number of limitations, including expense and risk (chronic infection, pulmonary collapse, or even death). Moreover, electronic pacemakers are palliative rather than curative. To create an alternative to electronic pacemakers, we sought to render electrically-quiescent myocardium spontaneously active.

Our strategy to effect such a conversion was based upon the premise that ventricular myocardium contains all it requires to pace, but that pacing is normally suppressed by an expressed gene. The reasoning is as follows. In the early embryonic heart, each cell possesses intrinsic pacemaker activity. The mechanism of spontaneous beating in the early embryo is remarkably simple.[23] The opening of L-type calcium channels produces depolarisation; the subsequent voltage-dependent opening of transient outward potassium channels leads to repolarisation. With further development, the heart differentiates into specialised functional regions, each with its own distinctive electrical signature. The atria and ventricles become electrically quiescent; only a small number of pacemaker cells, within compact 'nodes', set the overall rate and rhythm. Nevertheless, there is reason to wonder whether pacemaker activity may be latent within adult ventricular myocytes and masked by the differential expression of other ionic currents. Among these, the inward rectifier potassium current (I_{K1}) is notable for its intense expression in electrically-quiescent atria and ventricle, and for its absence in nodal pacemaker cells. I_{K1}, encoded by the Kir2 gene family,[24] stabilises a strongly negative resting potential and, thereby, would be expected to suppress excitability. We thus explored the possibility that dominant-negative suppression of Kir2-encoded inward rectifier potassium channels in the ventricle would suffice to produce spontaneous, rhythmic, electrical activity.

Replacement of three critical residues in the pore region of Kir2.1 by alanines (GYG144–146→AAA, or Kir2.1AAA) creates a dominant-negative construct.[25] The GYG motif plays a key role in ion selectivity and pore function.[26] Kir2.1AAA and GFP were packaged into a bicistronic adenoviral vector (AdEGI–Kir2.1AAA) and injected into the left ventricular cavity of guinea pigs during transient cross-clamp of the great vessels.[27] This method of delivery sufficed to achieve transduction of ~20% of ventricular myocytes. Myocytes isolated 3–4 days after *in vivo* transduction with Kir2.1AAA exhibited ~80% suppression of I_{K1}, but the L-type calcium current was unaffected.

Non-transduced (non-green) left ventricular myocytes isolated from AdEGI–Kir2.1AAA-injected animals, as well as green cells from AdEGI-injected hearts, exhibited no spontaneous activity, but fired single action potentials in response to depolarising external stimuli (Fig. 2A). In contrast, Kir2.1AAA myocytes exhibited either of two phenotypes: (i) a stable resting

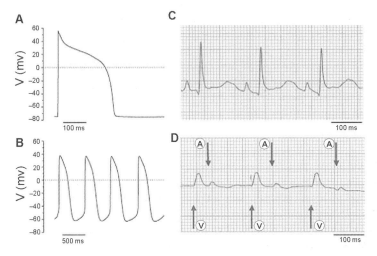

Fig. 2 Suppression of Kir2.1 channels unmasks latent pacemaker activity in ventricular cells. (A) Action potentials evoked by depolarising external stimuli in control ventricular myocytes. (B) Spontaneous action potentials in Kir2.1AAA-transduced myocytes with depressed I_{K1}. (C) Baseline electrocardiograms in normal sinus rhythm. (D) Ventricular rhythms 72 h after gene transfer of Kir2.1AAA. P waves (A and arrow) and wide QRS complexes (V and arrow) march through to their own rhythm.

potential from which prolonged action potentials could be elicited by external stimuli (7 of 22 cells, not shown); or (ii) spontaneous activity (Fig. 2B). The spontaneous activity, which was seen in all cells in which I_{K1} was suppressed below 0.4 pA/pF (at –50 mV; compared to. > 1.5 pA/pF in controls, or 0.4–1.5 pA/pF in non-pacing Kir2.1AAA cells), resembles that of genuine pacemaker cells; the maximum diastolic potential (–60.7 ± 2.1 mV; n = 15 of 22 Kir2.1AAA cells; $P < 0.05$ t-test) is relatively depolarised, with repetitive, regular and incessant electrical activity initiated by gradual 'phase 4' depolarisation and a slow upstroke.[21,28] Kir2.1AAA pacemaker cells responded to β-adrenergic stimulation (isoproterenol) just as sino-atrial nodal cells do, increasing their pacing rate.[28,29]

Electrocardiography revealed two phenotypes *in vivo*. What we most often observed was simple prolongation of the QT interval (not shown). Nevertheless, 40% of the animals exhibited an altered cardiac rhythm indicative of spontaneous ventricular foci. In normal sinus rhythm, every P wave is succeeded by a QRS complex (Fig. 2C). In two of five animals after transduction with Kir2.1AAA, premature beats of ventricular origin can be distinguished by their broad amplitude, and can be seen to 'march through' to a beat independent of, and more rapid than, that of the physiological sinus pacemaker (Fig. 2D). In these proof-of-concept experiments, the punctate transduction required for pacing occurred by chance rather than by design, in that the distribution of the transgene throughout the ventricles was not controlled. Nevertheless, ectopic beats, arising from foci of induced pacemakers, cause the entire heart to be paced from the ventricle.

Our findings provide new insights into the biological basis of pacemaker activity. The conventional wisdom postulates that pacemaker activity requires the highly localised expression in nodal cells of 'pacemaker genes', such as those of the HCN family,[30] although an important role for I_{K1} has also been recognised.[28] Exposure to barium induces automaticity in ventricular muscle and myocytes because of its time- and voltage-dependent block of I_{K1}.[31,32] However, barium also permeates L-type calcium channels in mixed solutions of Ca^{2+} (4 mM) and Ba^{2+} (1 mM)[33] and slows their inactivation,[34] effects which make it difficult to interpret barium-induced automaticity strictly in terms of I_{K1}. Our dominant-negative approach is durable and regionally-specific; the barium effect is not.

Thus, the specific suppression of Kir2 channels suffices to unleash pacemaker activity in ventricular myocytes. The crucial factor for pacing is the absence of the strongly polarising I_{K1}, rather than the presence of special genes (although such genes may play an important modulatory role in genuine pacemaker cells).[35] In addition to the conceptual insight into the genesis of pacing, our work implies that localised delivery of constructs such as Kir2.1AAA to the myocardium may be useful in the creation of biological pacemakers for therapeutic purposes. Focal injection into an area of the ventricle, possibly via an endocardial injection catheter, would be a logical means of trying to reduce this concept to practice in a larger animal.

BIOLOGICAL PACEMAKER DERIVED FROM HUMAN EMBRYONIC STEM CELLS

Human embryonic stem cells (hESCs) are pluripotent, clonogenic, and self-propagating.[36] Their versatility makes them one of the most effective supplies for cell-based therapies. Previous studies have demonstrated that spontaneously beating aggregates of myocytes, called embryoid bodies, could be generated from hESCs.[37–40] Although these spontaneously beating human embryoid bodies can be derived from hESCs *in vitro*, they need to integrate with recipient tissue in a syncytium in order to serve as a biological pacemaker. Thus, we set out to test if the spontaneously contracting human embryoid bodies could integrate with a host tissue and thus be used as biological pacemakers.[41] First, the hESCs were stably transduced with a lentiviral construct expressing GFP as a reporter in order to distinguish them from the recipient cells by fluorescence. An *in vitro* transplantation model was developed in which a single hESC-derived, spontaneously beating human embryoid body (about 500 µm in diameter) was transplanted on top of a quiescent monolayer of neonatal rat ventricular myocytes (NRVMs) serving as the recipient. After 2–3 days of co-culture, synchronous rhythmic contractions of the GFP-expressing human embryoid body and NRVM monolayer were observed at a rate of 49 ± 4 bpm ($n = 14$), which was similar to that of a spontaneously contracting human embryoid body cultured alone (Fig. 3A). Observing that the transplanted human embryoid body spontaneously contracted with the co-cultured NRVMs, we sought to examine the origin of conduction. Extracellular field potential recordings by multi-electrode array localised the site of pacemaker activity: rhythmic extracellular depolarisations were initiated from a region corresponding to the human embryoid body-transplantation site and spread to the rest of the NRVM monolayer. High-resolution optical mapping further revealed a consistent time delay in action potentials recorded from the human embryoid body to a region of NRVMs

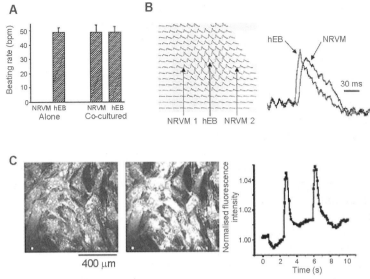

Fig. 3 (A) Spontaneously beating human embryoid body outgrowth, which stably expresses GFP, was microdissected and transplanted onto quiescent monolayer of NRVMs. Beating rate of spontaneously contracting human embryoid body exhibited similar beating rates before (alone, 47 ± 5 bpm) and after (co-cultured, 49 ± 4 bpm) transplantation onto monolayer of NRVMs. (B) Optical action potentials were mapped with a voltage-sensitive dye by photodiode array focused on a region containing spontaneously beating human embryoid body transplanted on a quiescent NRVM monolayer (left). NRVM1 and NRVM2 represent two distinct sites at 3.2 mm and 3.6 mm, respectively, away from pacing origin. Superimposed optical action potential profiles demonstrate delay of activation and slower rate of depolarisation of NRVMs (right). (C) Ca^{2+}-transient recording from NRVMs located 1 cm away from transplanted, beating human embryoid body, with rhod-2AM as indicator before (left) and during (middle) spontaneous contraction. Normalised fluorescence intensity was measured over 10 s in co-culture (right).

away from the transplantation site (Fig. 3B). Collectively, these observations demonstrated that the transplanted human embryoid bodies functioned as biological pacemakers driving the contraction of the recipient cells.

Since the co-culture system involved direct physical contact between the transplanted human embryoid bodies and the host NRVMs, it is possible that the rhythmic contraction of the whole co-culture was due to secondary effects rather than electrical conduction of pacemaker activity from the human embryoid bodies. We examined if influences such as electric field potential changes,[42] paracrine effects, or mechanical coupling were responsible for the electrical activities in the NRVM. First, when human embryoid bodies on a permeable plastic membrane were co-cultured with NRVMs without any physical contact, rhythmic contractions were observed only in human embryoid bodies and not in the NRVM monolayer. This excluded paracrine effects or long-range field potential changes as likely factors. Second, the contractility observed in the co-cultured NRVMs was not due to mere mechanical movement transduced from the spontaneously contracting human embryoid body; spontaneous Ca^{2+} transients, not seen in otherwise quiescent NRVMs, could be recorded from co-cultured NRVMs > 1 cm away from the human embryoid body (Fig. 3C). Use of 2,3-butanedione monoxime is known

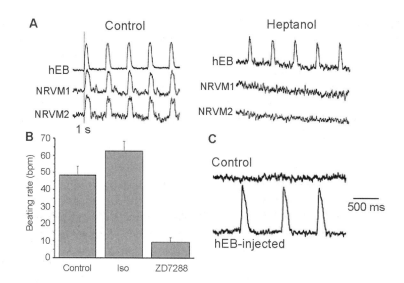

Fig. 4 (A) Gap-junction uncoupler heptanol reversibly eliminated action potential propagation to neighbouring NRVM sites but did not affect action potentials in pacing origin of human embryoid body at heptanol concentration of 0.4 mM. (B) β-Adrenergic stimulation with 1 μM isoproterenol (Iso) significantly accelerated spontaneous beating rate of human embryoid body ($P = 0.01$), whereas ZD7288 significantly attenuated the beating activity ($n = 9$ for each group). (C) Optical mapping of guinea pig left ventricle pre-injected with human embryoid bodies (bottom) or saline (top) after atrioventricular nodal cryo-ablation without external pacing.

to uncouple excitation–contraction coupling in myocytes.[43] Simultaneous contraction of the co-culture stopped altogether with an application of 1 mM 2,3-butanedione monoxime, but the electrical conduction persisted, eliminating mechanical coupling as a possible mechanism of electrical conduction from the human embryoid bodies to NRVMs.

How, then, are the spontaneous electrical depolarisations relayed to the neighbouring NRVMs? Gap-junction proteins are the molecular bridges for electrical communication between cardiac cells.[44,45] In order for the co-culture to contract spontaneously, the oscillating action potentials from the pacemaker (human embryoid body) need to communicate to the NRVMs via gap junctions. Immunostaining the co-culture with a primary antibody against the gap junction protein, connexin 43 showed expression of connexin 43 throughout human embryoid body and NRVMs and along their contact surface, demonstrating the substrate for gap-junctional coupling between the two tissue types. Furthermore, an application of 0.4 mM heptanol, a blocker of gap-junction proteins,[46] eliminated the spontaneous contractions in the NRVMs co-cultured with human embryoid bodies (Fig. 4A). Taken together, the data indicate that the spread of pacemaker activity from the human embryoid bodies to the recipient tissue proceeds via gap-junctional coupling.

β-Adrenergic stimulation is a potent physiological mechanism to accelerate cardiac pacing.[47] We asked if the rhythmic contractions in the syncytium formed between human embryoid bodies and NRVMs could adapt its beating rates in response to a β-adrenergic agonist, isoproterenol. Indeed, the beating frequencies of the co-culture increased significantly, from 48 ± 5 to 63 ± 8 bpm, after washing in 1 μM isoproterenol ($P < 0.05$), consistent with a previous finding that β-adrenergic receptors are already expressed in hESC-derived cardiomyocytes.[38] On the other hand, the bradycardic agent ZD7288 is a specific blocker of the pacemaker ion channels, HCN,[48] and would slow down the beating rate of the co-culture if the human embryoid bodies expressed the pacemaker ion channels. Addition of 100 μM ZD7288 significantly reduced the beating rate of the co-culture by 5-fold (Fig. 4B; $P < 0.05$). Addition of either isoproterenol or ZD7288 did not affect quiescent NRVMs without engrafted human embryoid bodies. The synchronous beating could be terminated by crushing or surgically excising the transplanted human cells ($n = 17$; analogous to ablation), further proving that human embryoid body pacemakers were indeed the origin of pacing.

We then went on to examine the biological pacemaker activity in a whole heart by injecting spontaneously beating human embryoid bodies into the left ventricular anterior wall of a guinea pig *in vivo*. In order to distinguish ectopic ventricular beats originating from the site of injection from the animal's own sinus rhythm, the animal's endogenous sino-atrial nodal pacemaker activity was terminated by cryo-ablation of the atrioventricular node. Upon ablation, *ex vivo* optical mapping of control (uninjected or saline-injected) guinea pig hearts exhibited complete electrical silence throughout the entire left ventricle ($n = 6$). However, spontaneous action potentials could be readily recorded from the epicardial surface of left ventricle of animals that had been transplanted with spontaneously beating human embryoid bodies *in vivo* ($n = 4$; Fig. 4C). Furthermore, the spontaneous action potentials initiated from the injection site, the origin of the spread of action potentials in the epicardium, coincided with the injection site of the spontaneously beating human embryoid bodies, as identified by their GFP fluorescence.

Taken together, this study demonstrates that biological pacemakers derived from hESCs are capable of pacing recipient ventricular cardiomyocytes *in vitro* and myocardium *in vivo*.

ADULT STEM CELL-DERIVED BIOLOGICAL PACEMAKER

As an alternative cell source, we used adult cardiac stem cells in order to derive biological pacemakers. The heart had long been thought to be a terminally differentiated organ incapable of regeneration. The view held that the cardiomyocytes that we are born with during embryonic and fetal development do not grow in numbers but only in size. Only recently, has this dogma been challenged and refuted to form a new paradigm by the discovery of cardiac stem cells.[49–54] The heart is now regarded as a self-renewing organ in which myocyte regeneration occurs throughout the organism's life-span.[55]

We have established a straightforward isolation technique that allows the retrieval and amplification of $> 10^6$ human adult cardiac stem cells in less than 4 weeks from a single endomyocardial biopsy specimen.[56] The adult cardiac stem cells differentiated into cardiomyocytes with cardiac-specific markers. These adult stem cells self-aggregate to form three-dimensional structures termed cardiospheres and, upon co-culturing with rat ventricular myocytes, could differentiate into a spontaneously contracting cardiac tissue with innate pacemaker function.[56] The use of adult stem cells circumvents complications associated with human embryonic stem cells such as obvious ethical concerns,[57] immunogenic reactions against the donor cells,[58] and a visible degree of teratoma formation.[59] The autologous cell therapy using adult cardiac stem cells thus presents a unique possibility in developing biological pacemakers.

CREATION OF A BIOLOGICAL PACEMAKER BY CELL FUSION

In a previous study, human mesenchymal stem cells (hMSCs) transfected with a mouse pacemaker ion channel gene, mHCN2, were shown to induce spontaneous pacing when injected into canine left ventricular wall.[60] A key prerequisite to this approach is a high degree of gap-junctional coupling between the donor (hMSCs) and the host tissue. However, such gap-junctional coupling may or may not be stable over time. Indeed, many of the major forms of human heart disease with increased arrhythmic risk coincide with gap junction remodelling and decreased cell–cell coupling.[61] In addition, frequency-tuning of the stem cell-derived biological pacemaker would require further genetic manipulations. Thus, we explored the feasibility of converting normally-quiescent ventricular myocytes into pacemakers by somatic cell fusion.[62]

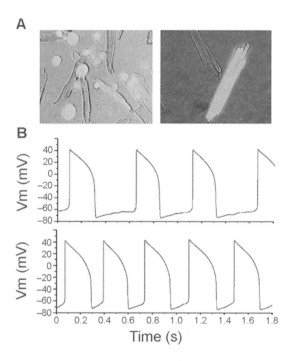

Fig. 5 (A) *In vitro* and *in vivo* fusion of myocytes with HCN1 fibroblasts. GFP-positive heterokaryons after *in vitro* (left) or *in vivo* (right) fusion of myocytes with HCN1 fibroblasts expressing GFP as a reporter. (B) Heterokaryon formed by *in vivo* fusion of HCN1 fibroblast and a myocyte displays spontaneous AP oscillations in normal Tyrode's medium (top). Presence of 1 mmol/l isoproterenol in the external solution increased the frequency of spontaneous action potential oscillation in the same heterokaryon (bottom).

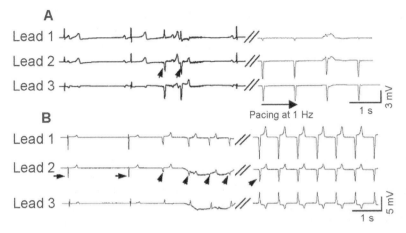

Fig. 6 ECGs from guinea pig hearts injected with HCN1 fibroblast cells. (A) The ectopic ventricular beats (diagonal arrows) are unleashed on slowing of the heart rate, which share the same polarity and morphology as the electrode-paced ECGs recorded at the site of HCN1 fibroblast injection. (B) In another animal, junctional escape rhythms (horizontal arrows) were overtaken by ectopic ventricular beats (diagonal arrows, 16 days after cell injection).

The idea was to create chemically-induced fusion between myocytes and syngeneic fibroblasts engineered to express pacemaker ion channels, HCN1. Upon establishing a guinea-pig lung fibroblast cell line stably expressing HCN1 channels with a GFP reporter (HCN1-fibroblasts), the fibroblasts were fused with freshly-isolated guinea-pig ventricular myocytes by using polyethylene glycol 1500 (PEG). In this study, a simple intracardiac, focal-injection of HCN1-fibroblasts suspended in 50% PEG into the apex of guinea-pig hearts verified *in vivo* fusion events (Fig. 5A). These heterokaryons formed by *in vivo* fusion of myocytes with HCN1-fibroblasts demonstrated pacemaker function by exhibiting spontaneous action potentials with a slow phase 4 depolarisation (Fig. 5B). *In vivo* biological pacemaker activities were also confirmed by electrocardiography in guinea pigs injected with HCN1-fibroblasts with PEG. In these animals, the biological pacemaker activity was demonstrated as early as 1 day after cell injection, and stable for at least 2 weeks after cell injection (Fig. 6).

The PEG-induced membrane fusion events have served as a model system to create mouse and human hybridomas,[63] to study eukaryotic cell–cell fusion events,[64] and to deliver outward K$^+$ currents into myocytes.[65] Furthermore, previous studies suggest that the *in vivo* fusion-induced heterokaryons can maintain the nuclei from each fusion partner separately and stably for at least several months.[66–69]

Straight injection of stem cells such as hMSC into heart does not guarantee that the injected cells will remain at the site of injection. Indeed, a recent study tracked the fate of hMSCs after injection into rat left ventricular free wall. One-hour after the cell injection, 50% of the injected cells were found to remain in the whole heart, and by 24-h post-injection, only 30% of the injected cells were found in the whole heart.[70] In contrast, the fusion approach implants the biological pacemakers to the site of injection by somatic cell fusion to cardiomyocytes thereby creating biological pacing at a specific site by design rather than by chance.

GENE TRANSFER OF A SYNTHETIC PACEMAKER CHANNEL INTO THE HEART

The HCN family of channel genes figures prominently in physiological automaticity,[71] and transfer of such genes into quiescent heart is an obvious way of creating a biological pacemaker. However, use of HCN genes may be confounded by unpredictable consequences of heteromultimerisation with multiple endogenous HCN family members in the target cell.[72,73] As I_f is expressed in ventricular myocytes and can contribute to arrhythmogenesis,[74,75] HCN gene transfer *in vivo* may have unpredicted consequences. Similarly, little flexibility with regard to frequency tuning would be achieved if the engineered pacemaker channels were to co-assemble with wild-type channels. A synthetic pacemaker channel with no affinity to co-assemble with HCN channels would circumvent

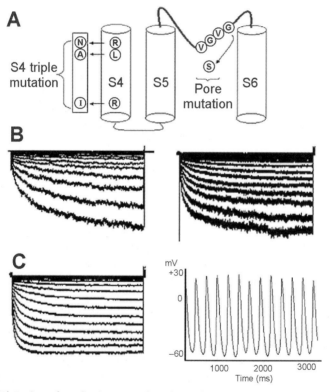

Fig. 7 (A) Design of synthetic pacemaker channel. To convert a human Kv1.4 channel into a pacemaker channel, three mutations (R447N, L448A, and R453I) in the S4 voltage-sensor and one pore mutation (G528S) were combined to render the channel activate upon depolarisation and permeate both Na+ and K+, respectively. (B) Representative raw current traces expressed from HEK cells expressing synthetic pacemaker channel (left) or wild-type HCN1 channels (right). (C) Current trace of an AdSPC-transduced myocyte in normal Tyrode's solution (external) with 0.5 mM BaCl₂ (left panel). Spontaneous action potential oscillation follows a triggered action potential with a brief depolarising current pulse in AdSPC-transduced myocyte. No such action potential oscillations were detected in control (GFP-alone) myocytes.

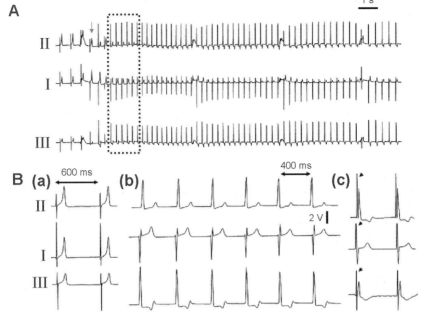

Fig. 8 (A) Overview of idioventricular rhythms. Arrows indicate start of idioventricular rhythms (150 bpm). (B,a) Junctional beats as intrinsic rhythms of guinea pig after methacholine injection. (B,b) A blown-up image of idioventricular rhythms indicated as a dashed-line square in (A,c). Pace-mapping of left ventricular free wall with hand-held electrode. Arrows indicate artefacts of pacing (150 bpm). Note that idioventricular rhythms were identical in polarity to paced beats, suggesting the idioventricular rhythms were originated from left ventricular free wall.

these limitations inherent with HCN gene transfer. To this end, we exploited accumulated knowledge regarding the biophysical properties of Shaker-type K$^+$ channels. First, depolarisation-activated Shaker K$^+$ channels had been shown to convert into hyperpolarisation-activated inward rectifiers by mutating three amino acid residues in the voltage sensor (S4) of the channel.[76] In addition, amino acid residues in the selectivity filter of Shaker K$^+$ channels were found to be critical for maintaining selectivity for K$^+$ over Na$^+$.[77] We combined the lessons from the two prior studies and converted the depolarisation-activated, potassium-selective human Kv1.4 channel into a hyperpolarisation-activated, synthetic pacemaker channel (AdSPC) suitable for biological pacing applications (Fig. 7A,B).[78] *In vivo* expression of synthetic pacemaker channel in a guinea-pig heart revealed robust hyperpolarisation-activated, inward currents (Fig. 7C,left panel) and demonstrated spontaneous action potentials from the AdSPC-transduced myocytes (Fig. 7C,right panel). Electrocardiography (ECG) taken from animals injected with AdSPC proved the *in vivo* pacemaker function of synthetic pacemaker channel; monomorphic idioventricular beats could be detected in animals 3–5 days after an intracardiac injection with AdSPC (Fig. 8), but not in control animals injected with adenovirus expressing GFP alone.

Given the sparse expression of Kv1 family channels in the human heart[79] and the capability of tuning the frequency of oscillation to any given desired rate range, the synthetic pacemaker channel based on Kv1 family has potentials to be a novel therapeutic tool for use in biological pacemakers.

CONVERSION OF NON-EXCITABLE CELLS TO SELF-CONTAINED BIOLOGICAL PACEMAKERS

Most gene- or cell-based approaches in creating a biological pacemaker centre around the idea of inducing spontaneous pacemaker activity in excitable, but quiescent, myocytes by adding pacemaker currents. An alternative is to create a pacemaker activity from non-excitable cells. We hypothesised that a non-excitable cell could be converted into a self-contained pacemaker by heterologous expression of a minimal complement of specific ion channels.[80] To this end, HEK293 cells were engineered to express the following ionic currents: (i) an excitatory current; (ii) an early repolarising current; and (iii) an inward rectifier current. For the excitatory current, the Na^+ channel from bacteria (NaChBac)[81] was chosen because of its slow gating kinetics and its compact cDNA. A repolarising current countering the depolarising effects of NaChBac was provided endogenously by the HEK293 cells. Repolarising currents were provided by a heterologous expression of Kir2.124 favouring a negative diastolic potential. With only two channel genes, NaChBac and Kir2.1, expressed in HEK293 cells, action potentials could be generated in response to depolarising external stimuli. The maximum diastolic potential (MDP) was -78 ± 7 mV with an action potential duration at 90% repolarisation (APD_{90}) value of 575 ± 33 ms ($n = 5$). In a previous study, mathematical modelling based on the Luo–Rudy guinea-pig formulation suggested that addition of I_f alone could trigger a ventricular myocyte to beat spontaneously.[82] Hence, we further co-expressed HCN1 providing I_f with NaChBac and Kir2.1. Whole-cell recordings from the triple-transfected HEK cells revealed spontaneous action potentials resembling the action potential morphology of ventricular myocytes but with slow phase-4 depolarisations, a hallmark of native cardiac pacemaker cells. The spontaneous action potentials exhibited an MDP of -81.5 ± 11.8 mV, maximum rate of rise (dV/dt_{max}) of 21.6 ± 8.6 V/s, APD_{90} of 660 ± 189 ms, and a rather slow frequency of 3 ± 1 bpm which was mainly due to the slow gating kinetics of NaChBac channels ($n = 4$). We further combined the three channel genes, HCN1, NaChBac, and Kir2.1-GFP in tandem via internal ribosome entry site (IRES) as a poly-cistronic vector in a single plasmid. Expectedly, current-clamp recordings of some of the triple-gene-transfected HEK293 cells exhibited spontaneously oscillating action potentials. Therefore, this study offers proof of the principle that a minimal set of ion channels can create spontaneous pacing activity even in non-excitable mammalian cells.

FUTURE DIRECTIONS

The concepts are generalisable to ventricular arrhythmias such as those associated with heart failure or heritable long QT syndrome. In heart failure, for example, over-expression of K channels can be used to antagonise the acquired long QT syndrome;[83,84] the attendant loss of contractility may be amenable to co-administration of a second gene to augment calcium cycling, in a dual gene therapy strategy. While such work is conceptually attractive, widespread delivery with long-term expression will be required before human trials can be anticipated.

Extensive further work will be required to optimise the frequency, evaluate the toxicology of the gene and cells used, to exclude potential tumorigenicity of transplanted stem cells, and to establish long-term stability of biological pacemakers. Nevertheless, given the promise, the effort to develop biological alternatives to the present therapies appears justified. The successful translation of these approaches to a clinical setting will actually cure the disease, representing a qualitative improvement over present approaches.

ACKNOWLEDGEMENTS

This work was supported by the Donald W. Reynolds Foundation and by a Heart Rhythm Society fellowship to HCC.

Key points for clinical practice

- The most tractable targets for near-term development are arrhythmias in which very local modifications of electrical properties suffice for effective treatment.

- Highly localised gene or cell delivery suffices to treat the problem. The amount of exogenous biological material delivered can be correspondingly reduced, and potential problems due to wide-spread dissemination can be more readily averted.

- Treated cells can remain responsive to endogenous nerves and hormones. Such was the case with G_i overexpression in the atrioventricular node: atrioventricular conduction remained responsive to β-adrenergic stimulation. Likewise, the induced pacemakers appropriately boosted their firing rate in response to β-adrenergic stimulation.

- Implantable hardware is avoided, obviating long-term risks and decreasing the expense and morbidity associated with battery and lead replacements.

- The localised coronary circulation may allow isolated delivery, as in the case of the atrioventricular node.

- The inner lining of the heart, the endocardium, is accessible by intracardiac injection, providing a potential alternative delivery route.

- The therapeutic effects can be readily detected by physical examination or by electrocardiography.

- Gene transfer-induced changes can be rescued by conventional electrophysiological methods (focal ablation and pacemaker implantation).

References

1. Thom T, Haase N, Rosamond W et al. Heart disease and stroke statistics – 2006 update: a report from the American Heart Association Statistics Committee and Stroke Statistics

Subcommittee. *Circulation* 2006; **113**: e85–e151.

2. Coplen SE, Antman EM, Berlin JA, Hewitt P, Chalmers TC. Efficacy and safety of quinidine therapy for maintenance of sinus rhythm after cardioversion. A meta-analysis of randomized control trials. *Circulation* 1990; **82**: 1106–1116.

3. Echt DS, Liebson PR, Mitchell LB *et al*. Mortality and morbidity in patients receiving encainide, flecainide, or placebo. The Cardiac Arrhythmia Suppression Trial. *N Engl J Med* 1991; **324**: 781–788.

4. Siebels J, Cappato R, Ruppel R, Schneider MA, Kuck KH. Preliminary results of the Cardiac Arrest Study Hamburg (CASH). CASH Investigators. *Am J Cardiol* 1993; **72**: 109F–113F.

5. Waldo AL, Camm AJ, deRuyter H *et al*. Effect of d-sotalol on mortality in patients with left ventricular dysfunction after recent and remote myocardial infarction. The SWORD Investigators. Survival With Oral d-Sotalol. *Lancet* 1996; **348**: 7–12.

6. Richardson AW, Josephson ME. Ablation of ventricular tachycardia in the setting of coronary artery disease. *Curr Cardiol Report* 1999; **1**: 157–164.

7. Falk RH. Atrial fibrillation. *N Engl J Med* 2001; **344**: 1067–1078.

8. Bernstein AD, Parsonnet V. Survey of cardiac pacing and implanted defibrillator practice patterns in the United States in 1997. *Pacing Clin Electrophysiol* 2001; **24**: 842–855.

9. Blaese RM, Culver KW, Miller AD *et al*. T lymphocyte-directed gene therapy for ADA–SCID: initial trial results after 4 years. *Science* 1995; **270**: 475–480.

10. Losordo DW, Vale PR, Symes JF *et al*. Gene therapy for myocardial angiogenesis: initial clinical results with direct myocardial injection of phVEGF165 as sole therapy for myocardial ischemia. *Circulation* 1998; **98**: 2800–2804.

11. Rosengart TK, Lee LY, Patel SR *et al*. Six-month assessment of a phase I trial of angiogenic gene therapy for the treatment of coronary artery disease using direct intramyocardial administration of an adenovirus vector expressing the VEGF121 cDNA. *Ann Surg* 1999; **230**: 466–470, discussion 70–72.

12. Ohno T, Gordon D, San H *et al*. Gene therapy for vascular smooth muscle cell proliferation after arterial injury. *Science* 1994; **265**: 781–784.

13. Mann MJ, Whittemore AD, Donaldson MC *et al*. *Ex-vivo* gene therapy of human vascular bypass grafts with E2F decoy: the PREVENT single-centre, randomised, controlled trial. *Lancet* 1999; **354**: 1493–1498.

14. Chugh SS, Blackshear JL, Shen WK, Hammill SC, Gersh BJ. Epidemiology and natural history of atrial fibrillation: clinical implications. *J Am Coll Cardiol* 2001; **37**: 371–378.

15. Khand AU, Rankin AC, Kaye GC, Cleland JG. Systematic review of the management of atrial fibrillation in patients with heart failure. *Eur Heart J* 2000; **21**: 614–632.

16. Blackshear JL, Safford RE. AFFIRM and RACE trials: implications for the management of atrial fibrillation. *Card Electrophysiol Rev* 2003; **7**: 366–369.

17. Pelargonio G, Prystowsky EN. Rate versus rhythm control in the management of patients with atrial fibrillation. *Nat Clin Pract Cardiovasc Med* 2005; **2**: 514–521.

18. Donahue JK, Heldman AW, Fraser H *et al*. Focal modification of electrical conduction in the heart by viral gene transfer. *Nat Med* 2000; **6**: 1395–1398.

19. Donahue JK, Kikkawa K, Thomas AD, Marban E, Lawrence JH. Acceleration of widespread adenoviral gene transfer to intact rabbit hearts by coronary perfusion with low calcium and serotonin. *Gene Ther* 1998; **5**: 630–634.

20. Nagata K, Marban E, Lawrence JH, Donahue JK. Phosphodiesterase inhibitor-mediated potentiation of adenovirus delivery to myocardium. *J Mol Cell Cardiol* 2001; **33**: 575–580.

21. Brooks CM, Lu H-h. *The sinoatrial pacemaker of the heart*. Springfield, IL: Charles C. Thomas, 1972.

22. Kusumoto FM, Goldschlager N. Cardiac pacing. *N Engl J Med* 1996; **334**: 89–97.

23. Wobus AM, Rohwedel J, Maltsev V, Hescheler J. Development of cardiomyocytes expressing cardiac-specific genes, action potentials, and ionic channels during embryonic stem cell-derived cardiogenesis. *Ann NY Acad Sci* 1995; **752**: 460–469.

24. Kubo Y, Baldwin TJ, Jan YN, Jan LY. Primary structure and functional expression of a mouse inward rectifier potassium channel. *Nature* 1993; **362**: 127–133.

25. Herskowitz I. Functional inactivation of genes by dominant negative mutations. *Nature* 1987; **329**: 219–222.

26. Slesinger PA, Patil N, Liao YJ, Jan YN, Jan LY, Cox DR. Functional effects of the mouse

weaver mutation on G protein-gated inwardly rectifying K$^+$ channels. *Neuron* 1996; **16**: 321–331.

27. Miake J, Marban E, Nuss HB. Biological pacemaker created by gene transfer. *Nature* 2002; **419**: 132–133.

28. Irisawa H, Brown HF, Giles W. Cardiac pacemaking in the sinoatrial node. *Physiol Rev* 1993; **73**: 197–227.

29. Brown HF, McNaughton PA, Noble D, Noble SJ. Adrenergic control of cardiac pacemaker currents. *Philos Trans R Soc Lond B Biol Sci* 1975; **270**: 527–537.

30. Santoro B, Tibbs GR. The HCN gene family: molecular basis of the hyperpolarization-activated pacemaker channels. *Ann NY Acad Sci* 1999; **868**: 741–764.

31. Imoto Y, Ehara T, Matsuura H. Voltage- and time-dependent block of i_{K1} underlying Ba^{2+}-induced ventricular automaticity. *Am J Physiol* 1987; **252**: H325–H333.

32. Hirano Y, Hiraoka M. Barium-induced automatic activity in isolated ventricular myocytes from guinea-pig hearts. *J Physiol* 1988; **395**: 455–472.

33. Rodriguez-Contreras A, Nonner W, Yamoah EN. Ca^{2+} transport properties and determinants of anomalous mole fraction effects of single voltage-gated Ca^{2+} channels in hair cells from bullfrog saccule. *J Physiol* 2002; **538**: 729–745.

34. Campbell DL, Giles WR, Shibata EF. Ion transfer characteristics of the calcium current in bull-frog atrial myocytes. *J Physiol* 1988; **403**: 239–266.

35. Brown HF, Kimura J, Noble D, Noble SJ, Taupignon A. The ionic currents underlying pacemaker activity in rabbit sino-atrial node: experimental results and computer simulations. *Proc R Soc Lond B Biol Sci* 1984; **222**: 329–347.

36. Hoffman LM, Carpenter MK. Characterization and culture of human embryonic stem cells. *Nat Biotechnol* 2005; **23**: 699–708.

37. Xu C, Police S, Rao N, Carpenter MK. Characterization and enrichment of cardiomyocytes derived from human embryonic stem cells. *Circ Res* 2002; **91**: 501–508.

38. Kehat I, Kenyagin-Karsenti D, Snir M *et al*. Human embryonic stem cells can differentiate into myocytes with structural and functional properties of cardiomyocytes. *J Clin Invest* 2001; **108**: 407–414.

39. He JQ, Ma Y, Lee Y, Thomson JA, Kamp TJ. Human embryonic stem cells develop into multiple types of cardiac myocytes: action potential characterization. *Circ Res* 2003; **93**: 32–39.

40. Mummery C, Ward-van Oostwaard D, Doevendans P *et al*. Differentiation of human embryonic stem cells to cardiomyocytes: role of coculture with visceral endoderm-like cells. *Circulation* 2003; **107**: 2733–2740.

41. Xue T, Cho HC, Akar FG *et al*. Functional integration of electrically active cardiac derivatives from genetically engineered human embryonic stem cells with quiescent recipient ventricular cardiomyocytes: insights into the development of cell-based pacemakers. *Circulation* 2005; **111**: 11–20.

42. Sperelakis N. An electric field mechanism for transmission of excitation between myocardial cells. *Circ Res* 2002; **91**: 985–987.

43. Wier WG, Blatter LA. Ca^{2+}-oscillations and Ca^{2+}-waves in mammalian cardiac and vascular smooth muscle cells. *Cell Calcium* 1991; **12**: 241–254.

44. Barr L, Dewey MM, Berger W. Propagation of action potentials and the structure of the nexus in cardiac muscle. *J Gen Physiol* 1965; **48**: 797–823.

45. Loewenstein WR. Junctional intercellular communication: the cell-to-cell membrane channel. *Physiol Rev* 1981; **61**: 829–913.

46. Jalife J, Sicouri S, Delmar M, Michaels DC. Electrical uncoupling and impulse propagation in isolated sheep Purkinje fibers. *Am J Physiol* 1989; **257**: H179–H189.

47. Lakatta EG, Maltsev VA, Bogdanov KY, Stern MD, Vinogradova TM. Cyclic variation of intracellular calcium: a critical factor for cardiac pacemaker cell dominance. *Circ Res* 2003; **92**: e45–e50.

48. Robinson RB, Siegelbaum SA. Hyperpolarization-activated cation currents: from molecules to physiological function. *Annu Rev Physiol* 2003; **65**: 453–480.

49. Beltrami AP, Barlucchi L, Torella D *et al*. Adult cardiac stem cells are multipotent and support myocardial regeneration. *Cell* 2003; **114**: 763–776.

50. Oh H, Bradfute SB, Gallardo TD *et al*. Cardiac progenitor cells from adult myocardium: homing, differentiation, and fusion after infarction. *Proc Natl Acad Sci USA* 2003; **100**:

12313–12318.
51. Matsuura K, Nagai T, Nishigaki N *et al.* Adult cardiac Sca-1-positive cells differentiate into beating cardiomyocytes. *J Biol Chem* 2004; **279**: 11384–11391.
52. Martin CM, Meeson AP, Robertson SM *et al.* Persistent expression of the ATP-binding cassette transporter, Abcg2, identifies cardiac SP cells in the developing and adult heart. *Dev Biol* 2004; **265**: 262–275.
53. Pfister O, Mouquet F, Jain M *et al.* CD31⁻ but not CD31⁺ cardiac side population cells exhibit functional cardiomyogenic differentiation. *Circ Res* 2005; **97**: 52–61.
54. Messina E, De Angelis L, Frati G *et al.* Isolation and expansion of adult cardiac stem cells from human and murine heart. *Circ Res* 2004; **95**: 911–921.
55. Anversa P, Kajstura J, Leri A, Bolli R. Life and death of cardiac stem cells: a paradigm shift in cardiac biology. *Circulation* 2006; **113**: 1451–1463.
56. Smith RR, Barile L, Cho HC *et al.* Regenerative potential of cardiosphere-derived cells expanded from percutaneous endomyocardial biopsy specimens. *Circulation* 2007; **115**: 896–908.
57. Robertson JA. Human embryonic stem cell research: ethical and legal issues. *Nat Rev Genet* 2001; **2**: 74–78.
58. Gerecht-Nir S, Itskovitz-Eldor J. Cell therapy using human embryonic stem cells. *Transpl Immunol* 2004; **12**: 203–209.
59. Odorico JS, Kaufman DS, Thomson JA. Multilineage differentiation from human embryonic stem cell lines. *Stem Cells* 2001; **19**: 193–204.
60. Potapova I, Plotnikov A, Lu Z *et al.* Human mesenchymal stem cells as a gene delivery system to create cardiac pacemakers. *Circ Res* 2004; **94**: 952–959.
61. van der Velden HM, Jongsma HJ. Cardiac gap junctions and connexins: their role in atrial fibrillation and potential as therapeutic targets. *Cardiovasc Res* 2002; **54**: 270–279.
62. Cho HC, Kashiwakura Y, Marban E. Creation of a biological pacemaker by cell fusion. *Circ Res* 2007; **100**: 1112–1115.
63. Shirahata S, Katakura Y, Teruya K. Cell hybridization, hybridomas, and human hybridomas. *Methods Cell Biol* 1998; **57**: 111–145.
64. Lentz BR, Lee JK. Poly(ethylene glycol) (PEG)-mediated fusion between pure lipid bilayers: a mechanism in common with viral fusion and secretory vesicle release? *Mol Membr Biol* 1999; **16**: 279–296.
65. Hoppe UC, Johns DC, Marban E, O'Rourke B. Manipulation of cellular excitability by cell fusion: effects of rapid introduction of transient outward K⁺ current on the guinea pig action potential. *Circ Res* 1999; **84**: 964–972.
66. Gibson AJ, Karasinski J, Relvas J *et al.* Dermal fibroblasts convert to a myogenic lineage in mdx mouse muscle. *J Cell Sci* 1995; **108**: 207–214.
67. Gussoni E, Bennett RR, Muskiewicz KR *et al.* Long-term persistence of donor nuclei in a Duchenne muscular dystrophy patient receiving bone marrow transplantation. *J Clin Invest* 2002; **110**: 807–814.
68. Alvarez-Dolado M, Pardal R, Garcia-Verdugo JM *et al.* Fusion of bone-marrow-derived cells with Purkinje neurons, cardiomyocytes and hepatocytes. *Nature* 2003; **425**: 968–973.
69. Weimann JM, Johansson CB, Trejo A, Blau HM. Stable reprogrammed heterokaryons form spontaneously in Purkinje neurons after bone marrow transplant. *Nat Cell Biol* 2003; **5**: 959–966.
70. Rosen AB, Kelly DJ, Schuldt AJ *et al.* Finding fluorescent needles in the cardiac haystack: tracking human mesenchymal stem cells labeled with quantum dots for quantitative *in vivo* three-dimensional fluorescence analysis. *Stem Cells* 2007; **25**: 2128–2138.
71. DiFrancesco D. The pacemaker current (I(f)) plays an important role in regulating SA node pacemaker activity. *Cardiovasc Res* 1995; **30**: 307–308.
72. Ulens C, Tytgat J. Functional heteromerization of HCN1 and HCN2 pacemaker channels. *J Biol Chem* 2001; **276**: 6069–6072.
73. Brewster AL, Bernard JA, Gall CM, Baram TZ. Formation of heteromeric hyperpolarization-activated cyclic nucleotide-gated (HCN) channels in the hippocampus is regulated by developmental seizures. *Neurobiol Dis* 2005; **19**: 200–207.
74. Cerbai E, Pino R, Porciatti F *et al.* Characterization of the hyperpolarization-activated current, I(f), in ventricular myocytes from human failing heart. *Circulation* 1997; **95**: 568–571.

75. Hoppe UC, Jansen E, Sudkamp M, Beuckelmann DJ. Hyperpolarization-activated inward current in ventricular myocytes from normal and failing human hearts. *Circulation* 1998; **97**: 55–65.
76. Miller AG, Aldrich RW. Conversion of a delayed rectifier K$^+$ channel to a voltage-gated inward rectifier K$^+$ channel by three amino acid substitutions. *Neuron* 1996; **16**: 853–858.
77. Heginbotham L, Lu Z, Abramson T, MacKinnon R. Mutations in the K$^+$ channel signature sequence. *Biophys J* 1994; **66**: 1061–1067.
78. Kashiwakura Y, Cho HC, Barth AS, Azene E, Marban E. Gene transfer of a synthetic pacemaker channel into the heart: a novel strategy for biological pacing. *Circulation* 2006; **114**: 1682–1686.
79. Wang Z, Feng J, Shi H, Pond A, Nerbonne JM, Nattel S. Potential molecular basis of different physiological properties of the transient outward K$^+$ current in rabbit and human atrial myocytes. *Circ Res* 1999; **84**: 551–561.
80. Cho HC, Kashiwakura Y, Marban E. Conversion of non-excitable cells to self-contained biological pacemakers. *Circulation* 2005; **112**: II-307.
81. Ren D, Navarro B, Xu H, Yue L, Shi Q, Clapham DE. A prokaryotic voltage-gated sodium channel. *Science* 2001; **294**: 2372–2375.
82. Azene EM, Xue T, Marban E, Tomaselli GF, Li RA. Non-equilibrium behavior of HCN channels: insights into the role of HCN channels in native and engineered pacemakers. *Cardiovasc Res* 2005; **67**: 263–273.
83. Nuss HB, Johns DC, Kaab S *et al*. Reversal of potassium channel deficiency in cells from failing hearts by adenoviral gene transfer: a prototype for gene therapy for disorders of cardiac excitability and contractility. *Gene Ther* 1996; **3**: 900–912.
84. Nuss HB, Marban E, Johns DC. Overexpression of a human potassium channel suppresses cardiac hyperexcitability in rabbit ventricular myocytes. *J Clin Invest* 1999; **103**: 889–896.

Yvonne Alexander   Anthony Heagerty
Daniel Keenan

2

Vascular calcification: characteristics and pathological mechanisms

Vascular calcification has a major impact on mortality. There are a number of reports suggesting it could act as an independent prognostic indicator for an increased risk of adverse cardiovascular outcomes, over and above the traditional Framingham score. There is no single theory to describe the aetiology and pathogenesis of vascular calcification. We will give an insight into the various theories derived from experiments and observations in relation to arterial calcification. Many factors have been implicated in vascular calcification including: (i) a change in gene expression in smooth muscle cells driving them towards an osteogenic phenotype; (ii) a release of cytokines and growth factors that influence vascular cell dynamics; (iii) smooth muscle cell apoptosis; (iv) an increased deposition of extracellular matrix; and (v) alterations in mineral metabolism. There is limited clinical management of vascular calcification; however, we are beginning to unravel some of the molecular and cellular mechanisms underpinning this process, opening up the potential for the identification of novel therapeutic strategies for this devastating pathology. This review will focus on the recent use of imaging of calcification as a prognostic tool in the clinic, the recent insights into the dynamic vascular remodelling which occurs in response to injury and altered mineral

M Yvonne Alexander DSc PhD (for correspondence)
Lecturer and Postgrduate Tutor in Cardiovascular Medicine, Cardiovascular Research Group, School of Clinical and Laboratory Sciences, Core Technology Facility (3rd Floor), University of Manchester, 46 Grafton Street, Manchester M13 9NT, UK. E-mail: yvonne.alexander@manchester.ac.uk

Anthony Heagerty MD FRCP FMedSci
Professor of Medicine, Cardiovascular Research Group, Core Technology Facility (3rd Floor), University of Manchester, 46 Grafton Street, Manchester M13 9NT, UK
E-mail: tony.heagerty@manchester.ac.uk

Daniel Keenan BSc MB BCh FRCS
Consultant Cardiothoracic Surgeon, Manchester Royal Infirmary, Oxford Road, Manchester M13 9WL, UK. E-mail: Daniel.Keenan@cmmc.nhs.uk

metabolism, drawing on the links between vascular calcification and bone metabolism.

Vascular calcification occurs during the development of atherosclerosis and many reports have shown an up-regulation of bone-related proteins, implicating similarities with bone formation. Developments in imaging technology, such as multirow detector computed tomography (MDCT), have stimulated an interest in the relationship between arterial calcification and coronary heart disease (CHD). Increasing evidence from these studies has shown that coronary artery calcium (CAC) is increased in the presence of atherosclerosis and diabetes. Furthermore, reports demonstrate a link between calcium burden and the future occurrence of myocardial infarction and stroke. The use of CAC measurements for the prediction of future cardiovascular events can provide additional prognostic information beyond that obtained from traditional CHD risk factors.[1] These findings provide the impetus to move from current observational studies to unravel the complexities underpinning calcium deposition in the vessel wall so that novel therapeutic targets, for diagnosis or treatment aimed at modulating vascular calcification, can be developed.

CLINICAL PRESENTATION

MEASURING CALCIFICATION

Imaging
Vascular calcification exists in the vasculature as calcium phosphate deposits and calcium hydroxyapatite, which has been confirmed by x-ray diffraction analysis. Accurate measurement of calcification is important for identifying factors associated with this process and, ultimately, for elucidating the mechanism(s) of calcification. A number of non-invasive imaging techniques are available to screen for the presence of ectopic calcification including: (i) X-rays of the abdominal aorta and peripheral arteries to visualise macroscopic calcifications of aorta and peripheral arteries (Fig. 1);[2] (ii) echocardiography (valvular calcification); (iii) two-dimensional ultrasound (carotid arteries, femoral arteries and aorta); and (iv) computed tomography (CT). All these technologies are now routine strategies for the quantification of coronary artery and aortic calcification. Improvements are such that CT scanning technologies have the potential to monitor calcification progression over a 3–7-year time-frame, evaluated as a percentage of a baseline calcium score value. This yields the potential to assess the effect of different therapeutic strategies directed at modifying calcification progression.

Calcium scores
MDCT is being used, in addition to electron beam CT (EBCT), for quantitation of CAC. Quantitative analysis of calcification using MDCT in cardiology has been described recently,[3] where assessment of coronary artery calcification is expressed as an Agatston score.[4] Coronary calcium can also be measured in terms of mass and volume, known as the volumetric score. Both quantitative measures are recognised as a valuable parameter in assessing the likelihood of the presence of a coronary stenosis, for use in cardiovascular risk stratification

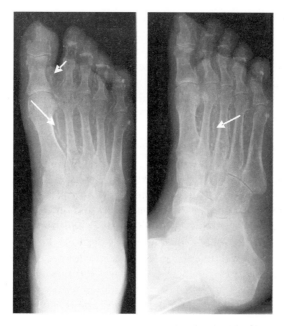

Fig. 1. Plain X-ray of the foot showing tramline/pipe stem calcification of the metatarsal and digital arteries.

and for identification of high-risk patients requiring aggressive treatment. MDCT uses thin slice CT imaging, and fast scan speeds to reduce motion artefacts. Thirty to forty adjacent axial scans are analysed and the calcium scoring system is based on the CT number measured in Hounsfield units, together with the area of calcium deposits (Fig. 2).[4] A fast CT study for coronary artery calcium measurement can be completed within 10–15 min and only requires a few seconds of scanning time. CAC score in the general population correlates with atherosclerotic plaque burden and predicts future

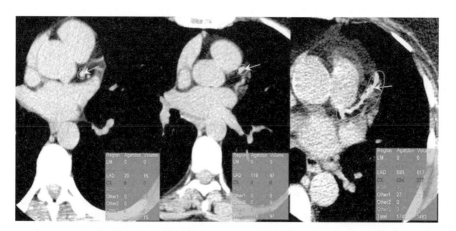

Fig. 2. Axial images taken using a Toshiba 64-slice CT scanning system 3 demonstrating the presence of coronary calcification along the lengths of the anterior descending branch of the left coronary artery (LAD) (arrows). This radiograph was taken by Melanie Greaves.

fatal and non-fatal cardiovascular outcomes. A patient with an intermediate Framingham risk score and a coronary calcium score of > 300 would be classified as being in a high-risk group for coronary heart disease. The clinical utility of MDCT combined with measurement of blood biomarkers and markers of subclinical disease is an appealing future strategy to integrate information on structural or functional vascular wall pathology and systemic 'activity' of the disease.

PATHOPHYSIOLOGY

The pathological changes in the vessel wall associated with vascular calcification result from structural alterations in the tunica media, brought about by a reprogramming of gene expression and extracellular matrix deposition. The calcified matrix can be deposited at various sites within different vascular beds, either as large calcific deposits or as spotty calcification – for example: (i) obstruction of arteries by calcification can occur in the arterial intima or media and can lead to a coronary thrombosis and/or stroke; (ii) calcium deposition in heart valves and arteries reduces valvular or arterial wall elasticity, which can result in stenosis and aneurysm respectively; and (iii) mineralisation in the femoral or tibial arteries can cause intermittent claudication in the legs. The loss of calcium from bone by osteoporosis can occur in conjunction with calcium accumulation in arteries. Whether there is a link between the two processes is unclear, but this is an area worthy of further study as it could have significant clinical impact, not only for bone-related

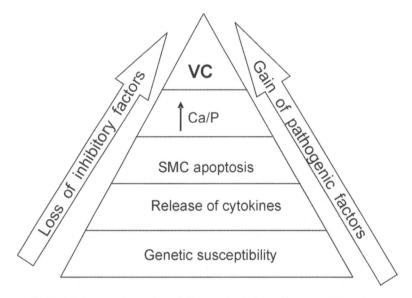

Fig. 3. The determinants of vascular calcification (VC), from the appearance of spotty calcification to the development of large calcified deposits, include a loss of inhibitory agents, such as matrix Gla protein or fetuin, and a gain of pathogenic factors, such as elevated alkaline phosphatase activity and increased calcium and phosphate concentrations. A disturbance in the balance of these agents is a consequence of a complex interplay of micro-environment influences such as pH, oxidative stress and release of cytokines in the vessel wall, a disturbed mineral homeostasis, all of which may cause smooth muscle cell (SMC) apoptosis and a complete reprogramming of gene expression.

disorders but other inflammatory diseases. In this regard, studies from this laboratory have shown that treatment of vascular cells *in vitro* with the anti-inflammatory agent dexamethasone, accelerated their mineralisation with a concomitant down-regulation of osteogenic inhibitor molecules.[5] These findings pose important questions about the consequences of corticosteroid treatment on the progression of vascular calcification *in vivo*. The data could also suggest that the potential protective effects of calcification inhibitory molecules may be obliterated *in vivo*, when certain treatment strategies are in use. Our data would support the proposal that protective factors are up-regulated, either in serum or in calcified tissue, to prevent mineralisation (Fig. 3). It has been suggested that calcification results from an imbalance of promoting and regulatory factors which exist in the vasculature. Therefore, modulating local expression of these proteins could potentially reduce/prevent the development of calcification in the vessel wall.

MODELS TO STUDY CALCIFICATION

IN VITRO MODELS

In vitro models of calcification have been established where distinct populations of human and bovine vascular smooth muscle cells (VSMCs), pericytes and calcifying vascular cells (CVCs) express osteoblastic and chondrocytic markers and form mineralised bone-like nodules *in vitro*.[6] To induce human vascular smooth muscle cells to calcify *in vitro*, elevated concentrations of phosphorous, calcium or both are often added to the culture media.[7] Cell calcium content, and alkaline phosphatase activity are measured as indices of calcification. The matrix deposited by these vascular cells *in vitro* resembles that present in calcified vessels *in vivo*, namely hydroxyapatite (Fig. 4).

In vitro models have been used to demonstrate the regulation of vascular calcification by many proteins and stimuli involved in both skeletogenesis and atherosclerotic plaque progression, including steroid hormones, oxidised lipids and inflammatory cytokines.[8]

IN VIVO MODELS

The characterisation of knockout mouse models with deletions in osteogenic genes has provided an understanding into the common signalling pathways involved in both skeletal and vascular calcification. For example, mice that lack the cytokine decoy receptor osteoprotegerin (OPG) display a combined osteoporosis–arterial calcification phenotype. The OPG anti-calcification activity in the aorta of these mice is thought to be caused by the down-regulation of alkaline phosphatase activity[9] and a prevention of the osteoclast-release of calcium and minerals from bone. Knockout mouse models of alkaline phosphatase, fetuin, ostepontin, and matrix Gla protein also display extensive calcification of the arteries. In addition, apolipoprotein E-deficient ageing mice (between 45–75 weeks) show evidence of calcified lesions in their innominate arteries. It has been suggested that since ApoE is involved in plasma transport of vitamin K, it may be that the mice suffer mild vitamin K deficiency and, consequently, have inadequate carboxylation of MGP.

Immunocytochemical analyses have identified one of the cell types involved in the deposition of hydroxyapatite in arteries as chondrocytes, using antibodies against recognised chondrocyte proteins, such as Runx2, Sox9 and MEF2C.[10] Chondrocyte-driven calcification resembles endochondral bone formation, whereby chondrocytes proliferate, undergo hypertrophy and die and the extracellular cartilage matrix they deposit is replaced by bone formed

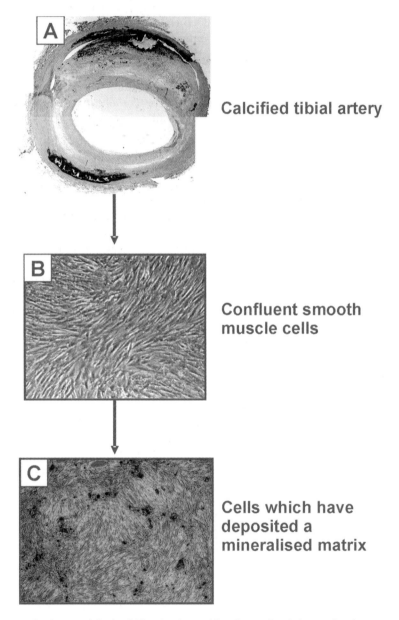

Calcified tibial artery

Confluent smooth muscle cells

Cells which have deposited a mineralised matrix

Fig. 4. An *in vitro* model of calcification is used for the study of the mechanisms involved in this pathogenesis. Vascular cells are explanted from calcified tissue (A). They are grown to confluency *in vitro* (B) and exposed to high phosphate conditions. These culture conditions induce the cells to deposit a mineralised matrix, which is identified using an Alizarin Red stain to indicate calcium deposition (C).

by osteoblasts. All of these structural and cellular changes in the vessel wall are controlled by intracellular signalling and systemic factors (including growth and thyroid hormone) and locally secreted factors (such as parathyroid hormone-related peptide and fibroblast growth factor,[11] and hepatocyte growth factor[12]).

The use of these respective models holds promise for the further elucidation of the pathophysiology of calcification mechanisms and for the potential design of effective treatments.

MOLECULAR AND CELLULAR ASPECTS OF VASCULAR CALCIFICATION

Numerous elegant studies have defined the key factors and cell types involved in vascular calcification, with evidence for common mechanisms underlying both vascular calcification and bone remodelling.[13,14] A number of risk factors such as ageing, oestrogen deficiency, abnormalities in vitamins D and K, chronic inflammation and oxidative stress have been proposed to cause the formation of bone mineral in vascular walls with simultaneous loss from bone.

Cells which have been shown to differentiate into osteoblasts and deposit a mineralised matrix *in vitro* have been isolated from human arteries, and have been identified in the tunica media,[15] by immunostaining using a surface marker characteristic of microvascular pericytes.[16] Some reports suggest these cells migrate from the adventitia or from the circulating blood (Fig. 5) and differentiate into cells which exhibit similar characteristics to osteoblasts. We[12,16,17] and others[18–20] have used histological analysis of calcified plaques in vessels obtained from patients with either diabetes or end-stage renal disease (ESRD) to demonstrate an up-regulation of several osteogenic proteins, at sites of intimal and medial calcification, such as elevated alkaline phosphatase, increased collagen type I, osteonectin, osteocalcin, the bone matrix protein, osteopontin, matrix Gla protein and bone morphogenetic protein-2a, together with a novel vascular calcification associated factor (VCAF) (the boxed area in Fig. 6i is enlarged in Fig. 6ii–vi).[16,17] These osteogenic proteins are generally found in close association with macrophages which can be identified with surface markers, such as CD68 as illustrated in Figure 6v.

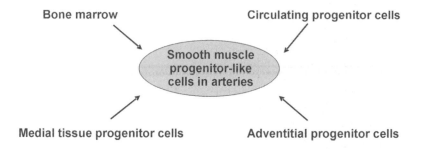

Fig. 5. The origin of the cells involved in vascular calcification is still unclear. There are reports to suggest that they are derived from the bone marrow, or as circulating progenitor cells. There is evidence that progenitor-like cells exist in the medial layer or that they migrate from the adventitial layer in the vessel wall and differentiate along an osteogenic lineage.

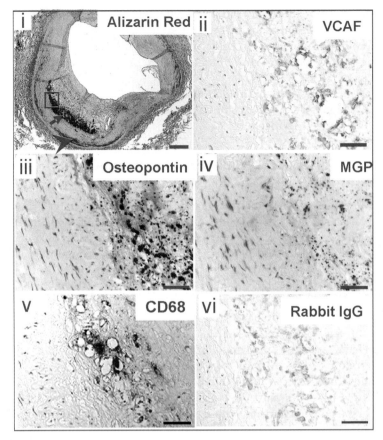

Fig. 6. Calcification-associated proteins and macrophages in calcified regions of plaques in tibial arteries. (i) Tibial artery stained with Alizarin Red to show calcification in the base of a plaque (long arrow) and in the medial layer (arrowhead). Bar = 500 mm. The box area in (i) is enlarged in (ii–vi). Consecutive sections were stained with VCAF (ii), osteopontin (iii), matrix Gla protein (iv), a macrophage marker, CD68 (v), and IgG negative control (vi). Bars = 50 mm.

PHENOTYPIC HETEROGENEITY OF SMOOTH MUSCLE CELL SUBPOPULATIONS

Adult human smooth muscle cells (SMCs) exhibit extensive phenotypic diversity during development, in different vascular beds in the adult, during repair after vascular injury and in disease states. Although isolation of distinct SMC sub-populations has proved difficult, many reports demonstrate morphologically and functionally distinct characteristics of isolated clonal populations of SMCs when grown in culture.[21] Demer and colleagues[18] have termed these cells 'calcifying vascular cells' (CVCs), since they express osteoblastic markers and form mineralised nodules *in vitro*. These studies have identified SMCs as having either a spindle-shaped contractile phenotype or an epitheloid, secretory phenotype. The determining factors distinguishing these phenotypes are a complex interaction of several positive and negative-acting regulatory molecules, including a range of osteogenic transcription factors, such as cbfa1, binding to a multiplicity of gene promoter control regions.[22]

CELL PROLIFERATION

A number of studies have identified differentially expressed genes during the transition of cells from a proliferative to differentiation status. Proliferating VSMCs, lymphocytes and macrophages have been detected in the arterial intima using immunohistochemical staining for cell-and proliferation-specific antigens (smooth muscle α-actin, CD45, cyclin D1 and proliferating cell nuclear antigen). After an initial vascular insult, SMCs alter their gene expression profile, contributing to the characteristic remodelling which occurs in the vessel wall. Sub-populations of SMCs engage in a programme of cell proliferation, migration, hypertrophic differentiation, apoptosis and, finally, osteogenic differentiation, depositing a bone-like matrix, in a process now defined as vascular calcification.

The intracellular signal transduction pathways and the triggering factors controlling these processes are slowly being defined. Data from *in vitro* proliferative studies, using [³H]-thymidine incorporation, bromodeoxyuridine incorporation and cell counting, suggest that IGF-I, IL-1β and high glucose all induce proliferation involving the ERK, the Ras-mitogen-activated protein kinase and the phosphatidylinositol-3-kinase–Akt pathways, as well as the β-catenin signalling pathway.

CELL DIFFERENTIATION

When cells in the vessel wall commit to an osteogenic differentiation programme, proliferative genes, including smooth muscle α-actin, desmin, CD45, cyclin D1 and proliferating cell nuclear antigen are down-regulated, in conjunction with an up-regulation of differentiation markers including smoothelin, a recently described late differentiation marker of vascular SMCs. RANK-L has been shown to stimulate osteogenic differentiation and calcification of vascular smooth muscle cells.[23] Up-regulation of the receptor activator of nuclear factor κ-B-ligand (RANK-L) is triggered by pro-inflammatory cytokines like IL-1, TNF-α, and IL-6 and may be viewed as part of the immuno-inflammatory milieu associated with advanced plaques (Fig. 7). Natriuretic peptides have also been shown to have paracrine effects on the development of calcification. *In vitro* studies lend credence to the idea that plaque calcification develops when a signal from an atherosclerotic plaque induces expression of osteogenic factors. Osteogenic differentiation of pluripotent cells located in the arterial intima is then induced, resulting in the deposition of a bone-like matrix and hydroxyapatite mineral. These findings add to the continuing debate over the use of osteogenic-promoting factors in the management of osteoporosis, which could in fact have detrimental effects on the development of calcification. As cells undergo apoptosis, smooth muscle cells fragment into apoptotic bodies which play a key role in triggering the onset of vascular calcification,[24] possibly brought about by impaired phagocytosis of the membrane-bound vesicles. For example, acetylated LDL may increase calcification by competing with apoptotic bodies for phagocytosis by VSMCs. Lipid-rich, membrane-bound vesicles have been found to take up calcium and phosphorous and are similar to the skeletal matrix vesicles which provide a paracrine signal and induce an epithelial–mesenchymal transition during skeletal development.

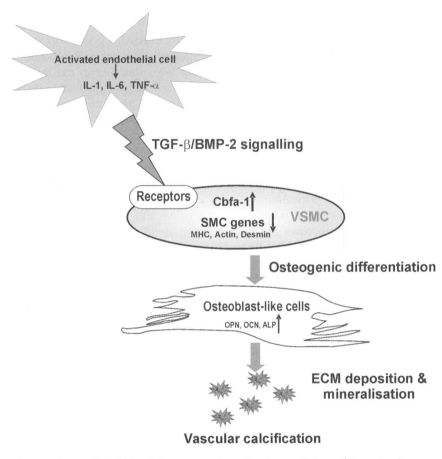

Fig. 7. When endothelial cells become activated under conditions of hypoxia, shear or oxidative stress, they release cyokines (*e.g.* IL-1, IL-6 and TNF-α). This activates signalling pathways involving transforming growth factor (TGF)-β or bone morpho-genetic protein (BMP)-2 which triggers the vascular smooth muscle (VSMC) cell to down-regulate SMC-specific genes, such as myosin heavy chain (MHC), smooth muscle actin and desmin and switch to an osteogenic lineage by expressing osteogenic proteins like cbfa1, osteopontin (OPN), osteocalcin (OCN) and alkaline phosphatase (ALP). The cells deposit matrix proteins which become mineralised. This constitutes one aspect of pathological vascular calcification in the vessel wall.

OSSIFICATION OF VASCULAR CELLS

Matrix vesicles are extracellular, 100 nM in diameter, membrane-invested particles detected at sites of initial calcification in cartilage and bone. Matrix vesicles are formed by a blebbing and pinching-off of vesicles from specific regions of the outer plasma membranes of differentiating chondrocytes and osteoblasts; it is within the inner surfaces of these membranes that the first crystals of apatitic bone mineral are formed (Fig. 8). Matrix vesicles have been shown to contain calcification inhibitors like MGP, fetuin and pyrophosphate[25] and can act as a nidus for calcium crystal formation. After mineral initiation, the mineral crystals can act as a nidus for further growth,[26] the development of which may require the presence of other promoting factors (such as

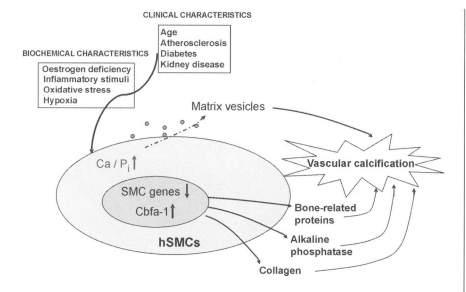

Fig. 8. Vascular calcification is associated with diseases such as atherosclerosis, diabetes and end-stage renal failure. Inflammatory cytokines, oxidative stress and hypoxia activate cells and trigger a reprogramming of gene expression. Smooth muscle cell genes are down-regulated, while osteogenic genes, such as Cbfa1 and bone-related proteins, such as the osteogenic transcription factor cbfa1, osteopontin and alkaline phosphatase are up-regulated, ultimately resulting in the deposition of a bone matrix in the vasculature. (Human smooth muscle cells [hSMCs].)

hypercalcaemia and/or hyperphosphataemia) and/or a deficiency in calcification inhibitor molecules (cellular protective mechanisms). Deregulation of intracellular calcium and phosphate homeostasis is thought to be one of the underlying pathophysiological mechanisms of calcification. High phosphate levels in hyperphosphataemia, uraemic conditions and high glucose levels have all been shown to promote an organised deposition of hydroxyapatite. Giachelli et al.[27] have described the role of sodium-dependent phosphate transport mechanisms in SMCs in the pathogenesis of vascular calcification via sodium/phosphate transporters, Pit1 and Pit2, although SMCs also exhibit a sodium-independent transport system.

The mineral deposited by the smooth muscle cells has been investigated using X-ray diffraction studies and is not just an amorphous calcium phosphate product, but occurs as very small, dispersed crystals of hydroxyapatite,[28] similar to the mineral formed in bone. Of note, calcification is often described as occurring in two distinct locations, First, intimal calcification, which is associated with lipid-filled foam cells at the base of the plaque (Fig. 9A), and possibly driven by inflammatory mediators. Second, medial calcification, located around the elastic lamina which can occur independently of atherosclerosis, and is generally associated with ageing, diabetes and renal failure (Fig. 9B). Non-inflammatory agents, such as inorganic pyrophosphate deficiency and hyperphosphataemia, may possibly drive medial calcification. However, in respect of the clinical phenotype, the boundaries between Monckeberg's sclerosis and micro-calcification are

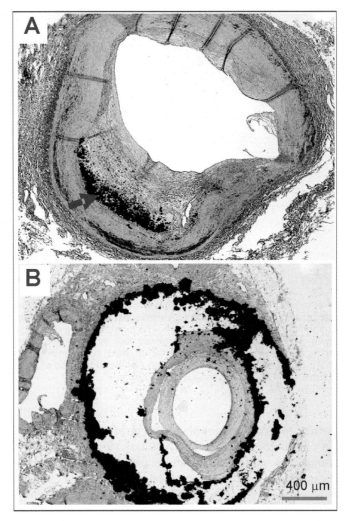

Fig. 9. Cross-section through representative tibial arterial segments which have been stained with Alizarin Red to show areas of intimal calcification from a non-diabetic patient (A) showing a large calcium deposit at the base of the plaque (arrow; bar = 500 μm). In contrast, (B) shows medial calcification has occurred independently of athero-sclerosis and clearly demonstrates the tramline pattern which is evident in patients with diabetes.

indistinct, and whether the deposition of a mineralised matrix in these different locations reflects endochondral ossification, intramembranous ossification or dystrophic calcification remains to be clearly defined.

GENETIC CHARACTERISTICS

A few studies are emerging to suggest that heritable factors may play a role in the presence and extent of abdominal aortic calcification (AAC). In relation to valve calcification, using population-based samples and genome-wide linkage analysis, a large family has been identified with autosomal-dominant aortic valve disease consisting of aortic valve calcification. The affected individuals have a nonsense mutation in NOTCH1.[29] The findings were given further support by the discovery of a NOTCH1 frameshift mutation in an unrelated family with similar aortic valve disease, suggesting that NOTCH1 haploinsufficiency is a genetic cause of aortic valve malformations and calcification.[30] The NOTCH signalling pathway represses activation of Runx2 – a transcription factor which is critical for osteogenic differentiation.[29]

Other studies on the molecular genetics of vascular calcification have shown that a polymorphism in the promoter of the MGP gene has a significant association with myocardial infarction in low-risk individuals and femoral calcification in the presence of atherosclerotic plaques, suggesting involvement of this mutation in coronary artery disease.[31] A recent population-based multi-ethnic study has also shown an association of a family history of premature CHD and the presence of CAC.[32] It is possible that the proportion of the variation detected in aortic valve and coronary calcification is due to an additive effect of genes, many of which have yet to be characterised.

VASCULAR CALCIFICATION AND CARDIOVASCULAR DISEASE

Vascular calcification is associated with advancing age and various diseases such as atherosclerosis, diabetes mellitus and end-stage renal disease. It has important clinical implications, especially in coronary arteries.

ATHEROSCLEROSIS

Atherosclerosis is recognised as an inflammatory disorder with oxidised lipids playing a major role in plaque development; there is evidence that these inflammatory agents may act as stimuli for the progression of vascular calcification.[8] Furthermore, sporadic resorptive osteoclast-like cells have been found in calcified atherosclerotic plaques, with the RANK-L signalling pathway being associated with the active resorption of ectopic vascular calcification,[33,34] thus lending credence to the concept of treatment strategies to prevent and/or retard the rate of progression of vascular calcification.

Increasing reports show an association between atherosclerosis and osteoporosis; for example, a study has shown routine lateral lumbar spine radiographs with osteopenic vertebrae lying adjacent to dense calcium mineral deposition in the aorta.[35] Osteoporosis and atherosclerosis are both chronic degenerative diseases, both are independent of each other, and are both prevalent in the ageing population. However, growing evidence suggests a correlation between cardiovascular disease and osteoporosis, irrespective of age.

DIABETES

Diabetes is associated with an increased incidence of atherosclerotic vascular disease and cardiovascular mortality. In general, patients with diabetes exhibit more vascular calcification than age- and gender-matched non-diabetic patients with peripheral vascular disease. Ectopic calcification appears to be a strong independent predictor of cardiovascular mortality, and occurs particularly in those with diabetes and neuropathy. In the condition known as Charcot neuroarthropathy, a complication of diabetes, there is a combination of dense peripheral neuropathy, increased bone resorption with destruction of the architecture of the foot and simultaneous bone matrix deposition in the peripheral vasculature. This paradox is poorly understood, and clearly further studies are needed to understand the link between the factors or mechanisms that predispose to vascular calcification with those that cause bone disease. In addition, 90% of those with diabetic Charcot neuroarthropathy have evidence of vascular calcification in vessels of the foot even on plain X-rays (Fig. 1),[2] while slightly less calcification is detected in ordinary diabetic neuropathy.[36] The reason for the elevated calcification in association with Charcot neuroarthropathy versus diabetic neuropathy is unclear. There is some emerging circumstantial evidence suggesting that, in diabetic patients, there is an accentuation of the RANK-L/osteoprotegerin (OPG) signalling pathway. Mechanistically, neuropathy and altered blood flow are also thought to be key pathogenetic factors involved in bone resorption and vascular calcium deposition and are areas worthy of further investigation.

KIDNEY DISEASE

Vascular calcification has long been recognised as a complication of chronic renal disease, and the availability of sensitive imaging technology (such as electron beam computed tomography (EBCT) and MDCT) has made it possible to conduct population-based investigations of the problem. These studies have demonstrated a link between calcium burden and the future occurrence of cardiovascular events. Patients on haemodialysis experience a mortality rate of 20% per year, driven primarily by a 30–100-fold increase in cardiovascular death (adjusted for age, gender and ethnicity).[37] CVD mortality is approximately 15 times higher in dialysis patients than in the general population.[38] Such patients, in general, exhibit more vascular calcification than age- and gender-matched controls without kidney disease. Indeed, in comparison with patients with established coronary artery disease and normal kidney function, dialysis patients show a 5-fold increase in coronary artery calcium scores. However, on initiation of dialysis, vascular calcification is only present in about a third of patients and progresses at a variable rate over subsequent years.[14]

Recent studies among patients undergoing maintenance dialysis have demonstrated a relationship between various measures of disordered mineral homeostasis (*e.g.* serum calcium, phosphorus and parathyroid hormone levels, and use of calcium-based phosphate binders) and the severity of vascular and valvular calcification.[14,39] However, while disturbances in divalent ion homeostasis have been proposed to play a role in calcification of the tunica media of patients with chronic kidney disease, patients with diabetes have an apparently intact bone and mineral metabolism, clearly implying that other factors are involved. Chronic kidney disease as well as diabetes are now recognised as pro-inflammatory states. It has been suggested that inflammation may be the mechanistic link to explain the similarities in phenotypic and molecular characteristics of medial calcification in patients with either renal failure or patients with diabetes mellitus.

AORTIC VALVE STENOSIS

Aortic valve stenosis is a major reason for valve replacement surgery and is often associated with ectopic calcification. It has similarities to both intimal and medial calcification and may result from both mechanical stress and inflammation in the valve. Studies have shown an involvement of transforming growth factor-β1 (TGF-β1)-related mechanisms with calcific aortic valve disease and an association with apoptotic events.[40] The mechanism of valvular heart disease involves an endochondral bone process that is expressed as cartilage in the mitral valves and bone in the aortic valves. Molecules such as Lrp5 have been shown to be up-regulated, thus implicating this pathway in the development of calcific valve stenosis.[41]

TRANSPLANT ARTERIOSCLEROSIS

Transplant vasculopathy, accelerated atherosclerosis and extensive calcification are all major causes of graft failure after transplant surgery. TUNEL- and Fas-positive cells have been shown to accumulate in the media, adding further strength to the involvement of apoptosis in the development of calcification. There is also an increase in expression of fibronectin and osteopontin, and an accumulation of macrophages. All these cellular and structural changes result in the deposition of a mineralised matrix and calcification around the graft site. Current interest in tissue engineering, for the creation of a functional, living, and non-immunogenic tissue substitute, demands an understanding of the fibrotic and calcification problems that may arise from their use in graft surgery. For this reason, a useful mouse model of vein graft disease with evidence of accelerated atherosclerosis and calcification has been generated, enabling investigative functional studies to be carried out.[42] Another recent study using elastin tubes with sustained release of β-FGF, shows a cellular coverage of an elastin scaffold *in vivo*, while inhibiting calcification.[43]

CURRENT CLINICAL MANAGEMENT

Therapies to correct mineral metabolism disturbances have been associated with some clinical benefit in a number of observational studies. Evidence is accumulating that phosphate control interventions and a number of serum biomarkers are associated with rate of progression of calcification. To reduce the negative impact of high phosphate, serum phosphate levels should be < 5 mg/dl and serum calcium < 10 mg/dl. This allows the calcium x phosphate product to be maintained at < 50 mg/dl, reducing the risk of vascular, valvular, and extraskeletal calcification. Since hydroxyapatite is an insoluble material, removing it from arteries could have serious implications on the skeleton. Therefore, a preventative targeted approach to the progression of calcification in arteries is necessary, if demineralising the bone is to be avoided.

Anticalcifying agents, like the bisphosphonates, have been developed as analogues of pyrophosphate and are resistant to chemical and enzymatic hydrolysis. They bind strongly to hydroxyapatite crystals, inhibiting their formation and dissolution. This physicochemical effect on crystal growth

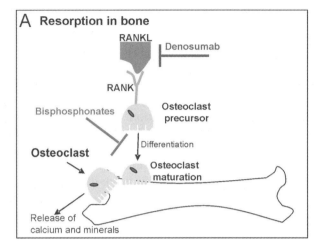

A Resorption in bone

RANKL

Denosumab

RANK

Bisphosphonates

Osteoclast precursor

Differentiation

Osteoclast

Osteoclast maturation

Release of calcium and minerals

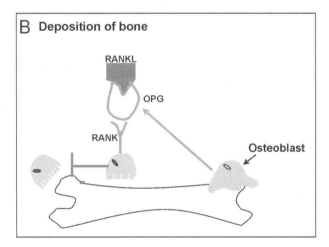

B Deposition of bone

RANKL

OPG

RANK

Osteoblast

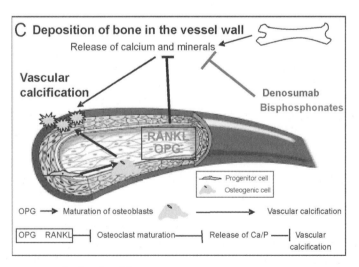

C Deposition of bone in the vessel wall

Release of calcium and minerals

Vascular calcification

Denosumab
Bisphosphonates

RANKL
OPG

Progenitor cell
Osteogenic cell

OPG → Maturation of osteoblasts → Vascular calcification

OPG RANKL ⊣ Osteoclast maturation ⊣ Release of Ca/P ⊣ Vascular calcification

Fig. 10. (see page opposite for details).

Fig. 10. Resorption of bone in the skeleton co-exists with the deposition of bone in the vasculature. (A) Binding of the receptor activator of nuclear factor-κB ligand (RANK-L) to the receptor activator of nuclear factor-κB (RANK) stimulates osteoclast maturation and loss of bone. (B) Osteoblasts express osteoprotegerin (OPG) the natural decoy receptor for RANK-L, inhibiting activation of RANK, preventing maturation of osteoclasts and preventing bone resorption. An increased availability of OPG and the block on RANK-L signalling supports osteoblast differentiation, maturation and function allowing the deposition of bone. (C) Elevated OPG in the vasculature and increased Ca/P products marks a commitment of progenitor cells in the vessel wall towards an osteogenic phenotype and the subsequent deposition of a calcified matrix. See text for details of bisphosphonates and denosumab prevention of osteoporosis and vascular calcification.

prevents soft tissue calcification although, in large doses, it may also prevent normal bone metabolism. The main effect of inhibiting bone resorption is a cellular and not a physicochemical mechanism. Bisphosphonates act directly on osteoclasts, which become inhibited after engulfing the compounds during the process of dissolution of the drug-containing mineral, and they may also have an inhibitory effect on the recruitment of osteoclasts. Price and colleagues[44] have demonstrated that the bisphosphonates Alendronate and Ibandronate suppressed the development of uraemia-related vascular calcification in 42-day-old male rats treated with warfarin. The bisphosphonates are widely administered for treatment of osteoporosis where it is important to prevent bone resorption (Fig. 10A). A recent randomised control trial has shown that specific blockage of RANK-L by the monoclonal antibody denosumab is more effective in increasing bone mineral density in postmenopausal women with osteopenia, compared to placebo and treatment with Alendronate.[45] The denosumab binds RANK-L, mimicking the effect of OPG. It is currently being tested to stop bone loss in postmenopausal osteoporosis, bone metastasis, and rheumatoid arthritis in phase II and III trials.[45]

In normal bone physiology, bone deposition by osteoblasts is in balance with bone resorption by osteoclasts (Fig. 10B). In the case of bone deposition in the vessel wall, with the excess calcium and mineral being released from bone, signalling events trigger an osteogenic differentiation programme whereby progenitor cells residing in the vessel wall differentiate into osteoblast-like cells depositing a mineralised matrix. Protection against mineralisation in the vessel wall is achieved by cells increasing their expression of OPG and RANK-L, which inhibit osteoclast maturation and prevent the subsequent release of calcium and mineral from bone (Fig. 10C). The protective effects of the bisphosphonates and denosumab may also be attributed to the inhibition of osteoclastogenesis. RANK-L antagonism may well become included in the care of patients with these acute vascular syndromes in the near future. The next steps will be to reproduce key findings in independent studies, to elaborate the effects of RANK-L in advanced atherosclerosis and vascular calcification, and to test RANK-L antagonism in appropriate animal models. These data support the link between bone disease and vascular calcification in the context of chronic renal failure, opening perspectives toward novel therapeutic strategies.[46]

Treatment with sevelamer, a non-calcium-based phosphorus binder, has shown an attenuation of the progression of valvular calcification and a significant survival benefit compared to treatment with calcium-containing phosphate binders,[47] suggesting that sevelamer may have important actions in

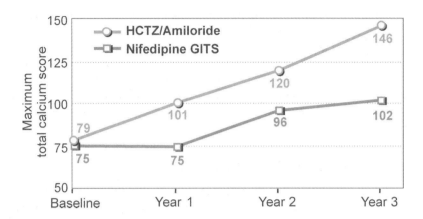

Fig. 11. The effect on maximum total calcium score in the left anterior descending coronary artery (LAD) in patients treated with Nifedipine GITS or HCTZ/Amiloride.

decreasing diabetic and uraemic vasculopathy. Two-hundred patients on haemodialysis were treated with either sevelamer or calcium-based phosphorus binders. Calcification was assessed using electron beam computed tomography (EBCT) and changes in valvular calcification were assessed over a year. Significantly more sevelamer-treated subjects experienced an arrest or regression in total valvular and vascular calcification, suggesting that sevelamer treatment, plus intensive control of calcium and phosphorus levels, may attenuate progression of vascular calcification,[48] in the context of renal disease where vascular calcification can occur independently of atherosclerosis and is thought to occur as a result of disturbed mineral metabolism.

There is growing evidence that control of conventional risk factors may have beneficial effects on delaying the progression of calcification. The statins inhibit cholesterol biosynthesis and are used for the treatment of atherosclerosis. Studies suggest that the mechanism of actions of both statins and bisphosphonates at the cellular level may not be mutually exclusive. There are some early clinical data to suggest that statins increase bone density and bisphosphonates may have a beneficial effect *in vivo* on plasma lipid levels and on the atherosclerotic process. A recent study correlated the effects of statins on the progression of calcification and showed that the inflammatory status of the patient determined the outcome of the progression of coronary artery calcification.[49] Furthermore, data from a subanalysis of a calcification side-arm study from the INSIGHT (International Nifedipine once daily Study Intervention as a Goal in Hypertension Treatment) trial investigated the protective ability of a calcium antagonist-based treatment regimen in high-risk hypertensive patients.[50] A total of 7434 patients were enrolled in the study, with 6321 patients deemed eligible for analysis in the trial. Of these, 3157 patients were treated with the calcium channel blocker nifedipine GITS (Gastrointestinal Therapeutic System), while 3164 patients received a diuretic combination of hydrochlorothiazide and amiloride as an active control. These studies showed that one of the effects of the antihypertensive drug nifedipine was a reduction in calcium scores in these patients, suggesting beneficial effects beyond blood pressure lowering and a potential for long-term cardiovascular protection (Fig. 11).[5]

Properly designed prospective studies that examine the effect of statins on bone density and fractures, as well as the effects of bisphosphonates and antihypertensive treatments on cardiovascular outcomes, lipid profiles, atherosclerotic progression and cardiovascular morbidity and mortality are needed to define clearly the clinical effects and potential new roles for these drugs.

DIRECTIONS FOR FUTURE RESEARCH

There appears to be some potential to either prevent the deposition of a mineralised matrix or to improve outcomes for patients with ectopic calcification. Future studies may include combination therapy, addressing the issues of vitamin D deficiency, parathyroid hormone and phosphorus excess. More investigation is needed to identify novel agents or strategies that could modulate circulating promoters and inhibitors of calcification. There is likely to be further research focusing on the identification and characterisation of as yet unidentified or uncharacterised, disease-causing and susceptibility genes, which may help in the development of prevention strategies. This is clearly an exciting, growing field and with further analysis of the molecular pathways involved in the process of calcification, we can envisage the development of effective therapeutic strategies to intervene with this process. Studies to date have provided new insights into the molecular and cellular regulation of calcification and provide hope for the design of effective therapeutic strategies to intervene with calcific vasculopathies.

Key points for clinical practice

- Multi-row detector computed tomography (MDCT) is a valid method for quantitative assessment of coronary artery calcium and can identify patients at risk of future coronary events.

- Vascular calcification is pathologically linked to bone destruction.

- Vascular calcification is a regulated process with potential for preventative therapeutic intervention.

- Modulation of promoters or inhibitors of calcification may attenuate the progress of vascular calcification.

- In end-stage renal disease, altered calcium and phosphate metabolism and the use of calcium-containing phosphate binders can result in progression of vascular calcification and an adverse outcome.

- Patients with bone disease should be screened for cardiovascular disease and treatment should be carefully monitored, especially those being administered calcium salts.

References

1. ACCF/AHA 2007 Clinical Expert Consensus Document on Coronary Artery Calcium Scoring by Computed Tomography in Global Cardiovascular Risk Assessment and in Evaluation of Patients With Chest Pain. *Circulation* 2007; **115**: 402–426.

2. Young MJ, Adams JE, Anderson GF, Boulton AJ, Cavanagh PR. Medial arterial calcification in the feet of diabetic patients and matched non-diabetic control subjects. *Diabetologia* 1993; **36**: 615–621.

3. Greaves M, Rowlands DJ. Coronary angiography by CT: is it now feasible? Achievements, limitations, future possibilities. In: Rowlands D, Clarke B. (eds) *Recent Advances in Cardiology*, vol. 14. London: Royal Society of Medicine Press, 2007; 149–172.

4. Agatston AS, Janowitz WR, Hildner FJ, Zusmer NR, Viamonte M, Detrano R. Quantification of coronary-artery calcium using ultrafast computed-tomography. *J Am Coll Cardiol* 1990; **15**: 827–832.

5. Kirton JP, Wilkinson FL, Canfield AE, Alexander MY. Dexamethasone downregulates calcification-inhibitor molecules and accelerates osteogenic differentiation of vascular pericytes: implications for vascular calcification. *Circ Res* 2006; **98**: 1264–1272.

6. Doherty MJ, Ashton BA, Walsh S, Beresford JN, Grant ME, Canfield AE. Vascular pericytes express osteogenic potential *in vitro* and *in vivo*. *J Bone Miner Res* 1998; **13**: 828–838.

7. Reynolds JL, Joannides AJ, Skepper JN *et al*. Human vascular smooth muscle cells undergo vesicle-mediated calcification in response to changes in extracellular calcium and phosphate concentrations: a potential mechanism for accelerated vascular calcification in ESRD. *J Am Soc Nephrol* 2004; **15**: 2857–2867.

8. Demer L, Tintut Y, Radcliff K. Regulation of vascular calcification and osteolysis by inflammatory lipids. *Atherosclerosis Suppl* 2003; **4**: 270.

9. Orita Y, Yamamoto H, Kohno N *et al*. Role of osteoprotegerin in arterial calcification. Development of new animal model. *Arterioscler Thromb Vasc Biol* 2007; **27**: 2058–2064.

10. Rattazzi M, Bennett BJ, Bea F *et al*. Calcification of advanced atherosclerotic lesions in the innominate arteries of ApoE-deficient mice: potential role of chondrocyte-like cells. *Arterioscler Thromb Vasc Biol* 2005; **25**: 1420–1425.

11. Mackie EJ, Ahmed YA, Tatarczuch L, Chen KS, Mirams M. Endochondral ossification: how cartilage is converted into bone in the developing skeleton. *Int J Biochem Cell Biol* 2008; **40**: 46–62.

12. Liu Y, Wilkinson FL, Kirton J *et al*. Hepatocyte growth factor and its receptor c-Met are expressed in human atherosclerotic lesions and induce pericyte migration *in vitro*. *J Pathol* 2007; **112**: 12–19.

13. Demer LL, Tintut Y. Mineral exploration: search for the mechanism of vascular calcification and beyond. *Arterioscler Thromb Vasc Biol* 2003; **23**: 1739–1743.

14. Raggi P, Giachelli C, Bellasi A. Interaction of vascular and bone disease in patients with normal renal function and patients undergoing dialysis. *Nat Clin Pract Cardiovasc Med* 2007; **4**: 26–33.

15. Abedin M, Tintut Y, Demer LL. Mesenchymal stem cells and the artery wall. *Circ Res* 2004; **95**: 671–676.

16. Wilkinson FL, Liu Y, Rucka AK *et al*. Contribution of VCAF-positive cells to neovascularisation and calcification in atherosclerotic plaque development. *J Pathol* 2006; **211**: 362–369.

17. Alexander MY, Wilkinson FL, Kirton JP *et al*. Identification and characterization of vascular calcification-associated factor, a novel gene upregulated during vascular calcification *in vitro* and *in vivo*. *Arterioscler Thromb Vasc Biol* 2005; **25**: 1851–1857.

18. Bostrom K, Watson KE, Horn S, Wortham C, Herman I, Demer LL. Bone morphogenetic protein expression in human atherosclerotic lesions. *J Clin Invest* 1993; **91**: 1800–1809.

19. Shanahan CM, Cary NRB, Metcalfe JC, Weissberg PL. High expression of genes for calcification-regulating proteins in human atherosclerotic plaques. *J Clin Invest* 1994; **93**: 2393–2402.

20. Canfield AE, Farrington C, Dziobon MD *et al*. The involvement of matrix glycoproteins in vascular calcification and fibrosis: an immunohistochemical study. *J Pathol* 2002; **196**: 228–234.

21. Tintut Y, Alfonso Z, Saini T *et al.* Multilineage potential of cells from the artery wall. *Circulation* 2003; **108**: 2505–2510.
22. Yoshida T, Owens GK. Molecular determinants of vascular smooth muscle cell diversity. *Circ Res* 2005; **96**: 280–291.
23. Kiechl S, Werner P, Knoflach M, Furtner M, Willeit J, Schett G. The osteoprotegerin/RANK/RANKL system: a bone key to vascular disease. *Expert Rev Cardiovasc Ther* 2006; **4**: 801–811.
24. Proudfoot D, Skepper JN, Hegyi L, Bennett MR, Shanahan CM, Weissberg PL. Apoptosis regulates human vascular calcification *in vitro* – Evidence for initiation of vascular calcification by apoptotic bodies. *Circ Res* 2000; **87**: 1055–1062.
25. Ketteler M, Westenfeld R, Schlieper G, Brandenburg V. Pathogenesis of vascular calcification in dialysis patients. *Clin Exp Nephrol* 2005; **9**: 265–270.
26. Nadra I, Mason JC, Philippidis P *et al.* Proinflammatory activation of macrophages by basic calcium phosphate crystals via protein kinase C and MAP kinase pathways: a vicious cycle of inflammation and arterial calcification? *Circ Res* 2005; **96**: 1248–1256.
27. Li X, Yang HY, Giachelli CM. Role of the sodium-dependent phosphate cotransporter, Pit-1, in vascular smooth muscle cell calcification. *Circ Res* 2006; **98**: 905–912.
28. Jeziorska M, McCollum C, Woolley DE. Observations on bone formation and remodelling in advanced atherosclerotic lesions of human carotid arteries. *Virchows Arch* 1998; **433**: 559–565.
29. Garg V, Muth AN, Ransom JF *et al.* Mutations in NOTCH1 cause aortic valve disease. *Nature* 2005; **437**: 270–274.
30. Mohamed SA, Aherrahrou Z, Liptau H *et al.* Novel missense mutations (p.T596M and p.P1797H) in NOTCH1 in patients with bicuspid aortic valve. *Biochem Biophys Res Commun* 2006; **345**: 1460–1465.
31. Herrmann SM, Whatling C, Brand E *et al.* Polymorphisms of the human matrix Gla protein (MGP) gene, vascular calcification, and myocardial infarction. *Arterioscler Thromb Vasc Biol* 2000; **20**: 2386–2393.
32. Nasir K, Budoff MJ, Wong ND *et al.* Family history of premature coronary heart disease and coronary artery calcification: Multi-Ethnic Study of Atherosclerosis (MESA). *Circulation* 2007; **116**: 619–626.
33. Collin-Osdoby P. Regulation of vascular calcification by osteoclast regulatory factors RANKL and osteoprotegerin. *Circ Res* 2004; **95**: 1046–1057.
34. Simpson CL, Lindley S, Eisenberg C *et al.* Toward cell therapy for vascular calcification: osteoclast-mediated demineralization of calcified elastin. *Cardiovasc Pathol* 2007; **16**: 29–37.
35. Kiel DP, Kauppila LI, Cupples LA, Hannan MT, O'Donnell CJ, Wilson PWF. Bone loss and the progression of abdominal aortic calcification over a 25 year period: The Framingham Heart Study. *Calcif Tissue Int* 2001; **68**: 271–276.
36. Clouse ME, Gramm HF, Legg M, Flood T. Diabetic osteoarthropathy. Clinical and roentgenographic observations in 90 cases. *AJR Am J Roentgenol* 1974; **121**: 22–34.
37. Moe SM, Drueke T, Lameire N, Eknoyan G. Chronic kidney disease-mineral-bone disorder: a new paradigm. *Adv Chronic Kidney Dis* 2007; **14**: 3–12.
38. Block GA, Spiegel DM, Ehrlich J *et al.* Effects of sevelamer and calcium on coronary artery calcification in patients new to hemodialysis. *Kidney Int* 2005; **68**: 1815–1824.
39. Block GA, Klassen PS, Lazarus JM, Ofsthun N, Lowrie EG, Chertow GM. Mineral metabolism, mortality, and morbidity in maintenance hemodialysis. *J Am Soc Nephrol* 2004; **15**: 2208–2218.
40. Clark-Greuel JN, Connolly JM, Sorichillo E *et al.* Transforming growth factor-beta1 mechanisms in aortic valve calcification: increased alkaline phosphatase and related events. *Ann Thorac Surg* 2007; **83**: 946–953.
41. Caira FC, Stock SR, Gleason TG *et al.* Human degenerative valve disease is associated with up-regulation of low-density lipoprotein receptor-related protein 5 receptor-mediated bone formation. *J Am Coll Cardiol* 2006; **47**: 1707–1712.
42. Xu QB. Mouse models of arteriosclerosis – From arterial injuries to vascular grafts. *Am J Pathol* 2004; **165**: 1–10.
43. Kurane A, Simionescu DT, Vyavahare NR. *In vivo* cellular repopulation of tubular elastin scaffolds mediated by basic fibroblast growth factor. *Biomaterials* 2007; **28**: 2830–2838.

44. Price PA, Faus SA, Williamson MK. Bisphosphonates Alendronate and Ibandronate inhibit artery calcification at doses comparable to those that inhibit bone resorption. *Arterioscler Thromb Vasc Biol* 2001; **21**: 817–824.
45. McClung MR, Lewiecki EM, Cohen SB *et al*. Denosumab in postmenopausal women with low bone mineral density. *N Engl J Med* 2006; **354**: 821–831.
46. Persy V, De BM, Ketteler M. Bisphosphonates prevent experimental vascular calcification: treat the bone to cure the vessels? *Kidney Int* 2006; **70**: 1537–1538.
47. Block GA, Raggi P, Bellasi A, Kooienga L, Spiegel DM. Mortality effect of coronary calcification and phosphate binder choice in incident hemodialysis patients. *Kidney Int* 2007; **71**: 438–441.
48. Mathew S, Lund RJ, Strebeck F, Tustison KS, Geurs T, Hruska KA. Reversal of the adynamic bone disorder and decreased vascular calcification in chronic kidney disease by sevelamer carbonate therapy. *J Am Soc Nephrol* 2007; **18**: 122–130.
49. Mohler III ER, Wang H, Medenilla E, Scott C. Effect of statin treatment on aortic valve and coronary artery calcification. *J Heart Valve Dis* 2007; **16**: 378–386.
50. Brown MJ, Palmer CR, Castaigne A *et al*. Morbidity and mortality in patients randomised to double-blind treatment with a long-acting calcium-channel blocker or diuretic in the International Nifedipine GITS study: Intervention as a Goal in Hypertension Treatment (INSIGHT). *Lancet* 2000; **356**: 366–372.
51. Motro M, Shemesh J. Calcium channel blocker nifedipine slows down progression of coronary calcification in hypertensive patients compared with diuretics. *Hypertension* 2001; **37**: 1410–1413.

Petra Jenkins   Vaikom S. Mahadevan

3

Emergencies in adult congenital heart disease

Congenital heart disease (CHD) occurs in about 0.8% of newborn infants.[1] With the continued development and success of paediatric cardiology and surgery, up to 85% of children with CHD can expect to live into adulthood.[2]

One of the large centres in Canada reported a near 3-fold increase in outpatient activity during the nineties and 69% of these patients had had a previous surgical repair, indicating the increasing prevalence and complexity of adults with congenital heart disease (ACHD).[3] A recent European study demonstrated an overall mortality of 3% on 5-year follow-up in ACHD patients. However, mortality varies appreciably among the conditions and was markedly higher for patients with cyanotic heart disease (at 12.6%) and those with a Fontan circulation (at 8%; Table 1). Arrhythmias were the most common cause for hospitalisation.[4]

In one reported series over a period of 1 year, 22% of all admissions in ACHD patients were unplanned and 83% of these were for cardiovascular causes. Many of these admissions were patients in their third decade of life and 70% of these patients had a history of previous cardiac surgery for congenital heart disease.[5,6] The mortality for ACHD patients having an unscheduled admission ranges from 5–7%.[5,6] With increasing longevity, 30% of admissions for ACHD patients are over 40 years of age, and 5% are over the age of 60 years.[7]

The modes of presentation, management and prognosis of this heterogeneous group depend on the pathophysiological substrate, the co-morbidities and the treatment received. On admission, the management of the

Petra Jenkins MB ChB MRCP
Specialist Registrar in Cardiology, Manchester Heart Centre, Manchester Royal Infirmary, Oxford Road, Manchester M13 9WL, UK

Vaikom S. Mahadevan MD MRCP (for correspondence)
Consultant Cardiologist and Interventionist in Adult Congenital Heart Disease, Manchester Heart Centre, Manchester Royal Infirmary, Oxford Road, Manchester M13 9WL, UK
E-mail: vaikom.mahadevan@cmmc.nhs.uk

43

Table 1 5-year survival rates from study entry date for eight common ACHD conditions

Adult congenital heart disease	Percentage Survival at 5 years (Kaplan-Meier)
Coarctation of the aorta	99.3
Atrial septal defect	98.9
Tetralogy of Fallot	98.7
Ventricular septal defect	98.4
Marfan's syndrome	98.3
Transposition of the great arteries	97.1
Fontan procedure	91.8
Cyanotic defect	87.4

Produced with data from The Euro Heart Survey on Adult Congenital Heart Disease (*Eur Heart J* 2005; **26**: 2325–2333).

Table 2 Primary reasons for cardiovascular emergency admissions in ACHD

Cardiovascular emergency	Percentage of total
Arrhythmia	53
Supraventricular arrhythmias	47
Acute congestive heart failure	19
Infectious emergencies	6
Ventricular tachycardia	3
Symptomatic bradycardia	2
Syncope	2
Cerebral ischaemia	2
Pacemaker problems	2
Acute aortic dissection	2
Pericardial tamponade/effusion	2
Sudden cardiac death	1
ICD burst	1

Modified from Kaemmerer H *et al.* Emergency hospital admissions and 3 year survival of adults with and without cardiovascular surgery for congenital heart disease. *J Thorac Cardiovasc Surg* 2003; **126**: 1048–1052.

majority of these patients requires collaboration with another speciality.[6] To avert iatrogenic exacerbation or escalation of an emergency situation, all unscheduled admissions should be discussed with the ACHD specialist team. This applies in non-emergency scenarios as well. Table 2 shows the primary reason for emergency cardiovascular admission in ACHD patients from one reported series.[5]

This chapter is intended to provide a brief overview of the salient cardiac and related vascular emergencies in this patient group and their management.

ARRHYTHMIAS

Arrhythmias constitute the majority of causes for unscheduled hospital admissions in ACHD patients.[6] The underlying structural abnormalities associated with previous surgical procedures create a unique substrate for arrhythmias in this patient group. Although the anatomical classification of congenital heart defects is complex, the categories constituting the majority of arrhythmias include patients with repaired Fallot's tetralogy, Fontan type of circulation with single ventricular physiology and patients who have a systemic right ventricle with a previous Mustard or Senning type of repair for transpositions. The spectrum of clinical consequences of arrhythmia in ACHD ranges from clinically occult arrhythmia to sudden death. Incessant or recurrent arrhythmia may cause gradual haemodynamic deterioration, and *vice versa*, often resulting in a vicious cycle of clinical decompensation and poor outcome.[8]

Thrombosis and thrombo-embolic events may also occur in association with tachycardia.[9]

Frequent hospitalisation, the management of cardiac devices (including access issues), anatomical complexities, sepsis, emboli, replacements, upgrade considerations, side effects of anti-arrythmics and refractoriness of many arrhythmias in this cohort to therapy together constitute a significant burden on quality of life and health economics.[10] The modern management of arrhythmias in ACHD requires the full expertise of a specialist ACHD unit with appropriate electrophysiology support.

TACHYARRHYTHMIAS

Supraventricular tachycardia

Supraventricular tachycardias (SVTs) are the most commonly encountered overall. In the European Heart Survey,[4] they occurred in 18% of patients compared with 5% for ventricular arrhythmias. SVT is common in patients who have undergone atrial surgery and in the presence of atrial morphological remodelling as in patients with a Fontan circulation.[11,12]

Intra-atrial re-entrant tachycardia

Intra-atrial re-entrant tachycardia (IART) is the most often encountered SVT.[13] Risk factors for development of IART are older age at surgery and longer follow-up. Its prevalence among patients who have undergone surgical procedures involving extensive atrial dissection and repair (*e.g.* Mustard and Fontan procedures) indicates a particular dependence on surgical injury. Evolution in surgical techniques, such as the development of the total cavopulmonary connection (TCPC), instead of the classical right atrial to pulmonary artery Fontan circuits, have been associated with lower incidence of IART.[14] Reports of stroke after cardioversion of IART in ACHD patients are rare. However, intravascular and intracardiac thromboses are associated with IART, and a prevalence of intracardiac thrombi in 42% of patients undergoing echocardiography before cardioversion has been reported.[9] Indeed, the frequent occurrence of thrombosis in patients with ACHD and atrial tachycardia suggests that warfarin or other potent anticoagulant treatment is indicated in most of these patients. Atrial antitachycardia pacing alone sometimes results in symptomatic improvement and a decrease in tachycardia frequency.[15] Current management aims at curative radiofrequency ablation.[14] If this is unsuccessful, surgical intervention should be considered to target the anatomical substrate and modify the pathophysiological residua.[16] The first large follow-up study of IART after CHD surgery revealed a mortality rate over 6.5 years of 17%, with 10% experiencing sudden death.[17] Patients with Ebstein's anomaly can have accessory conduction pathways and present with arrhythmias. Ablation therapy should be considered in suitable patients although this may be challenging since multiple accessory pathways may exist.

Atrial flutter

Atrial flutter is a common cause of problems after tetralogy of Fallot surgery.[18] Haemodynamically, this is not well-tolerated, especially in the setting of rapid AV conduction. The treatment considerations are as for IART.

Atrial fibrillation

Atrial fibrillation is not uncommon in this population group. The principles of management are those drawn from the general adult population, including anticoagulation and rate control. Sinus rhythm is haemodynamically preferable, and cardioversion, prophylactic anti-arrhythmic drugs, and atrial pacing have all been used to prevent, if possible, the establishment of permanent atrial fibrillation. The occurrence of atrial fibrillation in patients who also have IART reduces the likelihood that ablation will be beneficial, and may prompt consideration of a surgical maze procedure, though the efficacy of this approach to atrial fibrillation in ACHD has not yet been assessed in detail.

Late-onset ventricular tachycardia

Late-onset ventricular tachycardia (VT) is a major problem in patients who have undergone an otherwise successful repair of Fallot's tetralogy. Major risk factors for the development of VT are: (i) duration of follow up;[19] and (ii) QRS prolongation to greater than 180 ms, especially if associated with pulmonary regurgitation and RV dilatation.[20,21] Anti-arrhythmic therapy may be effective in suppressing ventricular arrhythmias, but has not been associated with improved survival.[10] Implantable defibrillator (AICD) therapy is feasible in these patients, and its use is increasing. Catheter ablation of VT has been successful in a small series of patients in this situation, and may be appropriate for patients with sustained, monomorphic VT that is haemodynamically tolerated.[22] When patients warrant surgery for haemodynamic reasons, attempts to resect potential critical zones for VT may be considered. The underlying structural issues need to be evaluated in these patients. Correction of severe pulmonary regurgitation along with intra-operative ablation has been shown to stabilise QRS duration and to reduce the incidence of arrhythmias.[23] VT can also occur in patients with previous other congenital surgery (Fig. 1) and can be associated with impaired ventricular function which requires appropriate electrophysiological management (Fig. 1B).

FONTAN CIRCULATION

Patients with a classical Fontan surgical connection between the right atrium and the pulmonary artery develop progressive increase in right atrial dimensions and are prone to atrial arrhythmias including flutter and fibrillation. It has been shown that macro re-entry is the commonest mechanism for this arrhythmia.[24] These patients can present as an emergency with symptoms of palpitations with heart rates of up to 200 bpm (Fig. 2A). Although they may initially be haemodynamically stable, rapid deterioration

A

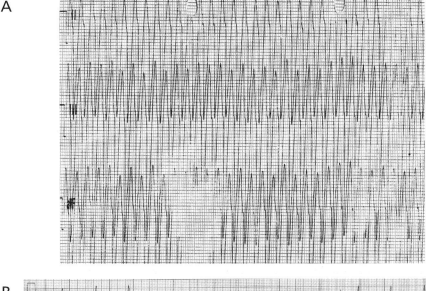

B

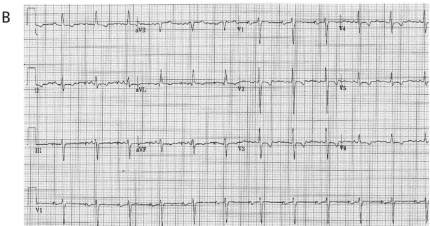

Fig. 1 (A) ECG showing ventricular tachycardia in a 25-year-old patient with poor left ventricular function with three previous surgeries for congenital mitral stenosis. (B) ECG from the same patient following insertion of a biventricular pacemaker with an AICD implant.

in ventricular function can occur. Patients require emergency assessment by an ACHD expert and often require a transoesophageal echocardiogram to ensure there are no thrombi in the enlarged right atrium prior to cardioversion, since up to 33% of patients have silent thrombi.[26] All these procedures should be performed only with support from an experienced anaesthetist involved in caring for patients with congenital heart disease. These patients may have sinus node dysfunction; hence, facilities for temporary pacing should be ensured prior to cardioversion in case of prolonged asystole (Fig. 2B). These patients should be routinely anticoagulated if they are not already on warfarin. Patients with recurrent arrhythmias should be considered for electro-physiological studies and ablation. Suitable patients should be considered for

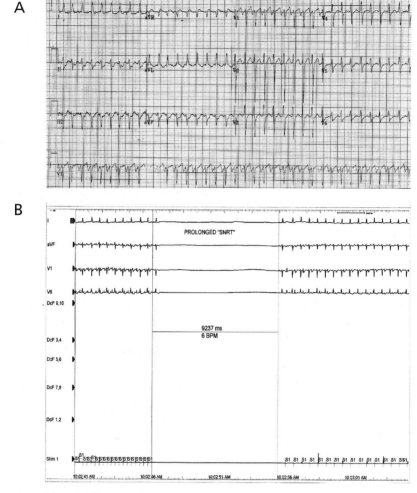

Fig. 2 (A) Atrial flutter with rapid ventricular response in 24-year-old patient with an atriopulmonary Fontan. (B) Prolonged sinus node pauses following successful ablation of atrial arrhythmia for which pacemaker insertion was successfully performed.

conversion into a total cavopulmonary connection to reduce the risk of arrhythmias.

Sudden cardiac death is the most common cause of death in adults with ACHD with a reported incidence of 26% in one series.[26] The average annualised risk of sudden death in patients with a Fontan connection has recently been reported to be around 0.15%, which is broadly similar to those with corrected Fallot's tetralogy and aortic coarctation.[27]

Simple models of risk stratification for sudden death do not exist for ACHD patients. Assessment of the risk of sudden death caused by arrhythmias requires an understanding of the limited predictive values of commonly used diagnostic tests in this population. Although Holter monitoring, exercise testing, and programmed ventricular stimulation are useful for recording and provoking clinically documented arrhythmias, their value as screening tests is not well established. Risk assessment is further complicated by the occurrence of atrial tachycardia, which may also cause symptoms and sudden death.[10] AICD therapy should be considered on an individual case basis in these situations since the indications for implantation of these devices in this population group are not well established, compared with patients having non congenital cardiac conditions.

BRADYARRHYTHMIAS

Gradual loss of sinus rhythm occurs after the Mustard and Senning and all varieties of Fontan procedures.[29] The incidence of this was found to be 17% in the Euro Heart survey in patients with transposition.[4] Patients with heterotaxy syndromes, particularly left atrial isomerism, may also have congenital abnormalities of the sinus node, independent of the effects of their surgical procedures. Paroxysmal atrial tachycardia is frequently associated with sinus node dysfunction, and loss of sinus rhythm may increase risk of sudden death.

Heart block is not uncommon in patients with transposition anatomy. In the recent European series, the incidence of this was 7%.[4] Heart block is not uncommon in patients with previous surgery or isolated congenitally corrected transposition and has been reported to be 39% in one series.[29] Intraventricular conduction abnormalities are common in ACHD and do not require specific treatment on their own. In many of these patients, bradycardia and heart block tend to occur over a period of time and permanent pacing is required. This should be done in specialised ACHD units by operators with experience in dealing with congenital cardiac abnormalities.

Patients with Fontan circuits do not have percutaneous access into the subpulmonary ventricle; hence, temporary pacing wire insertion in emergencies is not possible. These patients will require emergency external pacing until a stable rhythm can be restored.

SYNCOPE

The occurrence of syncope should trigger comprehensive investigation in the ACHD population, especially in cyanotic patients. Although benign, vasovagal syncope can occur, it is important other causes are excluded.

The aetiology of syncope is very varied and includes the tachy- and brady-arrhythmias alluded to earlier. Specific to the ACHD patient is the need to establish the cause of decompensated haemodynamics, including causes such worsening cyanosis due to occlusion of shunts, obstructed baffles, pulmonary embolism, systemic ventricular failure, prosthetic valve dysfunction and aortic root problems. Detailed haemodynamic and electrophysiological assessments may be required based on individual patient needs.

HEART FAILURE

Adult patients with congenital heart disease have previously been described as having a chronic heart failure syndrome. Decompensated heart failure has been reported to account for about 20% of unscheduled admissions in ACHD.[5] The rate of admissions caused by heart failure in the ACHD population is expected to increase because adults with univentricular physiology with a

Fontan circuit or morphological right ventricles subtending the systemic circulation are ageing.[30] In the Euro Heart Survey on ACHD over a follow-up period of at least 3 years,[4] NYHA class worsened in 6% overall and 17% and 21% in the Fontan and cyanotic cohorts, respectively.

Poor functional class, clinical signs of heart failure and arrhythmias have been reported to be predictors of death in patients with Eisenmenger's syndrome.[8] The usual management principles of heart failure[31] apply in most cases of ACHD. The precipitating causes of decompensation must be sought (for example, baffle obstruction, arrhythmia, progression of systemic ventricular dysfunction) and reversible causes treated aggressively.

Neurohormonal activation in adult congenital heart disease bears the hallmarks of chronic heart failure, relating to symptom severity and ventricular dysfunction and not necessarily to anatomical substrate. Neurohormonal antagonism across this large and anatomically diverse population should be considered.[32] Evidence for pharmacological intervention has been extrapolated from the non-ACHD heart failure arena and the evidence of benefit for angiotensin converting enzyme inhibitors in patients with systemic right ventricles and those with Fontan type of circulation is not convincing at the present time Indeed, care must be taken in the use of vasodilators in this group. Excessive diuresis should be avoided especially in the polycythaemic patient to reduce the risk of precipitating hyperviscosity symptoms.

Cardiac resynchronisation therapy is feasible, although its indications and benefits are yet to be established. While it has been shown to be of benefit,[33] there are no randomised control trial data in this population group for such therapy. There is little evidence in the literature of ventricular assist device use in the ACHD population. Congenital heart disease represented only 2.7% of those patients who received heart transplantation in the period 2001–2003.[34] The number of heart and lung transplantations is very low overall currently in the UK.

ENDOCARDITIS

Most ACHD patients, but not all, have a life-long risk of infective endocarditis. Patients who are considered to be at a moderate or higher risk include those with significant aortic valve disease, surgical conduits, systemic atrioventricular valve regurgitation, prosthetic valves, unoperated ventricular septal defects, repair of Fallot's tetralogy, patent ductus and Eisenmenger's syndrome. Isolated lesions of the pulmonary valve which are not severe, the ductus which has been closed and secundum atrial septal defects are considered to be of low risk.

Infective endocarditis accounted for approximately 4% of admissions to a specialised unit for ACHD patients in the UK.[35] This is commensurate with other European data.[4] Education of the patient and of their physicians, about the risks and importance of early diagnosis, needs constant reinforcement.

In one reported series, 41% of patients had a precipitating event.[35] There may be a variety of portals for entry of infection, including dental, surgical procedures and intravenous administration of medications; hence, line filters should be used. Since many patients are young, other causes such as body piercing, tattooing and intravenous use of recreational drugs need to be considered in these patients. Interventional cardiac catheterisation is infrequently associated with endocarditis, but antibiotic prophylaxis is usually given. The issue of antibiotic prophylaxis in patients with congenital and structural heart disease is being reviewed by the UK National Institute for Health and Clinical Excellence (NICE) and final recommendations are expected in the near future.

Delay in diagnosis and in referral is common, and antibiotics are frequently prescribed before the diagnosis of endocarditis is considered or blood cultures are taken. The mean time lag between onset of symptoms and clinical diagnosis of infective endocarditis was 29–60 days in one series.[35] More than one set of blood cultures should be performed in patients with suspected endocarditis. It is easy to miss vegetations in adults using transthoracic echocardiography, particularly when operators inexperienced in the investigation of congenital heart disease perform this. The use of transoesophageal echocardiography considerably increases the rate of detection of vegetations.[36]

Prompt referral to the specialist unit is usually indicated since haemodynamic deterioration may be rapid. The cardiac surgeon needs to be involved early, as surgical replacement of infected prosthetic material may be required, and to reduce the on-going risk of embolic events. Mortality rates up to 10% have been reported in some series for ACHD patients with a diagnosis of endocarditis.[37] Antibiotic treatment and overall patient management should be undertaken in liaison with a microbiologist. Cyanotic patients and patients with a Fontan connection and protein-losing enteropathy are immuno-compromised and require very careful specialist management. Fungal endocarditis may be particularly difficult to treat and other unusual organisms may be responsible. The European Society of Cardiology and the American Heart Association have published specific antibiotic regimens.[36,38,39]

VASCULAR EMERGENCIES

CEREBROVASCULAR EVENTS

The cumulative incidence of thrombo-embolic events was 25% during a 10-year period of follow-up in the Fontan population in one study, indicating the burden of this illness in this population group.[40] The prevalence of a history of stroke or transient ischaemic attack was 10% in the cyanotic ACHD patient in the European Heart Survey.[4] This is commensurate with other studies with reported rates of 13.6%[42] and 7.9%.[37] The association of arrhythmias and coagulopathy seen in the Fontan group in particular seem to be a powerful causative factor for these events.[40] Venous thrombosis associated with cyanosis and polycythaemia and emboli from the heart are known to occur and there is a report of central retinal vein occlusion in a patient with Eisenmenger's syndrome.[42] Thrombotic and embolic complications associated with cardiac prostheses can occur and may require surgical intervention.

The coagulopathies, seen particularly in cyanotic ACHD, causes a therapeutic dilemma in the use of anticoagulants although most centres now would use some form of anticoagulant or antiplatelet therapy in patients with a Fontan type of circulation.

The important risk factors in adults for thrombotic cerebrovascular and cardiovascular disease (such as hypertension, diabetes, alcohol abuse, and smoking) will become increasingly relevant in an ageing ACHD population.

PULMONARY EMBOLISM/HAEMOPTYSIS

Silent right atrial thrombi are known to exist in the Fontan population;[25] in one reported series, up to 17% of these patients had silent pulmonary emboli.[43] Pulmonary artery thrombi can occur in 20% of patients with Eisenmenger's syndrome (related to slow pulmonary flow).[44] A high index of suspicion of pulmonary embolic disease is required in the Eisenmenger's syndrome patients with pulmonary hypertension and those with a Fontan connection if they present with worsening dyspnoea or haemoptysis.

Ventilation perfusion scans can be difficult to interpret in patients with complex ACHD and are often inconclusive. The investigation of choice in these conditions is computed tomography pulmonary angiography, which can also provide information regarding pulmonary haemorrhage or infraction and associated bronchopulmonary collaterals.

Eisenmenger's syndrome patients presenting with haemoptysis can be difficult to manage and can have recurrent symptoms. Anticoagulation will have be carefully evaluated in this group bearing in mind that haemoptysis may be the manifestation of underlying pulmonary emboli. In certain cases where there is evidence of bleeding from bronchopulmonary or aortopulmonary collaterals, embolisation of these vessels could be considered if the pulmonary circulation is not collateral-dependent.

AORTIC ROOT EMERGENCIES

While a detailed review of this is beyond the scope of this chapter, patients with Marfan's syndrome can present as an emergency with acute aortic dissection, even in the absence of significant aortic dilatation. One of the more recently recognised causes of aortic dilatation in the ACHD population is the group of patients with previous repair of Fallot's tetralogy and those with pulmonary stenosis or atresia. The ascending aorta in these patients has been shown to be histologically abnormal with fibrosis, cystic medial necrosis and elastic fragmentation as compared to normal controls.[45] There have reports of these patients presenting with aortic dissection.[46]

MANAGEMENT OF THE CYANOTIC PATIENT IN THE EMERGENCY ROOM

In the Euro Heart Survey, approximately 10% of ACHD patients had cyanotic heart disease[4] and the commonest diagnosis among these was Eisenmenger's syndrome. These patients presenting to the emergency department can cause considerable difficulties to physicians and others not routinely involved in the care of these patients. The general issues that need to be addressed in the emergency department while urgent ACHD input is sought are summarised in Table 3.

Table 3 Issues that need to be addressed in the emergency department while urgent ACHD input is sought

- **The rhythm should be monitored** – arrhythmias are fairly common in this group of patients

- **Care should be exercised in the use of anti-arrythmics** (pro-arrhythmic and chronotropic effects and lesion propensity to sino-atrial and AV nodal disease)

- If considering cardioversion in emergency cases, **anaesthetic support** personnel with experience in managing patients with congenital heart disease are required together with staff with the ability to establish temporary pacing (bearing in mind access and complex anatomical issues)

- Attempts should be made to **obtain a baseline ECG** from the patient or records if possible since many complex patients have quite abnormal ECGs

- **Adequate hydration should be ensured** to reduce the risk of hyperviscosity syndrome and worsening of low cardiac output states. Great care must taken in patients with significant systemic ventricular dysfunction

- **Care should be taken in insertion of central catheters** in view of risk of infection and embolism. Line filters should be used and bubble traps for patients with intracardiac shunts. Oxygen may be administered as required

- **Venesection should be avoided** – secondary erythrocytosis is usually compensatory and venesection can have quite deleterious effects

- There should be **a low threshold for ruling out pulmonary embolism** if clinically indicated and CT pulmonary angiography is preferable

- In the event of sudden **worsening of cyanosis**, the possibility of pulmonary embolism or of acute occlusion of shunts should be considered

- Urgent **ACHD specialist advice** should be obtained and transfer effected

---

Key points for clinical practice

- The vast majority of children born with congenital heart disease now survive into adulthood. This has created an increasing population of adults with congenital heart disease (ACHD).

- Arrhythmias are the most frequent cause of emergency admissions in this population group, followed by heart failure.

- Supraventricular tachycardias are the commonest arrhythmia in these patients and can be associated with very rapid ventricular rates and acute decompensation.

- If the clinical situation warrants urgent cardioversion, this should be done with anaesthetic support from personnel experienced in treating patients with congenital heart disease. Patients with Fontan type of circulation may have silent thrombi and should have transoesophageal echocardiography, if clinically stable, prior to cardioversion with appropriate anaesthetic support.

(continued)

Key points for clinical practice *(continued)*

- Since patients may have underlying sinus or AV nodal disease and have access issues owing to the cardiac anatomy, a clear plan should be in place for emergency pacing in patients requiring cardioversion. This is likely to be transthoracic external pacing in patients with a Fontan or total cavopulmonary connection.

- There is an increased risk of cerbrovascular events in cyanotic patients with associated polycythaemia.

- Pulmonary thrombo-embolism is not uncommon in patients with Eisenmenger's syndrome and may be the cause of haemoptysis in these patients.

- Venesection should be avoided in cyanotic patients with polycythaemia.

- Urgent specialist ACHD advice should be sought for all complex patients presenting with an emergency.

References

1. Gatzoulis MA, Webb GD. Adults with congenital heart disease: a growing population. In: Gatzoulis MA, Webb DG, Daubeney PF. (eds) *Diagnosis and Management of Adult Congenital Heart Disease*. New York: Churchill Livingstone, 2003; 3.
2. Perloff JK, Warnes C. Congenital heart diseases in adults: a new cardiovascular speciality. *Circulation* 1991; **84**: 1881–1890.
3. Gatzoulis MA, Hechter S, Sui SC, Webb GD. Outpatient clinics for adults with congenital heart disease: increasing workload and evolving patterns of referral. *Heart* 1999; **81**: 57–61.
4. Engelfriet P, Boersma E, Oechslin E *et al*. The spectrum of adult congenital heart disease in Europe: morbidity and mortality in a 5 year follow-up period. The Euro Heart Survey on Adult Congenital Heart Disease. *Eur Heart J* 2005; **26**: 2325–2333.
5. Kaemmerer H, Fratz S, Bauer U *et al*. Emergency hospital admissions and 3 year survival of adults with and without cardiovascular surgery for congenital heart disease. *J Thorac Cardiovasc Surg* 2003; **126**: 1048–1052.
6. Kaemmerer H, Bauer U, Pensl U *et al*. Management of emergencies in adults with congenital cardiac disease. *Am J Cardiol* 2008; **101**: 521–525.
7. Somerville J. Grown-up congenital heart disease – medical demands look back, look forward 2000. *Thorac Cardiovasc Surg* 2001; **49**: 21–26.
8. Diller GP, Dimopoulos K, Broberg CS *et al*. Presentation, survival prospects and predictors of death in Eisenmenger syndrome: a combined retrospective and case control study. *Eur Heart J* 2006; **27**: 1737–1742.
9. Feltes TF, Friedman RA. Transoesophageal echocardiographic detection of atrial thrombi in patients with nonfibrillation atrial tachyarrhythmias and congenital heart disease. *J Am Coll Cardiol* 1994; **24**: 1365–1370.
10. Triedman JK. Arrhythmias in adults with congenital heart disease. *Heart* 2002; **87**: 383–389.
11. Fishberger SB, Wernovsky G, Gentles TL *et al*. Factors that influence the development of atrial flutter after the Fontan operation. *J Thorac Cardiovasc Surg* 1997; **113**: 58–60.
12. Shirai LK, Rosenthal DN, Reitz BA *et al*. Arrhythmias and thromboembolic complications after the extracardiac Fontan operation. *J Thorac Cardiovasc Surg* 1998; **115**: 499–505.
13. Roos-Hesselink J, Perlroth MG, McGhie J, Spitaels S. Atrial arrhythmias in adults after repair of tetralogy of Fallot. Correlations with clinical, exercise and echocardiographic findings. *Circulation* 1995; **91**: 2214–2219.

14. Kannankeril PJ, Anderson ME, Rottman JN *et al.* Frequency of late recurrence of intra-atrial reentry tachycardia after radiofrequency catheter ablation in patients with congenital heart disease. *Am J Cardiol* 2003; **92**: 879–881.
15. Rhodes LA, Walsh EP, Gamble WJ *et al.* Benefits and potential risks of atrial antitachycardia pacing after repair of congenital heart disease. *PACE* 1995; **18**: 1005–1016.
16. Deal BJ, Mavrondisc SC, Backer CL. Beyond Fontan: surgical therapy of arrhythmias including the patients with associated complex congenital heart disease. *Ann Thorac Surg* 2003; **76**: 542–554.
17. Garson Jr A, Bink-Boelkens MTE, Hesslein PS *et al.* Atrial flutter in the young, a collaborative study of 380 cases. *J Am Coll Cardiol* 1985; **6**: 871–878
18. Chun DS, Schamberger MS, Flaspohler T *et al.* Incidence, outcome and risk factors for stroke after the Fontan procedure. *Am J Cardiol* 2004; **93**: 117–119.
19. Nollert G, Fischlein T, Bouterwek S *et al.* Long term survival in patients with repair of tetralogy of Fallot: 36 year follow-up of 490 survivors of the first year after surgical repair. *J Am Coll Cardiol* 1997; **30**: 1374–1383.
20. Gatzoulis MA, Balaji S, Webber SA *et al.* Risk factors for arrhythmia and sudden cardiac death late after repair of tetralogy of Fallot: a multi-centre study. *Lancet* 2000; **356**: 975–981.
21. Gatzoulis MA, Till JA, Somerville J *et al.* Mechanoelectric interaction in tetralogy of Fallot. QRS prolongation relates to right ventricular size and predicts malignant ventricular arrhythmias and sudden death. *Circulation* 1995; **92**: 231–237.
22. Gonska BD, Cao K, Raab J *et al.* Radiofrequency catheter ablation of right ventricular tachycardia late after repair of congenital heart defects. *Circulation* 1996; **94**: 1902–1908.
23. Therrien J, Siu SC, Harrish L *et al.* Impact of pulmonary valve replacement on arrhythmia propensity late after repair of tetralogy of Fallot. *Circulation* 2001; **103**: 2489–2494.
24. Abrams DJ, Earley MJ, Sporton SC *et al.* Comparison of noncontact and electroanatomic mapping to identify scar and arrhythmia late after the Fontan procedure. *Circulation* 2007; **115**: 1738–1746.
25. Balling G, Vogt M, Kamerrer H *et al.* Intracardiac thrombus formation after the Fontan operation. *J Thorac Cardiovasc Surg* 2000; **119**: 745–752.
26. Oechslin EN, Harrison DA, Connelly MS *et al.* Mode of death in adults with congenital heart disease. *Am J Cardiol* 2000; **86**: 1111–1116.
27. Khairy P, Fernandes SM, Mayer JE *et al.* Long-term survival, modes of death and predictors of mortality in patients with Fontan surgery. *Circulation* 2008; **117**: 85–92.
28. Duster MC, Bink-Boelkens MT, Wampler D, *et al.* Long term follow-up of dysrhythmias following the Mustard procedure. *Am Heart J* 1985; **109**: 1323–1326.
29. Presbitero P, Sommerville J, Rabajoli F *et al.* Corrected transposition of the great arteries without associated defects in adult patients: clinical profile and follow up. *Br Heart J* 1995; **74**: 57–59.
30. Stamm C, Friehs I, Mayer Jr JE *et al.* Long term results of the lateral tunnel Fontan operation. *J Thorac Cardiovasc Surg* 2000; **121**: 28–41.
31. Swedberg K, Cleland J, Dargie H *et al.* Guidelines for the diagnosis and treatment of chronic heart failure. Executive summary (update 2005). The Task Force for the diagnosis and treatment of chronic heart failure of the European Society of Cardiology. *Eur Heart J* 2005; **26**: 1115–1140.
32. Bolger AP, Sharma R, Wei L *et al.* Neurohormonal activation and the chronic heart failure syndrome in adults with congenital heart disease. *Circulation* 2002; **106**: 92–99.
33. Dubin A, Janousek E, Rhee M *et al.* Resynchronization therapy in paediatric and congenital heart disease patients an international multicentre study. *J Am Coll Cardiol* 2005; **46**: 2277–2283.
34. Taylor DO, Leah BE, Boucek MM *et al.* The Registry of the International Society for Heart Lung Transplantation: twenty first official adult heart transplant report 2004. *J Heart Lung Transplant* 2004; **23**: 796–803.
35. Li W, Somerville J. Infective endocarditis in grown-up congenital heart (GUCH) population. *Eur Heart J* 1998; **19**: 166–173.
36. Horstkotte D, Follath F, Gutschik E *et al.* Guidelines on prevention, diagnosis and treatment of infective endocarditis. Executive summary. The Task Force on Infective

Endocarditis of the European Society of Cardiology. *Eur Heart J* 2004; **25**: 267–276.

37. Anon. Eisenmenger syndrome: factors relating to deterioration and death. *Eur Heart J* 1998; **19**: 1845–1855.

38. Bonow RO, Carabello B, de Leon AC *et al.* ACC/AHA guidelines for the management of patients with valvular heart disease: executive summary: a report of the American College of Cardiology/American Heart Association Task Force on Practice Guidelines (Committee on Management of Patients With Valvular Heart Disease). *Circulation* 1998; **98**: 1949–1984.

39. Sugrue D, Blake S, Troy P, MacDonald D. Antibiotic prophylaxis against infective endocarditis after normal delivery: is it necessary? *Br Heart J* 1980; **44**: 499–502.

40. Van den Bosch AE, Roos-Hesselink JW, Van Domburg R *et al.* Long term outcome and quality of life in adult patients after the Fontan operation. *Am J Cardiol* 2004; **93**: 1141–1145.

41. Ammash N, Warnes CA. Cerebrovascular events in adults with cyanotic congenital heart disease. *J Am Coll Cardiol* 1996; **28**: 768–772.

42. Rodriguez N, Eliott D. Bilateral central retinal vein occlusion in Eisenmenger syndrome. *Am J Ophthalmol* 2001; **132**: 268–269.

43. Varma C, Warr MR, Hendler AL *et al.* Prevalence of 'silent' pulmonary emboli in adults after the Fontan operation. *J Am Coll Cardiol* 2003; **44**: 2252–2258.

44. Broberg CS, Ujita M, Prasad S *et al.* Pulmonary arterial thrombosis in Eisenmenger syndrome is associated with biventricular dysfunction and decreased pulmonary flow velocity. *J Am Coll Cardiol* 2007; **50**: 634–642.

45. Tan JL, Davlouros PA, McCarthy KP *et al.* Intrinsic histological abnormalities of aortic root and ascending aorta in tetralogy of Fallot: evidence of causative mechanism for aortic dilatation and aortopathy. *Circulation* 2005; **112**; 961–968.

46. Kim WH, Seo JW, Kim SJ *et al.* Aortic dissection late after repair of tetralogy of Fallot. *Int J Cardiol* 2005; **101**: 515–516.

Derek J. Rowlands Philip R. Moore

4

The electrocardiography of repolarisation

More than 100 years after its first use in man, the electrocardiogram (ECG) remains an essential part of any cardiological assessment whether for elective or emergency clinical use, for screening or for research. In the diagnosis of arrhythmias, the ECG is the clinical 'gold standard' (with electrophysiological study as the true gold standard) and, in relation to the morphological information it provides, it is the most readily available, least expensive and most extensively studied non-invasive cardiac investigative technique. It has been estimated that over 300 million 12-lead ECGs are recorded annually, world-wide.[1]

For many years, the main area of study and of diagnostic use of the ECG has been concentrated on the electrocardiographic manifestations of depolarisation (P waves and QRS complexes), with consideration of the manifestations of repolarisation being virtually confined to ischaemic ST segment change and to those changes secondary to primary depolarisation abnormalities (*e.g.* ST segment changes occurring in ventricular hypertrophy or in bundle branch block). In recent years, there has been rapid development in the understanding of the cellular processes involved in repolarisation of the myocardium, and developments in this area have occurred in parallel with increasing awareness of the importance and clinical significance of ventricular myocardial repolarisation in situations such as acute coronary syndromes, long QT syndrome, Brugada syndrome and arrhythmogenic right ventricular cardiomyopathy. This chapter considers most of the clinically important repolarisation patterns of the ECG and reviews what is known concerning the

Derek J. Rowlands BSc MD FRCP FACC FESC (for correspondence)
Consultant Cardiologist, The Beeches Consulting Centre, Mill Lane, Cheadle, Cheshire SK8 2PY, UK
E-mail: djr@djr12ecg.demon.co.uk

Philip R. Moore MRCP PhD
SpR in Cardiology, Harefield Hospital, Royal Brompton and Harefield NHS Trust, Hill End Road, Harefield, Middlesex UB9 6JH, UK
E-mail: prmoore@ukonline.co.uk

cellular mechanisms involved in the production both of the normal and also of abnormal appearances.

NORMAL POLARISATION AND DEPOLARISATION

RESTING MEMBRANE POTENTIAL

Under resting conditions, the cells of the atrial and ventricular myocardium are polarised, *i.e.* there is a difference of electrical potential across the cell membrane (the sarcolemma) such that the inside of the cell is negative with respect to the outside. This polarisation results from an imbalance in the distribution of ions (atoms or molecules having unequal numbers of protons and electrons) across the membrane. As a result of this imbalance, the total number of negative charges inside the cell exceeds that outside the cell. The imbalance is dependent upon the fact that the sarcolemma is differentially permeable to the intracellular and extracellular constituents, as a result of which a Donnan equilibrium exists.

The normal value of the resting membrane potential is closely approximated by the **Goldman–Hodgkin–Katz** equation for three ions – Na^+, K^+ and Cl^-:

$$E = \frac{RT}{F} \, \ln \, \frac{P_K[K^+]^o + P_{Na}[Na^+]^o + P_{Cl}[Cl^-]^i}{P_K[K^+]^i + P_{Na}[Na^+]^i + P_{Cl}[Cl^-]^o} \qquad \text{Eq. 1}$$

where E is the multi-ion equilibrium potential, R is the universal gas constant, T is the absolute temperature, F is the Faraday constant, ln is the natural logarithm, P_K, P_{Na} and P_{Cl} are the permeabilities of the cell membrane (at rest) to the three ions, $[K^+]^o$, $[Na^+]^o$, and $[Cl^-]^o$ are the extracellular concentrations of the three ions and $[K^+]^i$, $[Na^+]^i$, and $[Cl^-]^i$ are the intracellular concentrations of the three ions. Numerous experiments have been performed to demonstrate the usefulness and applicability of this equation in studies of membrane electrophysiology.[2] When the known normal values for the variables and the constants are introduced into the equation, the value calculated for E works out very close to the measured diastolic potential for human ventricular cells of –80 mV.[3]

It is clear from Equation 1 that, at any one instant in time, the trans-membrane voltage is determined both by the concentrations of all the relevant ions and by the permeabilities of the membrane to those ions at that instant. If, at any moment, the permeability of the membrane to a given ion species is zero, the ion, at that moment, plays no part in the resulting membrane potential (whatever its concentration) and need not, therefore, be represented in the equation.

In the resting state, the membrane is highly permeable to potassium ions and relatively impermeable to sodium ions and to chloride ions. P_K is, therefore, an order of magnitude greater than both P_{Na} and P_{Cl}. To a first order approximation, therefore, P_{Na} and P_{Cl} can be considered to be zero, in which case Equation 1 can be simplified to:

$$E = \frac{RT}{F} \, \ln \, \frac{P_K[K^+]^o}{P_K[K^+]^i} \; = \; \frac{RT}{F} \, \ln \, \frac{[K^+]^o}{[K^+]^i} \qquad \text{Eq. 2}$$

This is the **Nernst equation**. It gives the equilibrium potential for potassium (E_K), which indicates the value of the resting membrane potential which would obtain if the membrane were permeable only to a single ion, K$^+$. Again, insertion of the known normal values for the variants (in this case [K$^+$]^o and [K$^+$]^i) leads to a value close to the measured resting potential, the difference from the observed value being related to the fact that the permeabilities to Na$^+$ and Cl$^-$, whilst very small in the resting state of the membrane, are not truly zero.

The Nernst equation can, of course, be further simplified to:

$$E \text{ varies directly as } \quad \frac{[K^+]^o}{[K^+]^i} \qquad\qquad \text{Eq. 3}$$

Thus, the resting membrane potential is proportional to the ratio of the internal and external potassium ion concentrations. This is, of course, the result which would be obtained from Equation 1 if the membrane were permeable only to K$^+$.

Whilst this equation is widely quoted and is held to be consistent with experimental verification, its significance is often underestimated. It is important to understand that the fact that the Nernst equation gives almost exactly the same result as the Goldman–Hodgkin–Katz equation, relates not to the concentration of the various ions but to their respective permeabilities. When, in a condition of dynamic equilibrium, the permeability of one of the three ions is greatly in excess of that of the other two, it is the ratio of internal to external concentrations of that ion which determines the resting membrane potential. The significance of this will be apparent in relation to the onset of the action potential.

DEPOLARISATION OF THE CELL MEMBRANE

When the myocardial cell is stimulated, there is a major change in the properties of the cell membrane in the area of the stimulation. The change consists of a sudden dramatic reduction in the permeability of the membrane to K$^+$ and a very substantial increase in the permeability to Na$^+$. P_{Na} becomes very much greater than P_K and P_{Cl}. Consequently, for a brief period immediately following effective stimulation of the membrane, the Goldman–Hodgkin–Katz equation simplifies to:

$$E = \frac{RT}{F} \; \ln \frac{P_{Na}[Na^+]^o}{P_{Na}[Na^+]^i} \qquad\qquad \text{Eq. 4}$$

and, therefore, to:

$$E \text{ varies directly as } \quad \frac{[Na^+]^o}{[Na^+]^i} \qquad\qquad \text{Eq. 5}$$

It follows that, with the onset of the action potential, the transmembrane voltage is transiently determined by the ratio of the internal and external sodium ion concentrations. This equation gives the equilibrium potential for sodium (E_{Na}). In consequence, the transmembrane voltage ceases to be determined by the equilibrium potential for potassium (E_K) and transiently approximates to the equilibrium potential for sodium (E_{Na}).

It is important to stress that the ionic movements accompanying the waves of excitation spreading across the membrane involve only a minute number of ions, the total cell content of these ions remaining virtually unchanged.[4] Although the increase in membrane permeability to Na^+ during phase 0 of the action potential necessarily involves some movement of Na^+ ions, it is the change in permeability, rather than the actual movement of ions which creates the upstroke of the action potential. Inspection of Equation 1 reveals that the sudden change in the relative permeabilities of the membrane to sodium and potassium ions is in itself sufficient to account for phase 0 of the action potential. Thus, during phase 4, when P_K is high and P_{Na} is low Equation 1 approximates to the equilibrium equation for potassium (Eq. 2). The primary change at the onset of depolarisation (phase 0) is a dramatic increase in permeability of the membrane to sodium, so that, at the (transient) peak of the action potential, the transmembrane voltage briefly approximates to the voltage predicted by the Goldman–Hodgkin–Katz equation if Na^+ were the only ion to which the membrane were permeable (Eq. 4).

THE ACTION POTENTIAL

Under normal, resting conditions, the myocardial cell membrane potential is stable and the internal potential remains in the region of –80 mV to –90 mV with respect to the extracellular side of the membrane. Depolarisation has to be induced by an adjacent depolarised cell (the initial depolarisation emanating from a pacemaker cell). Once the process of depolarisation has been induced, a complex series of changes occurs, ultimately resulting in the

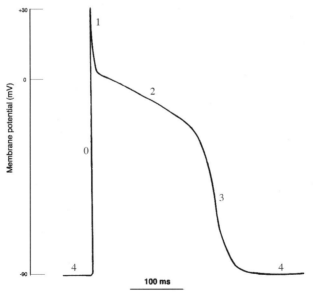

Fig. 1 Typical configuration of a ventricular myocardial action potential. During the resting phase (phase 4), the membrane potential is determined by the ratio of the internal and external K^+ concentrations. Transiently, at the onset of depolarisation (phase 0) the membrane potential rises so that at the peak of phase 0, it is determined by the ratio of the internal and external Na^+ concentrations ('equilibrium potential for sodium' – E_{Na}). During phases 1, 2 and 3, complex ionic movements occur involving K^+, Na^+, Ca^{2+} and Cl^-.

restoration of the resting membrane potential. The whole waveform, starting with the onset of depolarisation and ending with the completion of repolarisation is referred to as the action potential.

Figure 1 shows, in diagrammatic form, the main phases of the ventricular myocardial action potential. During the stable phase 4 there is equilibrium and the resting membrane potential is determined virtually exclusively by the ratio of the internal (intracellular) to the external (extracellular) potassium ion concentrations. During the (very brief) phase 0, the permeability to potassium suddenly falls and that to sodium suddenly rises. As a result, transiently (at the peak of phase 0) the membrane potential is determined virtually entirely by the ratio of the internal and external sodium ion concentrations. From the peak of phase 0 to the end of phase 3 the membrane potential changes continuously as a result of complex variations in the permeability of sodium, potassium, calcium and chloride ions.

THE REPOLARISATION PHASE OF THE ACTION POTENTIAL

Depolarisation is best regarded as ending at the peak of phase 0 of the action potential. As previously noted, the change from phase 4 to phase 0 relates virtually entirely to the sudden reversal of the differential permeabilities to Na^+ and K^+. During both phase 4 and then phase 0, the membrane is effectively permeable to a single ion (respectively, K^+ and then Na^+). From the peak of phase 0, however, and during the remainder of the action potential, multiple transient changes in the selective membrane permeability to various ions occur and, at any one time, significant permeability is not confined to a single ion. It follows that at no further point during the action potential is the instantaneous transmembrane voltage simply determined by the ratio of the internal and external concentrations of a single ion. Furthermore, during parts of the repolarisation phase, the membrane becomes highly permeable to Ca^{2+}, which is not even represented on the Goldman–Hodgkin–Katz equation (because P_{Ca} in the resting state of the membrane is effectively zero) and to Cl^-, to which the membrane is relatively impermeable during phase 4. This does not call into question the validity of the Goldman–Hodgkin–Katz concept or of the Nernst equation. The Nernst equation is valid (i) for K^+ in relation to the resting state of the membrane (phase 4) and (ii) for Na^+ in relation to phase 0 of the action potential, since in each of these situations the permeability to a single ion species is so much greater than that of all other ions that, during those periods, the internal and external concentrations of one specific ion (K^+ or Na^+) alone determines the transmembrane voltage. If the general form of the Goldman–Hodgkin–Katz equation were extended to include every ion species which at any point in the action potential had anything other than zero permeability and if the instantaneous concentrations and the instantaneous selective membrane permeabilities of all these ions were known and if these values were inserted into the (inevitably much extended) Goldman–Hodgkin–Katz equation, one would expect, on theoretical grounds, that the observed action potential could be replicated from these known values.

PERMEABILITY, CONDUCTANCE AND GATES

The term 'permeability' refers to the ease with which a given ion can cross the membrane at any instant. 'Conductance' is a measure of permeability. The rate of flow (*i.e.* current) of an ion across the membrane is determined by the product of the conductance of the membrane to the ion and the potential difference between the voltage across the membrane and the equilibrium or 'reversal' potential of the membrane in respect of that ion. Thus:

$$I_{Na} = gNa(V_m - E_{Na}) \qquad\qquad \text{Eq. 6}$$

where I_{Na} is the sodium current flow, gNa is the membrane conductance to sodium, V_m is the voltage across the membrane and E_{Na} is the sodium equilibrium or reversal potential.[5]

Ions pass through the cell membrane via channels. Each channel is operated by two or more gates which control the opening and closing of the channel. Thus, during phase 4 of the action potential the Na^+ gates are closed and the K^+ gates are open. With the onset of phase 0, this situation reverses. During phase 0 there is a minute flow of Na^+ ions across the membrane but, as noted above, it is not the extent of the movement of Na^+ ions (which is very small) but the fact that the permeability (conductance) of the membrane to Na^+ now suddenly exceeds that to K^+ which determines the dramatic change in the membrane voltage, in accordance with the Goldman–Hodgkin–Katz equation.

There are several (at least eight) different potassium gates, most of which are voltage activated, there are at least two calcium gates and a calcium exchanger. It is the intimate and precisely timed interplay of several potassium gates which ultimately results in the restoration of the resting membrane potential (phase 4).

ELECTROCARDIOGRAPHIC MANIFESTATIONS OF REPOLARISATION

VENTRICULAR REPOLARISATION

In clinical electrocardiography, ventricular repolarisation is traditionally held to commence with the onset of the ST segment, at the J point. Barr[6] defined the J point as 'the time when the tracing changes slope abruptly at the end of the S wave' and pointed out that the J point is sometimes used as a marker for the end of excitation. However, Spach *et al.*[7] have stated that overlap of potentials occurs at the end of depolarisation and the beginning of repolarisation. It is clear from inspection of the form of the action potential (Fig. 1) that, electrophysiologically, the repolarisation process begins at the peak of phase 0 of the action potential, which is very early during the QRS complex. Yan *et al.*[8] have stated that 'ventricular depolarisation (activation) is depicted by the QRS complex, whereas ventricular repolarisation is defined by the interval from the beginning of the QRS to the end of the T- or U-wave'. The components of the surface ECG which relate to ventricular myocardial repolarisation are the ST segments, the T waves, the U waves and the J waves. In most normal ECGs, the T waves are upright in the precordial leads and are generally concordant (in relation to the polarity of the deflections) with the QRS complexes both in the mid and left precordial leads and also in the limb leads (where, strictly speaking, normality of the T waves is defined by its having a frontal plane axis within $\pm 45°$ of the frontal plane QRS axis[9]).

ATRIAL REPOLARISATION

Electrocardiographically, atrial myocardial depolarisation gives rise to the P wave. Atrial myocardial repolarisation gives rise to the Ta wave. This is a low voltage wave with polarity opposite to that of the depolarisation wave in all leads. The Ta wave (which is inevitably present whenever there is a P wave) is usually obscured by the following QRS complex. It is most easily recognised when: (i) it is separated from the QRS by conduction delay (Figs 2 and Figure 3); or (ii) it is augmented in size as when there is sinus tachycardia (Fig. 4).

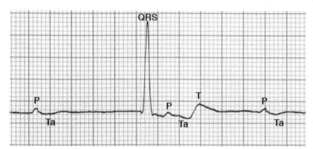

Fig. 2 Complete heart block, revealing concordance of the QRS and T wave polarities but discordance of the P and Ta wave polarities. This ECG is from a patient with complete heart block and a very slow idioventricular escape rhythm (27 per minute).

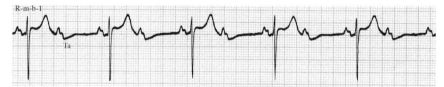

Fig. 3 Sinus rhythm with 2:1 atrioventricular block. The record clearly demonstrates how, in the conducted sinus beats the Ta waves are completely obscured. The Ta waves are clearly visible in relation to the non-conducted beats.

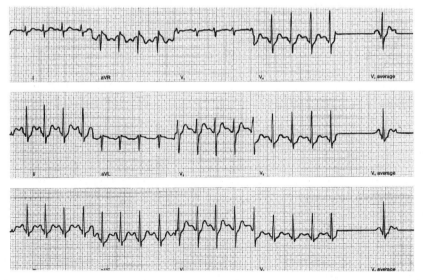

Fig. 4 Prominent Ta wave seen during an exercise stress test. Leads II, III and aVF show deep, broad, rounded negative waves beginning at the end of the P wave and extending into the proximal part of the (ventricular) T wave. The Ta waves are also well seen in V$_2$ to V$_6$. Upright Ta waves, as expected, are apparent in aVR. The (entirely normal) prominent Ta waves seen in the left precordial leads during peak exercise often give rise to the erroneous conclusion that the test is positive (*i.e.* abnormal).

ELECTRICAL HETEROGENEITY ACROSS THE VENTRICULAR WALL

In the early 1990s, Antzelevitch et al.[10–12] described three electrophysiologically distinct cell types at different levels within the wall of the left ventricle. These were: (i) cells from the endocardium; (ii) cells from the epicardium; and (iii) specialised cells situated in the region of the deep subendocardium to mid-myocardium. These latter cells were named the M cells (by Antzelevitch). The differing electrical behaviour of these three cell groups goes a long way to explaining the electrocardiographic manifestations of normal myocardial repolarisation as well as that in the various abnormal states in which repolarisation is altered. Cells with M-cell characteristics have been demonstrated in canine, guinea pig, rabbit, pig and human ventricles.[13,14] The extensive and imaginative work of this group of authors has revolutionised our understanding of the basic electrophysiological mechanisms underlying the appearances of the ECG in health and disease.

Examples of the action potentials from these three types of myocardial cells ('Epi', 'Endo' and 'M cells') are shown in Figure 5, which is taken, with permission, from the work of Antzelevitch et al.[15] The action potentials were recorded from arterially perfused canine ventricular wedge preparations, and transmural ECG recordings were made concurrently. It is clear from this figure that there are important morphological differences (particularly in respect of phase 1 and phase 3) between the action potentials of these three cell types.

The main differences between the three types of action potential are:

1. The epicardial and M cells display a prominent phase 1, giving a 'spike-and-dome' appearance to the action potential, whereas the endocardial cells do not have a prominent phase 1 and do not have the 'spike-and-dome' appearance (the difference between the endocardial and epicardial action potential configurations is shown more clearly in Fig. 9).

2. The M-cell action potential is significantly longer than that of the Epi or Endo cells.

3. Although myocardial depolarisation begins in the endocardium well before it starts in the epicardium, the difference in action potential durations is such that repolarisation is complete in the epicardium before it is complete in the endocardium, thus justifying to some degree the concept elucidated by early workers[16] that 'the direction of depolarisation is exactly opposite to that of the net direction of repolarisation', i.e. completion of depolarisation occurs sequentially from endocardium to epicardium, whereas completion of repolarisation occurs sequentially from epicardium to endocardium.

The main similarity between the repolarisation phases of the three types of action potential is that, during phase 2, the voltage levels of all three action potential types are similar. This accounts for the fact that the ST segment normally is iso-electric.

Those cells with a 'spike-and-dome' type of action potential have a prominent transient outward current (I_{to}). Differences in the magnitude of the action potential notch and corresponding differences in I_{to} have been observed between right and left ventricular epicardial cells and between epicardial cells and M cells.

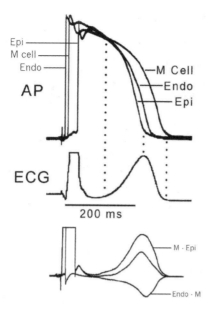

Fig. 5 (Top) Action potentials simultaneously recorded from endocardial, epicardial and M region sites of an arterially perfused canine left ventricular wedge preparation. (Middle) ECG recorded across the wedge. (Bottom) Computed voltage differences between the endocardial and M region action potential and between the M region and epicardial responses. If these traces are representative of the opposing voltage gradients on either side of the M region, responsible for the inscription of the T wave, then the weighted sum of the two traces should yield a trace (middle trace in the bottom grouping) resembling the ECG, which it does. Note that, although depolarisation spreads from the endocardium via the M cells to the epicardium, and is completed last in the epicardium, repolarisation is completed first in the epicardium. This figure was published by Elsevier © 2000 in Antzelevitch C, Yan G-X, Shimizu W, Burashnikov A.[15] and is reproduced and modified with permission.

What is not shown in Figure 5 is the typical action potential of a Purkinje cell. These cells have the longest action potential of all. Depolarisation begins in the Purkinje cells before that in the endocardium and continues until after the completion of M-cell repolarisation but makes no detectable contribution to the transmural ECG recording, presumably because of the small mass of the tissue involved.[14]

THE CELLULAR BASIS FOR THE QRS COMPLEX, S-T SEGMENT, T WAVE, J WAVE AND Ta WAVE

The transmural ECG reflects the time-varying potential difference across the myocardial wall. The morphology of the QRS complexes, ST segments and T waves can be understood by a consideration of the time relations between the onset and offset of the action potentials in the endocardial cells, M cells and epicardial cells (as noted above, the mass of the Purkinje tissue is insufficient for its activity to be detectable in the transmural ECG).

The QRS complex

Depolarisation of the ventricular myocardium spreads transmurally, from endocardium, through the M-cell region to the epicardium, as shown by the consecutive onsets of phase 0 of the action potentials of endocardial cells, M cells and epicardial cells (Fig. 5). The QRS complex therefore extends from the onset of phase 0 of the action potential of the endocardial cells to the completion of phase 0 of the action potential of the epicardial cells. The voltage at any instant in time during the QRS complex (Fig. 5, middle) is given by the sum of the two partial transmural voltages, M–Epi and Endo–M (Fig. 5, bottom). (The difference in morphology between the endocardial and the epicardial action potentials is more clearly seen in Fig. 9).

The ST segment

In the period immediately following phase 0 of the epicardial cells, the height of the plateau phase is similar in each of the three action potentials so there is no trans-myocardial gradient. During this period, therefore, the ECG shows zero voltage and the S-T segment is virtually iso-electric (Fig. 5).

The T wave

As the myocardium repolarises, the gradient in potential between the epicardium and the M region ('M–Epi', bottom section of Fig. 5) becomes increasingly positive at a faster rate than the gradient in potential between the endocardium and the M cells ('endo–M', bottom section of Fig. 5) becomes increasingly negative, thus giving rise to the ascending limb of the T wave. Therefore, the onset of the recognisable T wave (end of the S-T segment) occurs when the plateaux of the three action potentials begin to diverge (and, in particular, when the plateau of the epicardial action potential begins to diverge from that of the M cell). The peak of the T waves ('T peak') occurs with the completion of epicardial repolarisation and the T wave ends ('T end') with completion of M cell repolarisation. The interval T peak to T end corresponds to the time between the end of epicardial repolarisation and that of the M cells. The voltage at any instant in time during the T wave (Fig. 5, middle) is given by the sum of the two partial transmural voltages, M–Epi and Endo–M (Fig. 5, bottom).

The U wave

The normal U wave is best seen in the mid precordial leads and is more obvious during bradycardia. It is also augmented during exercise.

It is the least well understood of the ECG waves and no universally accepted explanation for its inception has so far emerged. Early theories suggested that U waves were created by delayed repolarisation of the His–Purkinje system but, as noted above, the mass of this tissue is very small and it is difficult to believe that such a small amount of tissue could generate some of the large U waves which can be observed. Furthermore, amphibia do not possess Purkinje fibres but do have U waves.[17]

In 1996, Antzelevitch and his group[18] suggested that the M cells, considerably greater in mass than the Purkinje cells and possessing delayed repolarisation characteristics similar to those of the Purkinje cells, might be involved in the inscription of the U wave but this does not fit well with the fact that separate (from the T waves), clear U waves are not apparent in most wedge preparation studies.[13] Yan et al.[8] demonstrated not only changes in the QT interval and in the T wave height but also the development of pathological

A ECG T Wave Shapes Clinically Recorded in Different Serum K$^+$ Concentrations

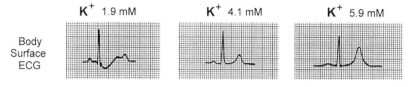

B Canine Ventricular Action Potentials and ECG

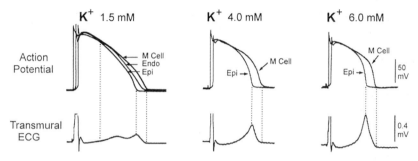

Fig. 6 (A) The ECG tracings were taken from patients with the serum potassium levels as shown. (B) Simultaneous recordings of action potentials from endocardial cells (Endo), M cells and epicardial cells (Epi), together with a transmural ECG all taken from a canine ventricular perfused wedge preparation. Interplay between the differing action potential morphologies at each of the three levels of potassium concentration determines the T wave shape in each case. The U wave is thought probably to be 'a second component of a bifid or notched T wave'. This figure was published by Elsevier [© 2003 American College of Cardiology Foundation] in Yan et al.,[8] with permission.

U waves in canine wedge preparations under conditions of varying potassium concentrations (Fig. 6). They found that, under conditions of hypokalaemia, the peak of the pathological U wave coincides with the completion of epicardial repolarisation (Fig. 6B, first set of traces) whereas the later completion of repolarisation of the endocardial and M cells contributes significantly to the descending limb of the pathological U wave (Fig. 6B, first set of traces). They concluded that the 'apparent T–U complex is, in fact, a T-wave whose ascending limb is interrupted'.

The concept of mechano-electrical feedback as a possible mechanism for the genesis of the U wave was first introduced by Lepeshkin in 1957.[19] This hypothesis emphasises the close temporal relationship between the *start* of the U wave and the second heart sound and suggests that stretch of the ventricular myocardium in the phase of rapid ventricular filling may generate delayed after potentials which could be responsible for the inscription of the U waves. Indirect evidence in support of this has been provided by the demonstration of clear separation of U waves from the preceding T waves in patients with the short QT syndrome (leads V$_2$–V$_4$ in Figure 4B of this reference).[20]

The mechanism of production of the U wave is not fully understood and it is likely that some U waves are actually modifications of the T wave morphology, whereas others are likely to be independent of those action potential variations which determine the form of the T waves.

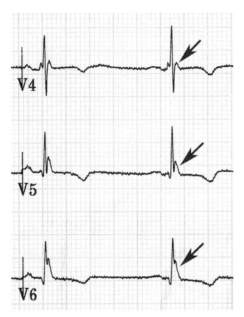

Fig. 7 J waves (arrowed) in the left precordial leads. The patient had angina and 3-vessel disease at angiography. There was a history of previous stroke. There was no hypothermia or biochemical abnormality and no recent infarction. No prior ECG recording was available.

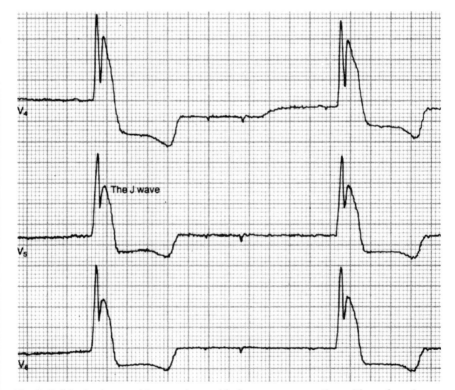

Fig. 8 Strikingly abnormal J waves in an elderly woman presenting with profound hypothermia.

The J wave

The J wave (also referred to as the J point wave, J deflection, camel hump sign, late delta wave and Osborn wave) is a wave occurring in relation to the terminal part of the QRS complex. Hurst[21] has written: 'the term J deflection has been used to designate the formation of the wave produced when there is a large, prominent deviation of the J point from the baseline'. It may be seen in association with hypothermia, hypercalcaemia, brain injury, subarachnoid haemorrhage, cardiopulmonary arrest from over-sedation and damage to the sympathetic nerves in the neck.[21] A prominent J wave is also seen in the early repolarisation syndrome, the Brugada syndrome and in those with idiopathic ventricular tachycardia.[8] Although the J wave appears as the terminal part of the QRS complex, it is clearly related to activity occurring after the peak of phase 1 of the action potential and is, therefore, properly considered as part of the repolarisation process. An example is shown in Figure 7.

Prominent J waves are thought to occur as a result of an increase in both the width and depth of the 'spike-and-dome' morphology of the action potential of the epicardial cells. Hypercalcaemic accentuation of the J wave is thought to be related to accentuation of the epicardial action potential notch, possibly as a result of an increased calcium-activated chloride current and a decrease in I_{Ca}. Hypothermia, in addition to inducing a more prominent notch, also produces slowing of conduction which results in occurrence of the epicardial notch clear of (following) the QRS complex.[13] Figure 8 shows an example of a very striking J wave in a patient presenting with profound hypothermia.

Yan and Antzelevitch,[22] using the arterially perfused canine right or left ventricular wedge preparation provided evidence that 'the transient outward current-mediated spike-and-dome morphology of the action potential across the ventricular wall underlies the manifestation of the electrocardiographic J wave'. They found that an I_{to}-mediated notch in the epicardial, but not in the endocardial, action potential was associated with a J wave. Yan et al.,[8] showed that a premature stimulus caused a parallel decrease in the amplitude of the epicardial action potential notch and in the size of the J wave. This is illustrated in Figure 9, which also shows the difference between the endocardial and epicardial action potential configurations more clearly than in Figure 5. They noted a highly significant correlation between the amplitude of the epicardial action potential notch and the amplitude of the J wave recorded during interventions that alter the electrocardiographic J wave appearances, such as hypothermia, premature stimulation, and drug-induced block of I_{to}.[13] Di Diego and Antzelevitch[23] showed that, in canine myocardium, hypercalcaemia-induced accentuation of the action potential notch in the epicardium can account for the appearance of the J wave, the slight slowing of conduction can account for the widening of the QRS and the disparate effects on the action potential duration in epicardium and endocardium for the flattening of the T wave.

The Ta wave

The atrial repolarisation wave (Ta wave) rarely receives much attention during ECG interpretation. It is, however, inevitably present following an atrial depolarisation wave. Examples have been shown in Figures 2–4, and a further example is shown in Figure 10. In all these examples, it is the separation of the P waves and Ta waves from the following QRS which facilitates the

A   J Wave in a Healthy Young Asian Male

Body Surface ECG (II)

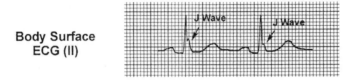

B   Canine Ventricular Action Potentials and ECG

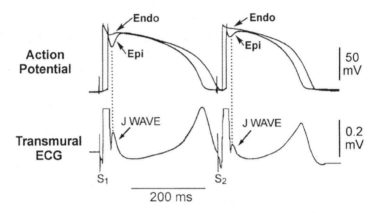

Fig. 9 Cellular basis for the J wave. The second stimulus is premature (S_1–S_2 interval 200 ms). Both the epicardial notch and the J wave are reduced, compared with the preceding beat. This figure was published by Elsevier [© 2003 American College of Cardiology Foundation] in Yan *et al.*,[8] with permission.

recognition of the Ta waves (which are normally obscured by the QRS complexes). The one common situation in which Ta waves are clearly recognisable during normal sinus rhythm is in relation to sinus tachycardia as a result of which the Ta waves increase substantially both in depth and in duration. When this occurs in the context of an exercise stress test, the (normal) exaggerated Ta wave can be misinterpreted as S-T segment depression (Fig. 4). The key to the recognition of the exaggerated Ta wave in this situation is that the depression begins before the QRS complex.

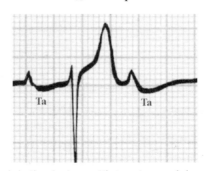

Fig. 10 The background rhythm is sinus with type I second degree atrioventricular block. The separation of the P waves from the QRS complexes facilitates the recognition of the Ta waves.

THE CONCORDANCE OF THE QRS COMPLEXES AND T WAVES

This was considered a puzzle in the early days of electrocardiography. Intuitively, one would expect the process of repolarisation to produce voltage changes opposite in direction to those of depolarisation (and, therefore, that the T waves would be opposite in polarity to the QRS). In repolarisation, the *changes in potential are reversed* compared with those of depolarisation, but, in addition, *the transmural direction of completion of repolarisation is opposite to that of depolarisation* so that the T waves are concordant with the QRS complexes. The key to the reversed direction of completion of depolarisation lies in (i) the transmural, *i.e.* centrifugal, (rather than longitudinal) transmission of myocardial depolarisation within the ventricles, together with (ii) the above noted differences in the action potentials of the three main cell types. As a result of these features, depolarisation commences in the endocardium (strictly speaking in the Purkinje tissue but activity within this tissue is not detectable from the surface ECG), spreads consecutively through the M-cell region to the epicardium and is completed when the cells of the epicardium commence phase 1 (Figs 1 and 5). Repolarisation, however, is completed first in the epicardium, then in the endocardium and finally (except for the Purkinje tissue) in the M cells. The M cells are close to the endocardium so *the wave of completion of repolarisation travels in the opposite direction to the wave of completion of depolarisation* and the two resulting deflections are concordant. The dominantly transmural spread of depolarisation is determined by the rapid longitudinal conduction through the (electrically silent) Purkinje network, which ensures rapid transmission to the endocardial cells in all areas, from which slower intramyocardial (transmural) spread then occurs.

DISCORDANCE OF THE P WAVE AND Ta WAVES

The structural feature most relevant to the difference between the mode of spread of excitation within the atria and within the ventricles is the specialised conducting tissue of the His bundle, bundle branches and Purkinje network. This structure facilitates rapid longitudinal transmission in advance of the much slower transmural transmission from endocardium to epicardium. For that reason, in relation to ventricular myocardial depolarisation and repolarisation, the surface ECG reflects predominantly radial (transmural) rather than longitudinal transmission, as explained above.

The atria, however, have no anatomically clear subendocardial network of rapidly conducting tissue (though there are functionally recognisable pathways of preferential conduction). Consequently, the spread of the activation process through the atrial myocardium is predominantly longitudinal rather than radial.[24] This results in a different relationship between depolarisation and repolarisation on the surface record, a difference which is magnified by virtue of the fact that the atrial myocardial wall is much thinner than that of the ventricles.

The ionic and electrical properties of atrial myocardium have been much less extensively studied than those of ventricular myocardium[25] but there is clear evidence of heterogeneity both regionally and transmurally. Avanzino *et al.*[26] reported the presence, in rabbit atria, of cells with properties similar to the now well-recognised M cells of ventricular myocardium but Burashnikov et al.[25] were unable to confirm this in the canine right atrium. The conditions which give rise to an upright repolarisation wave in the ventricle ([1] rapid longitudinal conduction along the Purkinje tissue (not recognisable on the surface ECG); [ii] the thick ventricular wall with slower, centrifugal conduction; [iii] clearly recognisable M cells on the subendocardial myocardium; and [iv] repolarisation finishing early in the epicardial cells) are either absent or not demonstrably present in the atrial myocardium and both depolarisation and repolarisation spread longitudinally. The electrocardiographic atrial repolarisation wave (Ta wave) is, therefore, in the opposite direction to the atrial depolarisation wave (P wave), which is what would be anticipated in the absence of the special features which obtain in relation to the ventricular myocardium.

IMPORTANT CLINICAL SYNDROMES INVOLVING ELECTROCARDIO-GRAPHIC MANIFESTATIONS OF ABNORMALITIES OF REPOLARISATION

In recent years, there has been a major and rapidly increasing realisation of the importance of electrocardiographic recognition of repolarisation abnormalities in a wide variety of clinical areas. These include the early repolarisation variant, ECG findings in athletes, the Brugada syndrome, arrhythmogenic right ventricular cardiomyopathy (dysplasia), the long and short QT syndromes, acute S-T elevation myocardial infarction, non-ST elevation acute coronary syndromes and drug- and electrolyte-induced QT prolongation. There are also, of course, the well-established and generally well-understood repolarisation changes secondary to primary QRS abnormalities (ventricular hypertrophy, bundle branch block, pre-excitation, etc.), but these latter features will not be discussed further.

EARLY REPOLARISATION SYNDROME (VARIANT)

The early repolarisation syndrome (ERS) has traditionally been regarded as being benign, although Gussak and Antzelevitch[27] point out that, in experimental models, 'the ECG signature of ERS can be converted to that of the

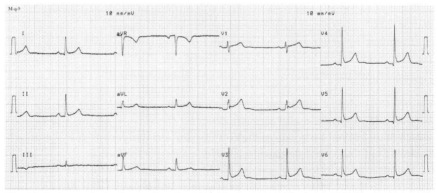

Fig. 11 Early repolarisation variant in a healthy 29-year-old. There is slight, concave ST elevation from V_2 to V_6, most marked from V_2 to V_4. The notch at the end of the QRS in V_2 and V_3 is a J wave.

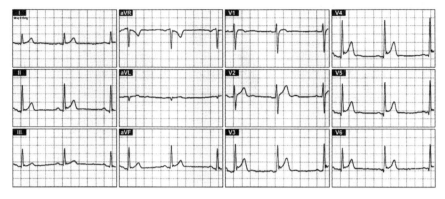

Fig. 12 Early repolarisation variant in a healthy 48-year-old. There is slight, concave ST elevation from V_3 to V_6, most marked in V_3 and V_4. The notch at the end of the QRS in V_3, V_4 and V_5 is a J wave. There is also slight ST elevation in II, III and aVF with 'reciprocal' ST depression in aVR. J waves are also seen in II, III and aVF.

Brugada syndrome'. Inevitably, its presence is a diagnostic challenge in anyone presenting with acute (potentially ischaemic) chest pain or pericarditis. Because of the similarity to the Brugada pattern it may also cause difficulty in patients presenting with ventricular arrhythmias. It is characterised by a mild degree (typically 1–2 mm) of ST segment elevation, concave upwards and ending in a positive T wave. It is usually most apparent in the mid precordial leads (V_2–V_4). There is frequently a distinct J wave in two or more of the precordial leads. Typical examples are shown in Figures 11 and 12. Mehta *et al.*,[28] in a review of 60,000 files of adult ECGs over a 5-year period, found the prevalence to be in the region of 1–2%, though the nature of the population is not made clear. The frequency of occurrence was greater in young subjects but there was no obvious racial difference. As will be seen later, the condition is present in the majority of athletes.

Cellular basis for the ECG appearances in the early repolarisation syndrome

Yan *et al.*[8] have suggested that the syndrome is the result of depression (*i.e.* partial loss) of the dome of the action potential (AP) of the left ventricular epicardial cells, bringing the plateau of the epicardial cell AP down to a lower level (see Fig. 5). This would account both for the J wave and for the ST elevation. As noted earlier, in relation to a single cell, repolarisation commences at the end of phase 0 of its action potential. In relation to the heart, therefore, ventricular repolarisation begins at the end of phase 0 of the action potential of the earliest ventricular cells to depolarise, the endocardial cells. Review of Figure 5 shows that this is significantly before the onset of phase 0 of the AP of the epicardial cells and is, therefore, early within the QRS.

Earlier, Yan and Antzelevitch[22] showed that the pronounced 'spike-and-dome' configuration seen in the epicardial cells (Epi; Fig. 5) plays an important part in the production of the J wave and the ST elevation. Action potential notches (from the spike and dome pattern) are also present in the endocardial cells (though much less pronounced than in the epicardium), but would not be expected to contribute to the J wave because their depolarisation is early and

73

the small notch is likely to be buried in the QRS complex. The notch of the M cells is larger than that of the endocardial cells but is still significantly earlier in the QRS than that of the epicardial cells (Fig. 5) and plays little part in the generation of the J wave.

Boineau,[29,30] in a recent, thought-provoking pair of communications has stressed the importance of QRS changes in the ERS (which he refers to as the 'early repolarisation variant [ERV]'). He reports that the QRS amplitude is often increased and that there is often slight initial slurring of the QRS ('subtly similar to the delta wave in Wolff–Parkinson–White'), that the rate of upstroke of the QRS is slightly reduced whereas the rate of descent of the intrinsic deflection is increased. He reports 'an anecdotal association' between ERV and sudden death but stresses that this is uncommon. An editorial[31] accompanying the articles emphasised that there is no evidence that ERV is related to the Brugada syndrome or to other channelopathies and in a letter to the journal in response to these papers, Liebman[32] also stresses the benign nature of the condition, which certainly is the currently accepted view.

REPOLARISATION ABNORMALITIES IN THE ATHLETE'S ECG

Minor repolarisation abnormalities are frequently seen in the ECGs of athletes. More marked repolarisation changes are also relatively common (Fig. 13). It should not, of course, be assumed that changes such as those shown in Figure 13 are acceptable as normal, just because the subject is an athlete. It remains essential to exclude prognostically significant abnormalities such as hypertrophic cardiomyopathy and arrhythmogenic right ventricular cardiomyopathy.

Bianco et al.[33] studied the electrocardiograms of 139 athletes and 50 sedentary controls and found the early repolarisation syndrome (≥ 1 mm ST elevation in two or more adjacent precordial leads) in 139 athletes (89%) and 18 controls (36%).

Marked repolarisation abnormalities (MRAs) are also common in athletes. Serra-Grima et al.[34] studied 26 athletes with MRAs (negative T waves ≥ 2 mm in three or more leads at rest). Four athletes with hypertrophic cardiomyopathy were excluded.

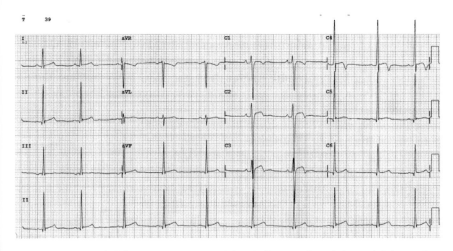

Fig. 13 ECG recorded from an international footballer. No clinical abnormalities and normal echocardiographic findings.

Clinical and physical examinations, echocardiographic studies, exercise tests and antimyosin studies were carried out in all cases and rest/exercise myocardial perfusion studies were performed in 17 cases. The investigations revealed no significant abnormality and the ECG appearances showed a tendency to 'normalise' during exercise.

Pelliccia et al.[35] found markedly abnormal ECG patterns in 14% and mildly abnormal patterns in 26% of athletes and concluded that bizarre ECG patterns may be part of the athlete's heart syndrome. *However, when abnormal repolarisation patterns are found in the ECG of athletes, it cannot be assumed that the hearts are normal. Full clinical and echocardiographic assessment is essential to exclude abnormalities such as hypertrophic cardiomyopathy, arrhythmogenic right ventricular cardiomyopathy (dysplasia), anomalous coronary arteries, etc.*

This view is supported by the recent publication by Pellicia et al.[112] They studied a database of 12,250 trained athletes. Eighty-one had diffusely distributed, deeply inverted T waves ($\geq$ 2 mm in at least 3 leads) with no clinical or echocardiographic abnormalities on serial studies. Outcomes were compared with 229 matched control athletes, with normal ECGs, from the same database. Of the 81 athletes with abnormal ECGs, 5 (6%) ultimately proved to have cardiomyopathy. Of these, one died suddenly (aged 24) from clinically undetected arrhythmogenic right ventricular cardiomyopathy, 3 developed clinical and phenotypic features of hypertrophic cardiomyopathy after 12 ±5 years (at ages 27, 32, 50) and one developed dilated cardiomyopathy after 9 years of follow-up. In contrast, none of the 229 athletes presenting with normal ECGs had major cardiac events or received a diagnosis of cardiomyopathy by 9 ±3 years after initial evaluation.

The clear message seems to be that, while sinus bradycardia, sinus arrhythmia, mildly prolonged P-R interval, Möbitz type I second degree atrioventricular block and satisfaction of the voltage criteria for left ventricular hypertrophy are all common findings in athletes and do not appear to predict significant future heart disease, marked repolarisation abnormalities give rise to more concern. Not only should athletes with such changes receive comprehensive clinical and investigative assessment, but they should also be kept under long-term review

THE BRUGADA SYNDROME

The Brugada brothers, in 1992, reported eight cases (six male and two female) with recurrent episodes of aborted sudden death.[36] The ECGs in sinus rhythm showed right bundle branch block, normal QT intervals and persistent ST elevation in V_1 and V_2 or V_1 to V_3 'not explainable by electrolyte disturbances, ischaemia or structural heart disease'. Since then there have been numerous further reports. In 2003, Antzelevitch et al.,[37] in an excellent review, summarised the understanding of the condition gained during the intervening decade.

The diagnosis of the condition presents a very real challenge since: (i) it occurs in subjects without evidence of structural heart disease; (ii) it is associated with sudden cardiac death; (iii) the prevalence in the population is low; (iv) the ECG may show any of three types of repolarisation pattern, not equally diagnostic; and (v) there is considerable time variation in the electrocardiographic appearances as well as significant modulation of those appearances by autonomic, metabolic and pharmacological factors. It is much commoner in males than in females, tends to have a familial incidence and is

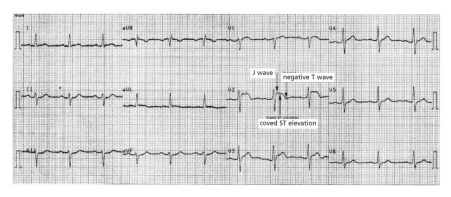

Fig. 14 Type 1 Brugada pattern (seen in V_2 and to a lesser extent in V_1). The patient presented with syncope. There is an S wave in V_6, but it is not the usual broad, slurred S wave of right-bundle branch block.

recognised as being significantly commoner in Southeast Asian men. In Japan and Southeast Asia, sudden and unexpected death of young adults during sleep is not uncommon. Autopsy findings are usually negative. The incidence is reported as being as high as 26 per 100,000 per year in some areas of Thailand.[38]

The prevalence of the condition in Western society is not reliably known. Hermida *et al.*[39] found one case among 1000 apparently health subjects (0.1%) and Monroe and Littman[40] found 52 cases among approximately 12,000 (0.43%) unselected non-cardiac patients (50 with the saddleback pattern, *i.e.* types 2 or 3, and only two with the type 1 [coved] pattern [0.017%]).

ECG characteristics of the Brugada syndrome

The ECG in Brugada syndrome shows both depolarisation and repolarisation abnormalities.

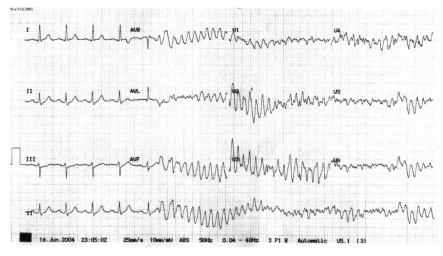

Fig. 15 Patient developed syncope whilst having a 12-lead ECG recorded in the emergency department. Sinus rhythm and full consciousness returned spontaneously after approximately 20 s. There was no history of chest discomfort. Clinical examination on recovery revealed no abnormality.

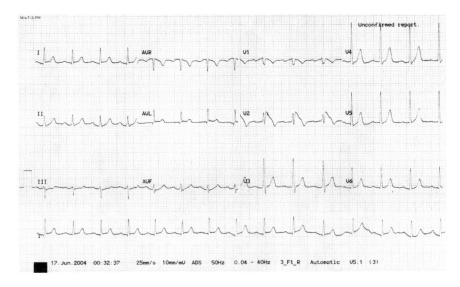

Fig. 16 An ECG from the same patient as in Figure 16. This trace was recorded about 90 min after the record in Figure 16 and shows type 1 Brugada pattern. Note especially the coved ST-T segment in lead V₂.

Depolarisation changes

The QRS pattern may show complete right-bundle branch block (RBBB), incomplete RBBB or 'focal' RBBB in which the QRS complex has what appears to be a terminal R' deflection in the right precordial leads but without the anticipated slurred S wave in the left precordial leads . The apparent terminal R' is probably best described as an exaggerated J wave.

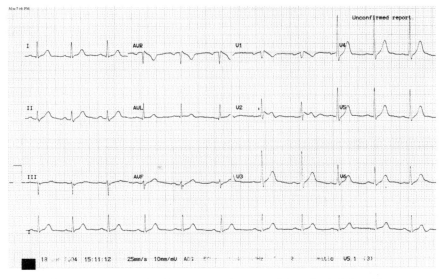

Fig. 17 The same patient as in Figure 16, on the second day of admission. The trace shows type 2 Brugada pattern.

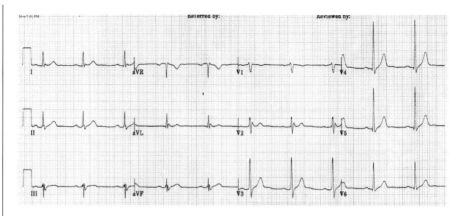

Fig. 18 The same patient as in Figure 16, on the fifth day of admission. The record shows type 3 Brugada pattern. This illustrates the considerable difficulties in relation to the electrocardiographic diagnosis of the Brugada syndrome.

Repolarisation changes
There are three recognised types of repolarisation change:

Type 1 The type described in the original paper[36] is characterised by: (i) prominent, coved ST elevation; (ii) a J wave or initial ST segment elevation ≥ 2 mm; (iii) a gradually down-sloping ST segment; followed by (iv) a small, brief negative T wave with little or no iso-electric separation from the ST segment.[42] Examples are shown in Figures 14 and 16.

Type 2 This type: (i) has a high J wave and ST segment takeoff, similar to type 1; (ii) following the J wave, the ST segment initially descends; (iii) the ST segment remains above the baseline; before (iv) ascending again as a positive or biphasic T wave. This gives a 'saddleback' appearance to the ST segment (Fig. 17).

Type 3 This is similar to type 2, the difference being that the nadir of the 'saddle' is less than 1 mm above the baseline (Fig. 18).

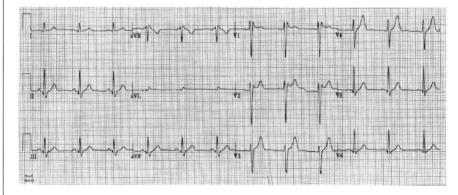

Fig. 19 Routine ECG in a healthy, asymptomatic subject, with no family history of heart problems.

As Surawicz has pointed out,[41] it can be very difficult to be confident about some of these minor changes and Gussak et al.[43] have listed 18 conditions associated with ST elevation in the right precordial leads. In most cases, the examples quoted would be unlikely to be confused with the Brugada syndrome, but the saddle back pattern is not infrequently found in otherwise normal records in asymptomatic subjects and in association with the early repolarisation syndrome. The possibility that the appearances might indicate the Brugada syndrome creates understandable anxiety in patient and doctor alike. Gussak et al.[43] have stated (and Surawicz has re-iterated[41]) that the diagnosis of the Brugada syndrome cannot be made on the basis of the ECG alone, though very clearly the ECG appearances are usually the starting point for the diagnosis. An example of a challenging ECG is shown in Figure 19. The appearances suggest minor delay in the right bundle branch system, but the appearances in V_2 raise the possibility of the Brugada syndrome. Clearly, if there were a personal or family history of sudden death (aborted or terminal), then the possibility of Brugada syndrome would have to be taken very seriously. This record, however, was taken from an asymptomatic male, with no family or personal history, with no abnormal clinical findings and with normal echocardiographic appearances.

Variability of the ECG findings in the Brugada syndrome

A major problem in the diagnosis of the Brugada syndrome is the appreciable variability of the electrocardiographic findings.[44] It is known, for example, that exercise and increasing heart rates tend to reduce the ECG changes and bradycardias to augment them. Sodium channel blocking drugs have a powerful effect in augmenting the appearances and play a role in the diagnostic process. Scheinman and Keung[45] have stressed that multiple ECG recordings are essential if the type I ECG phenotype is used to assess risk.

Figures 15–18 are taken from the records of a 40-year-old man who presented to the emergency department following an episode of syncope at home. He had been watching television with his wife. He recovered spontaneously and she took him to the accident and emergency department. Whilst having an ECG recorded there, he had a further episode of syncope, as a result of the onset of ventricular fibrillation (Fig. 16). Sinus rythm returned spontaneously after about 30 s. The subsequent ECGs were recorded on the first, second and fifth day after admission. During this 5-day period, the ECGs sequentially displayed all three Brugada patterns – type 1 (Fig. 16), type 2 (Fig. 17), and type 3 (Fig. 18). Further investigations (including coronary angiography and myocardial biopsy) showed no evidence of structural or coronary heart disease and biochemical parameters were normal. The only history of note was that, on the previous day, he had purchased antihistamine tablets (chlorphenamine, formerly known as chlorpheniramine) for mild hay fever. He had taken one tablet. An automated implantable cardioverter– defibrillator (AICD) was inserted. He remains well 3 years later and has received no appropriate device therapies.

A comparison of Figures 18 and 19 illustrates the enormous practical difficulty in knowing how to handle ECGs showing type 3 Brugada patterns. The patient with the ECGs shown in the last four figures clearly has the Brugada syndrome. Had he been asymptomatic and been found to have the

ECG shown in Figure 19, the probability of his having the Brugada syndrome would have been considered to be low and the patient whose ECG is shown in Figure 15 would have been considered a more likely candidate.

The diagnosis of Brugada syndrome: the concept of 'idiopathic Brugada ECG pattern'

The criteria for the diagnosis of Brugada syndrome are to some extent agreed but to a significant degree are still evolving. Although this chapter is primarily concerned with the electrocardiographic manifestations of the syndrome, the variability of the ECG appearances within a given subject and the uncertainties concerning the definitive application of the diagnosis are such that further comment on the significance or otherwise of the various ECG manifestations is appropriate.

Table 1 Brugada-type QRS and ST segment abnormalities seen in V_1-V_4. The 'terminal portion' of the ST segment refers to the latter half of this segment

	Type 1	Type 2	Type 3
J-wave amplitude	≥ 2 mm	≥ 2 mm	≥ 2 mm
T wave	Negative	Positive or biphasic	Positive
ST-T configuration	Coved type	Saddle back	Saddle back
ST segment (terminal portion)	Gradually descending	Elevated ≥ 1 mm	Elevated < 1 mm

Modified from the Consensus Report of the Study Group on the Molecular basis of Arrhythmias of the European Society of Cardiology.[42]

2002 Consensus Report

In 2002, a Consensus Report for the Study Group on the Molecular Basis of Arrhythmias of the European Society of Cardiology produced proposed diagnostic criteria for the Brugada syndrome.[42] Table 1 shows data from that report.

Significance of type 1 ECG
The recommendations of the 2002 Consensus Report included the suggestion that the 'Brugada syndrome should be strongly considered' when (in the presence or absence of sodium channel blocking drugs) the ECG appearance is of type 1 in more than one right precordial leads in the presence of one or more of:

- *documented ventricular fibrillation*
- *self-terminating ventricular tachycardia*
- *a family history of sudden cardiac death (< 45 years)*
- *coved-type ECGs in family members*
- *electrophysiological inducibility*
- *syncope or nocturnal agonal respiration*

and in the absence of any other factor accounting for the ECG.

The report also stated that the appearance of ECG features without any clinical symptoms should be referred to as 'idiopathic Brugada ECG pattern' and not as 'Brugada syndrome'.

Significance of type 2 ECG

The report concluded that the appearance of type 2 ECG changes (in more than one right precordial lead) which convert to type 1 following challenge with a sodium channel blocker should be considered to be equivalent to the finding of type 1 ECG. It was felt (in the light of information available at the time of writing of the report) that those with a negative response to drug challenge were unlikely to have Brugada syndrome and that a < 2 mm ST elevation response to drug challenge should be considered inconclusive.

Significance of type 3 ECG

The report concluded that the appearance of type 3 ECG changes (in more than one right precordial lead) which convert to type 1 following challenge with a sodium channel blocker should be considered to be equivalent to the finding of type 1 ECG. Drug-induced conversion of type 3 to type 2 should be considered inconclusive.

The report also recommended that patients 'who do not fully qualify the proposed criteria' should be 'considered seriously' and that a drug challenge or an electrophysiological study might be appropriate.

Second Consensus Report (2005)

A second Consensus Report (emanating from a second conference held in September 2003) was published in 2005.[46] The report stressed that the patients at highest risk of sudden death from ventricular tachyarrhythmia were those with a spontaneously appearing type 1 ECG. Patients in whom ST elevation appeared only after provocation with sodium channel blockers appeared to be 'at minimal or no risk for arrhythmic events'.[46] The report also commented that the role of electrophysiological study (EPS) in defining the on-going risk is controversial.

Further insights into the significance of Brugada patterns

Brugada *et al.*[47] reported on the follow up of 334 patients with type 1 Brugada phenotype ECG. In 71 patients, the ECG diagnosis was recognised after a cardiac arrest, in 73 after a syncopal episode and 190 were asymptomatic patients who had ECGs done during a routine examination (sometimes prior to surgery) or as part of a family screening after the diagnosis of Brugada syndrome had been made in a family member. Drug provocation was used as the means of revealing the characteristic type 1 ECG appearances when not initially present (these patients either had had normal ECGs or type 2 or 3 changes initially). The highest risk of sudden cardiac death or documented ventricular fibrillation during follow-up (62%) was in the 71 patients who had presented with a cardiac arrest and the second highest risk (19%) was in the 73 patients who presented with syncope. Of note is the fact that no arrhythmic events were observed during follow-up in any of the patients without initial type 1 Brugada appearances (whether or not arrhythmias were inducible by electrophysiological stimulation). Thus, the asymptomatic patients with type 2 or type 3 ECG changes appear to have a very good prognosis even if (as in all in this study) type 1 changes could be induced by drug provocation. Brugada *et al.*[47] suggested that, among asymptomatic patients with an initial type 1 pattern, the inducibility (or lack of it) of ventricular tachycardia or ventricular fibrillation (VT/VF) during EPS could be used to forecast risk; however, Priori et al.[48] failed to find an association between inducibility and occurrence of VT/VF in both symptomatic and asymptomatic patients with Brugada syndrome. It should be also noted that VF is inducible in 6–9% of apparently healthy individuals under aggressive electrical stimulation.[49] Junttila et al.[50] reported on the prevalence and prognosis of the Brugada ECG pattern among young and middle-aged males in the Finnish population. They noted the benign course of patients with the Brugada sign (provided they were of asymptomatic and had no family history of sudden cardiac death) and stated that the type 2 and 3 'Brugada patterns' were normal variants rather than predictors of life-threatening ventricular arrhythmias. Hermida et al.,[51] in a study of the prevalence in an apparently healthy population, estimated that an ECG compatible with Brugada syndrome can be found in 6 per 1000 of normal individuals. In 2005, Eckardt et al.[52] reported the longest follow-up (to date) of a large population (212 patients) with type 1 Brugada ECG pattern (either spontaneously or after provocation with a class 1 anti-arrhythmic drug). They demonstrated a very low incidence of severe arrhythmic events, particularly in asymptomatic individuals and that electrical stimulation 'showed very little accuracy in predicting outcome'. It also seems likely that asymptomatic patients with type 1 changes only after drug provocation also have a good outlook. However, Priori et al.[53] have stated that life-threatening cardiac events can occur in patients with the type 2 pattern with genetically confirmed diagnosis and have conceded that this creates 'diagnostic uncertainty'.

The overall impression is of a very broad range of outcomes across the spectrum of 'Brugada patterns' with the highest risk in groups with spontaneous type 1 ECGs and: (i) a prior cardiac arrest; (ii) prior syncope; or (iii) a family history of sudden arrhythmic death. The lowest risk is in those with none of these features and no more than type 2 or type 3 ECG changes.

Cellular basis for the ECG appearances in the Brugada syndrome

The mechanism responsible for the normal J wave and the slightly more prominent J wave associated with the early repolarisation syndrome has already been described. The cellular basis for the Brugada syndrome is thought to be an outward shift in the ionic current active during phase 1 of the right ventricular epicardial potential with consequent exaggeration of the 'spike-and-dome' potential. The spike-and-dome potentials of the normal right ventricular epicardium are more accentuated than those in the left ventricular epicardium but, in normal circumstances, because of the thinner right ventricular wall and the consequent briefer activation time, the right ventricular epicardial cells contribute little to the generation of the J wave. Under the pathological conditions of the Brugada syndrome, accentuation of the right ventricular epicardial notch is accompanied by increase in the transmural voltage gradient producing an exaggerated J wave and the saddleback repolarisation pattern (Fig. 20a–c).[54] With a progressive reduction in the plateau phase voltage of the epicardial cells, there is further ST elevation and marked transmural dispersion of repolarisation creating conditions in which a premature beat could initiate a re-entrant arrhythmia (Fig. 20d,e).[54] Under pathophysiological conditions, changes in membrane currents other than I_{to} can accentuate the spike-and-dome morphology. Antzelevitch[54] has

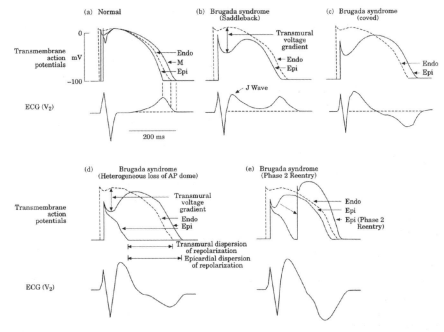

Fig. 20 Schematic diagram showing the changes in right ventricular epicardial potential thought to underlie the ECG appearances in the Brugada syndrome. From Antzelevitch,[54] [© 2007 European Society of Cardiology] with the permission of Oxford University Press.

shown that agents which reduce I_{Na} or I_{Ca} or agents that activate $I_{K\text{-}ATP}$ or augment I_{Kr}, $I_{Cl(Ca)}$ or I_{to} result in augmentation of the spike-and-dome morphology of the action potential of the canine ventricular epicardial cells.

It is thought that the development of polymorphic ventricular tachycardia in the Brugada syndrome occurs as a result of the amplification of heterogeneities in the early phase of the action potential (in the region of the phase-1 mediated notch) of cells in different layers of the right ventricular myocardium.[55]

ARRHYTHMOGENIC RIGHT VENTRICULAR DYSPLASIA (ARVD) – ARRHYTHMOGENIC RIGHT VENTRICULAR CARDIOMYOPATHY (ARVC)

This rare condition predominantly affects the right ventricle and is characterised, histologically, by the gradual replacement of myocytes by adipose and fibrous tissue.[56] Although both ventricles can be involved (and, in one series,[57] fibrofatty left ventricular involvement was demonstrable histologically in 76% cases), the condition typically dominantly or exclusively affects the right ventricle. It is associated with re-entrant arrhythmias arising from the affected areas. The associated arrhythmias are, therefore, of right ventricular origin and the QRS complexes have a left bundle branch block (LBBB) configuration during the episodes of tachycardia. The condition affects men more than women, in a 3:1 ratio. The age at presentation is most commonly in the range 20–40 years. The prevalence of the condition is impossible to establish with accuracy at the present time because the less striking cases are often undiagnosed in life or even at autopsy.

There is a wide spectrum of severity both between different patients and also in relation to any given patient. Thus the patient may have:

(i)   *isolated ventricular premature, ectopic beats*

(ii)   *non-sustained ventricular tachycardia*

(iii) *sustained ventricular tachycardia, or*

(iv)   *ventricular fibrillation, leading to sudden cardiac death.*

The arrhythmias are often precipitated by exercise and are thought to be to be catecholamine-induced. Arrhythmias are the main concern in ARVD, but a small minority of patients develop right ventricular dysfunction and a smaller proportion still develop biventricular dysfunction. There may be a family history of palpitations, sustained tachycardia, syncope or sudden death. Occasionally, family members are known to have 'minor' ECG abnormalities or abnormal echocardiograms.

Patients may present with 'palpitations' as a result of ventricular premature, ectopic beats or of sustained or non-sustained ventricular tachycardia. Since the ectopic rhythms most commonly arise from the region of the right ventricular outflow tract, they usually have a left bundle branch block configuration (because they arise to the right of the interventricular septum) and they have a vertical axis, most often +60° to +120° (because they arise from the superior part of the right ventricle). In more serious cases, the patient may present with syncope or cardiac arrest. The condition may also be discovered by accident in an asymptomatic person who has an ECG recorded.

Baseline ECG features of ARVC

The electrocardiographic abnormalities in this condition include both depolarisation and repolarisation changes. The 12-lead ECG is said to be abnormal in 'up to 90%' of cases with this condition.[58]

The electrocardiographic features of ARVD were described by Marcus *et al.*[59] in their original description of the disease in 1982. They recorded that the most frequent abnormalities on the resting ECG were T-wave inversion in the anterior precordial leads (V_1–V_4) and post-excitation waves. (Post-excitation waves are now referred to as epsilon waves).

In 2004, Nasir *et al.*[60] assessed the ECG features of the condition in a study of 50 patients with ARVD (11 with right bundle branch block and 39 without) and compared the findings with those of 50 age- and gender-matched controls and 28 consecutive patients presenting with right ventricular outflow tract tachycardia. In 4 cases there was complete RBBB (QRS duration [QRSd] ≥ 0.12 s and secondary R wave in right precordial leads) and in 7 cases there was incomplete RBBB (QRSd ≥ 0.10 s and < 0.12 s and secondary R wave in right precordial leads). They also noted prolongation of the S-wave upstroke in V_1–V_3 in 95% of those cases which did not have RBBB.

The ECG changes associated with ARVC are as follows.

T-wave inversion in the precordial leads

T-wave inversion in the right precordial leads is the most common ECG finding. Such repolarisation changes are not pathognomonic of ARVD, because they can occur as a normal variant in V_1 and V_2 (but not in V_3), especially in

Table 2 Frequency of T-wave inversion in precordial leads in ARVC

	T wave inversion
V_1–V_2	10%
V_1–V_3	59%
V_1–V_4	18%
V_1–V_5	5%
V_1–V_6	5%

women and in children less than 12 years of age. In their series of 50 proven cases of ARVD, Nasir et al.[60] found the frequency of T inversion shown in Table 2.

Epsilon waves

These are small electrical potentials that occur at the end of or immediately after the QRS complex in V_1 or V_2.[61] They are thought to be the result of late activation of a limited group of right ventricular fibres. An example is shown in Figure 21. Hurst[21] reports that it was Fontaine who named the epsilon wave. They were originally described (for self-evident reasons) as 'post-excitation waves'. Fontaine, in a letter to Hurst,[21] explained that he introduced the term epsilon 'because it occurs in the Greek alphabet after delta (the 'pre-excitation' wave) and because the small size of the wave seemed appropriate as 'epsilon is also used in mathematics to express a very small phenomenon'.

Of the original 24 cases described by Marcus et al.,[59] in 7 (24%) post excitation waves were 'suspected' on the resting ECG and were confirmed in all who had high amplitude and signal averaging techniques performed. In some cases, the waves became visible after increased magnification or gain of the ECG recording. The authors stated that the 'specificity of this finding is not certain' but they felt that, the later the delayed potential, the higher the specificity of the finding. Epsilon waves have subsequently been noted (rarely) in patients with posterior[63] and inferior myocardial infarction, in right ventricular infarction and in infiltrative disorders of the right ventricle such as sarcoidosis.[64,65] It seems probable that epsilon waves are the result of delayed depolarisation of small groups of right ventricular fibres. However, even though they are not absolutely specific in relation to the diagnosis of ARVC, they are considered to be a major diagnostic criterion for this condition. In a review article in 2001, Gemayel et al.[66] stated that they are 'highly specific for ARVC'.

Partial or complete right bundle branch block

This feature is not, of course, diagnostic of the condition. When present (and ARVD is diagnosed, for example by echocardiography), RBBB makes it more difficult to recognise the usual, more subtle, ECG changes. In the original description by Marcus et al.,[59] one of the 24 cases (4%) had complete, and 9 (38%) incomplete, RBBB. The corresponding frequencies in the series by Nasir et al.[60] were 8% and 14%, respectively.

Manifestations of prolongation of the QRS complex in the right precordial leads

The ECG in ARVC shows changes in depolarisation as well as changes in the repolarisation phase. Nasir et al.[60] listed the important findings (in cases of

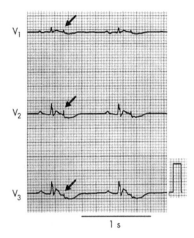

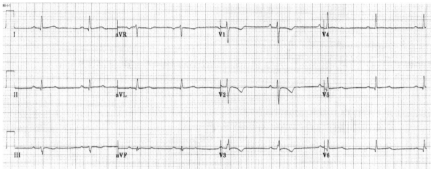

Fig. 21 Epsilon waves in V_1, V_2 and V_3. Reproduced from Anan *et al.*,[62] © 2007 BMJ Publishing Group Ltd with permission.

Fig. 22 The 12-lead ECG in a patient with echocardiographically proven ARVD. There is T wave inversion in V_1–V_3, the T waves are flat in V_4 and of low voltage in V_5 and V_6. The tiny positive notch at the end of the QRS in V_1 could be an epsilon wave, but there is no significant abnormality of the QRS complexes.

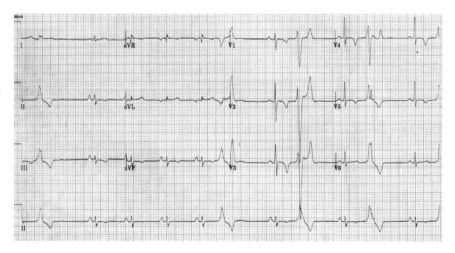

Fig. 23 The 12-lead ECG in a symptomatic patient with echocardiographically proven ARVD. There is T wave inversion in V_1–V_5, the T waves of low voltage in V_6. There is no significant abnormality of the basic QRS complexes. There are frequent unifocal (uniform) ventricular premature, ectopic beats, which all have the same LBBB configuration with a frontal plane QRS axis of +75°.

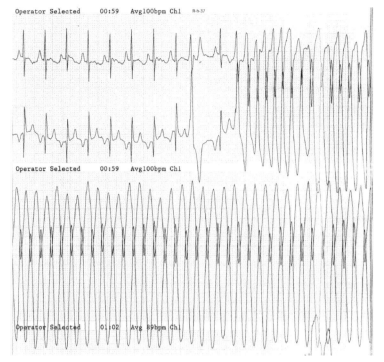

Fig. 24 The same patient as in Figure 23 showing onset of ventricular tachycardia at 00.59 h.

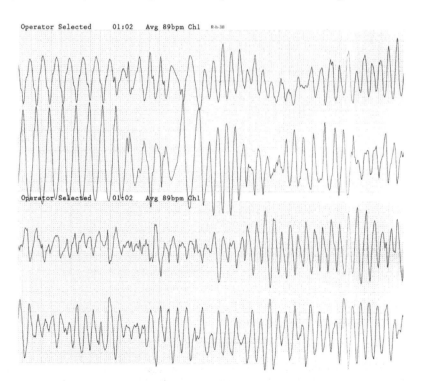

Fig. 25 The same patient as in Figure 23 showing onset of ventricular fibrillation at 01.02 h. The initial rhythm is ventricular tachycardia at 215 per min.

ARVD without BBB) as follows (the figures in brackets indicate the percentage frequency in their series):

1. QRS duration (QRSd) in V_1–V_3 ≥ 0.11 s (64%).

2. QRSd in V_1, V_2 or V_3 exceeds that in V_6 by 0.025 s, so called 'parietal block' (52%).

3. Ratio of sum of QRS durations in (V_1 + V_2 + V_3) to that sum in (V_4 + V_5 + V_6) ≥ 1.2 (77%).

4. S wave upstroke time in V_1–V_3 (time from nadir of S wave to iso-electric baseline) ≥ 0.055 s (95%).

5. Epsilon waves (see Fig. 21) (33%).

6. QRS dispersion (difference between maximum and minimum QRSd in different leads) ≥ 0.04 s (44%).

7. QT dispersion (difference between maximum and minimum QTd in different leads) ≥ 0.065 s (69%).

Epsilon waves are highly specific for the condition but are insensitive and are only present in 33% of patients (53% in those with diffuse RV involvement and 15% in those with localised involvement).[60]

An example of a 12-lead ECG taken from an asymptomatic patient with echocardiographically proven ARVD is shown in Figure 22.

A further illustration is shown in Figure 23. In this example, there are frequent unifocal ventricular premature beats, which have a left bundle branch block configuration and an inferiorly directed axis.

The patient whose ECG is shown in Figure 23 developed ventricular tachycardia (VT) during a period of ambulatory electrocardiography. He was alone in his home. VT developed at 00.59 hours (Fig. 24) and degenerated into VF 3 min later (Fig. 25). The patient described in this series was reported in 2000 by Aziz et al.[67] (He had been consecutively under the care of one of the authors (DJR) and then of C. Garratt, one of the authors of the report in 2000). The initial rhythm is sinus tachycardia at 125 per min. During ventricular tachycardia, the rate is approximately 250 per min.

The cellular basis for the ECG changes in ARVC

The cellular mechanisms responsible for the ECG changes in ARVC are not well defined. The depolarisation changes (regionally selective prolongation of QRS duration) are thought to be the result of slow conduction through the diseased right ventricular myocardium.[68] In ARVC, as in the Brugada syndrome, electrical abnormalities in the right ventricular outflow tract are important in the mechanism of arrhythmogenesis. It has been shown that the prolongation of the QRS complexes dominantly seen in the right precordial leads in the Brugada syndrome has different characteristics from that seen in ARVC, where the delay is thought to be the result of the fibrofatty replacement of the right ventricular myocardium.[69] The cellular mechanism for the right-sided precordial T-wave inversion has not been clearly elucidated.

THE LONG QT SYNDROME (LQTS)

The importance of this genetically determined 'channelopathy' in relation to arrhythmias giving rise to syncope or to sudden death has been increasingly recognised in recent years. Currently, more than 150 different mutations have been identified in 10 LQTS genes.[70,71] Distinctive T-wave patterns have been recognised in patients with each of the three major ECG phenotypical expressions of the LQTS gene mutations, which between them account for 95% of the identified mutations (LQT1, 43%; LQT2, 45%; LQT3, 7%).[72]

Sauer et al.[74] have recently risk-stratified adults with the long QT syndrome by genotype, gender, QTc (duration of measured QT interval 'corrected' to an equivalent value for a heart rate of 60 per min) and history of cardiac events, and found that: (i) female gender, QTc (increasing risk with increasing QTc for QTc > 440), LQTS genotype (risk for LQT2 > LQT1, risk for LQT3 > LQT1, risk for LQT2 > LQT3) and frequency of cardiac events before age 18 years were all associated with an increased risk of cardiac events between ages 18-40 years; and (ii) female gender, QTc > 500 ms and interim cardiac events during follow-up after age 18 years were associated with a significantly increased risk of life-threatening events in adulthood.

Measurement of the QT interval

With the rapidly increasing awareness of the importance of variations in the QT interval as a marker of fatal, or potentially fatal, arrhythmias, there has been much concern about how to correct the QT interval for variations in heart rate (QTc). The fact that there are considerable difficulties in the actual measurement of the QT interval in a given record often receives less attention. The latter difficulty, of course, consists entirely of deciding at which point the QT interval ends; there is no major practical difficulty in deciding where it starts. This issue was first addressed in detail in a classic paper by Lepeschkin and Surawicz in 1952.[74]

Goldberg et al.[75] have recently addressed this difficult issue and have pointed out that automatic measurements of the corrected QT (QTc) interval are of questionable accuracy. These authors recommend the use of a high-quality, but standard, 12-lead ECG recording at 25 mm/s recording speed, rightly pointing out that higher recording speeds distort the record and do not help – in fact, in terms of any time measurements made, doubling the recording speed doubles both the accuracy of any measurements made and also the difficulty of deciding at which points the measurements are to be made. They correctly state that the accuracy levels for manual determination with a pair of dividers is no more than 20–40 ms. We have been fortunate in obtaining loupes with specialised ECG reticles and 10x magnification from Ronald Prineas (Wake Forest University Health Service, Winston-Salem, NC, USA); with these loupes, there is no doubt that an accuracy of 10 ms is readily achievable. Goldberg et al.[75] recommend that the QT interval should be measured in leads II, V_5 and V_6 (using the mean of at least 3–5 cardiac cycles) with the longest value being used. When the T wave is not followed by a U wave, or when the T and U waves are distinct, they define the end of the T wave as being when its descending limb returns to the TP baseline (Fig. 26 [1,2]). When dual repolarisation deflections (T1 and T2 or T wave plus U waves) of equal, or near equal, amplitude are seen, the QT measurement is taken to the time of final return to the baseline (Fig. 26 [3]). When a second, low-amplitude repolarisation wave interrupts the terminal portion of the larger T wave (and it is not clear whether to label the deflections 'T1 and T2' or 'T and U'), they recommend recording both the QT interval with the T-wave offset measured to the nadir between the T and U waves (Fig. 26 [4], short arrow) and the QTU

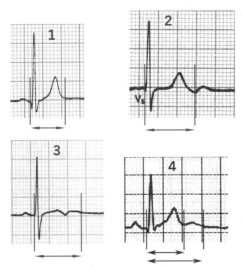

Fig. 26 QT interval measurements from V_5 using techniques for identifying the end of the period as suggested by Goldenberg *et al.*[75] Record 3 was taken from a patient with LQT2. Records 1, 2 and 4 were taken from normal subjects.

interval, with the repolarisation offset measured at the end of the second wave (Fig. 26 [4], long arrow).

The approach by Goldberg *et al.*[75] provides a useful discipline, but the issue remains problematical. Viskin *et al.*[76] presented the ECGs of two patients with the long QT syndrome and two from healthy females to 902 physicians from 12 countries. Twenty-five were 'world renowned QT experts', 106 were 'arrhythmia specialists', 329 were cardiologists and 442 were non-cardiologists. All were asked to measure the QT interval, calculate the QTc (see later) and determine whether or not the QT interval was prolonged. Correct classification of all four QT intervals as either 'long' or 'normal' was achieved by 96% of the QT experts (*i.e.* one got one wrong!), by 62% of the arrhythmia experts and by < 25% of the cardiologists and physicians.

Even in cases where there appears to be no problem in deciding what is a T wave and what is a U wave, there are still practical difficulties in measuring the QT interval. Marek,[77] in a disciplined article on 'errors and misconceptions' in relation to measurement of the QT interval, points out that the common recommendation to use leads II and V_5 is essentially arbitrary. As he correctly states, the result of the projection of the 3-dimensional T-wave loop on to any single ECG lead is dependent on the relationship of the T-wave axis to that lead. If the terminal part of the T-wave loop is at right angles to the chosen lead, that part of the T wave will be iso-electric on the given lead, leading to an underestimate of the T-wave duration, whether the measurement is made manually or automatically. The closest approximation to the true QT interval will be achieved by measuring from the earliest recognisable deflection of the QRS complex (in whichever lead it appears) to the latest recognisable component of the T wave (in whichever lead), provided all leads are recorded simultaneously. This, of course, calls into question the validity of the concept of 'QT dispersion' as measured by the difference between the longest and shortest QT measurements within the 12 ECG leads.

Rate correction of the QT interval (QTc)

It is well recognised that the QT interval varies significantly, and inversely, with the heart rate. In consequence, a number of formulae have been devised for 'correcting' (*i.e.* normalising to the value expected at a heart rate of 60 per min) the QT interval. The use of a formula does not, of course, guarantee that 'correction' is achieved. The criterion for successful correction is that there should be no significant correlation between the corrected QT intervals derived from the formula and the heart rate (or RR interval) at which the basic measurement was made.

The first formula developed was that of Bazett[78] and this is still the one most commonly used, although it is known to under-correct the QT interval at heart rates below 60 per min and to over-correct at heart rates above 60 per min.[79] The Fredericia formula (which is similar to the Bazett formula but uses the cube root, rather than the square root, of the RR interval) has the same limitations at slow heart rates but is considered to reflect a more accurate correction with rapid heart rates.[75] The Hodges formula[80] was shown by Macfarlane and Lawrie to give values of QTc which showed no correlation with the heart rate and which were, therefore, preferable to the Bazett formula.[79] Despite the fact that the Hodges formula is preferable, Bazett's formula remains the most widely used and is, therefore, associated with the largest available database. The properties of the four rate correction formulae can be summarised:

Bazett formula $\quad$ $QTc = QT \, (rate/60)^{1/2}$ or $QTc = QT/(RR \, interval)^{1/2}$

Fredericia formula $\quad$ $QTc = QT \, (rate/60)^{1/3}$ or $QTc = QT/(RR \, interval)^{1/3}$

Hodges formula $\quad$ $QTc = QT + 1.75 \, (rate - 60)$

Framingham formula $QTc = QT + 0.154 \times (1000 - RR)$

Goldenberg *et al.*[75] used digitised data files to obtain QT- and RR-interval measurements on 581 healthy subjects. There were 158 children aged 1–15 years (80 boys, 78 girls) and 423 adults aged 16–81 years (223 men and 200 women). There was no detectable gender difference in children for the Bazett QTc but there was a gender difference for adults. They therefore suggested a three level classification for the recognition of QT prolongation (Table 3).

Moss[81] has emphasised that the 'measurement of the QT interval is not an exact science'. His group have consistently demonstrated a significant increase for life-threatening cardiac events in LQTS subjects with QTc prolongation

Table 3 Bazett-corrected QTc values for the diagnosis of QT prolongation

	Child 1–15 years (ms)	Adult male (ms)	Adult female (ms)
Within normal limits	< 440	< 430	< 450
Borderline abnormal	440–460	430–450	450–470
Clearly prolonged	> 460	> 450	> 470

Adapted from Goldenberg *et al.*[75]

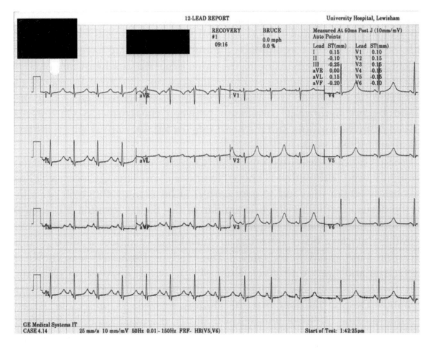

Fig. 27 The 12-lead ECG of an athlete demonstrating paradoxical QTc prolongation Reproduced with permission of Oxford University Press [© 2007 European Society of Cardiology] from Basavarajaiah *et al.*[83]

> 500 ms and in those with prior syncope (with a greater risk for adult women than for men).

The definition of an abnormally long QT interval is of significance in relation to the screening of high-performance athletes. In a proposed European protocol, the suggested guidelines for an abnormally long QTc interval were > 440 ms in males and > 460 ms in females.[82] Basavarajaiah *et al.*[83] have stressed that an isolated, prolonged QTc interval *per se* does not fulfil the proposed criteria for the congenital long QT syndrome, which is based on the triad of: (i) prolonged QTc interval; (ii) unheralded syncope or polymorphic VT; and (iii) a family history of sudden cardiac death or prolonged QT syndrome. Using the European criteria, they found 7 cases among 2000 elite athletes (a prevalence of 0.4%). Three of the seven exhibited one of: (i) paradoxical prolongation of QTc during exercise; (ii) a confirmatory genetic mutation; or (iii) prolonged QTc in a first degree relative. All three had a QTc > 500 ms. The four cases with a QTc < 500 ms had no other features to support a diagnosis of LQTS and they felt that, in the absence of symptoms of familial disease, a QT interval which is prolonged (but less than 500 ms) is unlikely to represent LQTS in elite athletes. An example of paradoxical QTc prolongation during the recovery period of exercise is shown in Figure 27.

With the multiplicity of criteria, the diagnosis of LQTS is not easy. What seems to be clear, however, is that a QTc of 500 ms is associated with a significant increase in risk and that this risk is greater still in females, in those with a family history of LQTS or sudden death, and in those with a personal history of prior syncope.

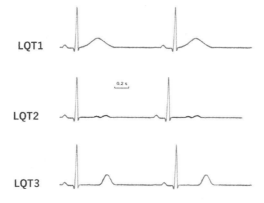

Fig. 28 Typical ECG phenotypes of the three common varieties of long QT.

Common electrocardiographic phenotypical expressions of the LQTS

Some 95% of patients with the long QT syndrome have one of three ECG phenotypes.[72] Examples of each of these ECG phenotypes are shown in Figure 28.

LQT1 The T waves begin early after the QRS and are broad-based.

LQT2 The T waves are of low amplitude and often notched or bifurcated.

LQT3 The T waves begin late after the QRS and are narrow.

Figure 29 shows an ECG obtained from a 39-year-old woman presenting with several episodes of syncope induced by the morning alarm and by being woken by the ringing of the telephone. The appearances are typical of LQT2. The risk is greater in females, in those with a family history of LQTS or of sudden death and in those with a prior history of syncope. Figure 30 shows the ECG from the same patient as Figure 29, after the insertion of a dual chamber pacemaker and the institution of β-blocking therapy (patient now asymptomatic).

Figure 31 shows an example of the ECG appearances in LQT3.

Cellular mechanisms involved in the long QT syndrome

As described earlier, and shown in Figure 5, the early repolarisation of the epicardium gives rise to the positive T wave. The onset of the T wave is the

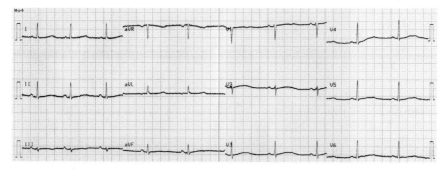

Fig. 29 Typical LQT2. Low-voltage T waves with broad terminal T2/U wave. Record taken from a 39-year-old woman presenting with episodes of syncope in response to early morning telephone calls or to the alarm ringing.

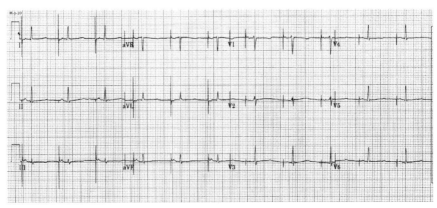

Fig. 30 Recording from same patient as in Figure 29. The patient is asymptomatic following insertion of dual chamber pacemaker and with continuing β-blocker therapy.

result of the more rapid decline of the plateau (phase 2) of the epicardial action potential and the peak of the T wave is reached when repolarisation of the epicardium is complete.

The unique characteristics of the M cells are central to the mechanism of the long QT syndrome. The striking property of these cells is the ability of their action potential to prolong more than that of the epicardial or endocardial cells in response to a slowing of the heart rate (Fig. 32).[84] This phenomenon gives rise to considerable accentuation of spatial dispersion (transmural, trans-septal and apico-basal) of repolarisation. The augmented spatial dispersion of repolarisation combined with the development of early-after-depolarisation induced triggered activity are thought to underlie the substrate and trigger for the development of torsade de pointes.[85]

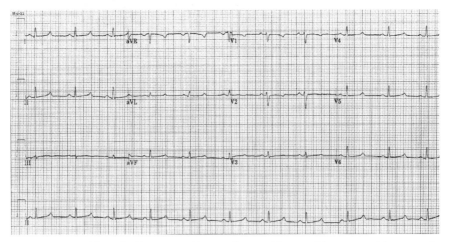

Fig. 31 LQT3, with typical late-onset T wave. From a 21-year-old woman with syncopal episodes. The measured QT interval is 500 ms. The RR interval is 0.98 s (heart rate is 62) and the Bazett-corrected QTc is 505 ms. The patient is asymptomatic but has two close family members with LQT3, ventricular arrhythmias and syncope. Both have had defibrillators implanted. The patient has confirmed LQT3 genotype and has opted to have a defibrillator.

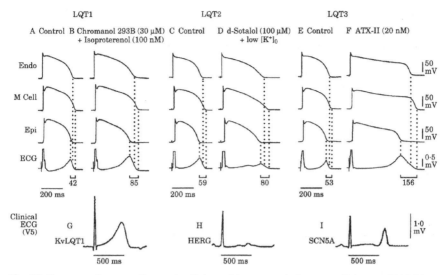

Fig. 32 Transmembrane action potentials and transmural electrocardiograms (ECGs) in control (A, C and E) and LQT1 (B), LQT2 (D) and LQT3 (F) models of LQT syndrome in arterially perfused canine left ventricular wedge preparations, clinical ECGs (lead V₅) from patients with LQT1, LQT2 and LQT3 syndrome (G, H and I). Reproduced from Antzelevitch.[84] [© 2001 European Society of Cardiology] with the permission of Oxford University Press.

It is thought that the principal arrhythmogenic substrate, both in congenital and in acquired long QT syndrome, is amplification of spatial dispersion of repolarisation within the ventricular myocardium.[55]

THE SHORT QT SYNDROME

The first suggestion of the occurrence of a congenital syndrome involving a short QT interval was made as recently as 2000,[86] whereas the congenital long QT syndrome was first described in 1957.[87] The initial report of the short QT syndrome (SQTS) described two siblings and their mother. The 51-year-old mother had a QT of 260 ms at a heart rate of 74 per min, her 21-year-old son had a QT of 272 ms (at a heart rate of 58 per min) and her 17-year-old daughter had a QT of 280 ms (at heart rate 69 per min). The daughter had several episodes of atrial fibrillation, requiring DC cardioversion. The article also referred to an unrelated 37-year-old who died suddenly and had similar ECG appearances. Gaita *et al.*[88] reported on six patients (from two families) with palpitations, syncope, cardiac arrest and sudden death. In all cases, the QT interval was ≤ 280 ms and the QTc was ≤ 300 ms. In no case was there evidence of structural organic heart disease. Four patients underwent electro-physiological testing and three were found to have increased susceptibility to ventricular fibrillation. Four of the patients went on to have ICD implantation.

ECG features of the short QT syndrome

The electrocardiographic appearances in the short QT syndrome consist essentially of an abnormally short QT interval (QTc ≤ 300 ms; QT ≤ 280 ms), with tall, pointed, symmetrically shaped T waves. Extramiana and Antzelevitch[89]

Table 4 The main electrocardiographic feature of the short QT syndrome

ECG feature	Details	Comments
Short QT interval	Absolute QT below 300 ms[90]	Absolute QT below 300–320 ms are strongly suggestive'[91]
		Measurement should be made at heart rates below 80 per min[91]
		Secondary causes of short QT should be excluded[91]
Tall T waves	Tall, peaked, symmetrical T waves in right precordial leads	Present in 50% or more[90]
Relatively prolonged T_{peak} to T_{end}	Measurements not yet precisely defined	Indicative of transmural dispersion of repolarisation.[89]
Absent ST segment	T wave starts immediately from the S wave[90]	All the ECGs in SQTS have this feature[90]

have pointed out that the time from the peak to the end of the T waves (T_{peak} to T_{end}) is relatively increased in the short QT syndrome. This electrocardiographic feature is a measure of the maximum transmural dispersion of repolarisation within the ventricular wall. Borggrefe et al.[90] list the ECG features as: (i) absolute QT interval below 300 ms (range, 220–300 ms); (ii) tall, symmetrically peaked T waves in the right precordial leads (this second feature is said to be present in about half of the patients); and (iii) absence of a clear ST segment, with the T wave beginning immediately after the S wave. These authors stress that 'all ECGs have in common that a clear ST segment is absent and the T wave initiates immediately from the S wave'. They emphasise that the QT interval should be measured, and corrected for heart rate, at rates below 80 per minute. Priori et al.[91] state that absolute values of QT interval below 300–320 ms should be considered as 'strongly suggesting' SQTS. They also stress the need to measure the QT interval at heart rates below 80 per min since one of the distinguishing features of the condition is an impaired QT adaptation to heart rate increases. They acknowledge that this introduces difficulty in identifying the SQTS in children. They also stress the importance of excluding known causes of a short QT interval such as hypercalcaemia, hyperthermia, acidosis and digoxin therapy. The main features of the SQTS are given in Table 4.

Possible cellular mechanisms involved in the short QT syndrome

The short QT syndrome has not been as extensively studied as the long QT syndrome but the canine ventricular wedge studies of Extramiana and Antzelevitch[89] suggest that augmented transmural dispersion of repolarisation (of which increased T_{peak} to T_{end} is a manifestation) is the probable mechanism of arrhthymogenesis in this condition.

Brugada *et al.*[92] demonstrated a gain in function of the cardiac I_{Kr} channel HERG (KCNH2) and Bellocq and co-workers[93] have described the case of a 70-year-old man who presented with ventricular fibrillation (from which he was resuscitated), had a QT of 290 ms (QTc 302 ms), with no abnormality on clinical examination, echocardiography, exercise testing, coronary angiography, right and left ventricular angiography, ergonovine coronary spasm test or electrophysiological study. Their studies showed a gain of function of KCNQ1, the gene that encodes for I_{Ks}.

DRUG-INDUCED AND ELECTROLYTE-RELATED CHANGES IN REPOLARISATION

DRUG-RELATED QT PROLONGATION

Anti-arrhythmic drugs

The development and initially relatively enthusiastic use of anti-arrhythmic drugs (particularly class III anti-arrhythmics) gave rise to cases of sometimes fatal ventricular arrhythmias and, in turn, to a general awareness of the important pro-arrhythmic potential of QT prolongation. Whilst sotalol and amiodarone have the same potent effects on QT prolongation, the incidence of torsade de pointes with amiodarone is much lower than that with sotalol[94] and, in the case of sotalol, the incidence is dose-related. Torsade de pointes can occur with most class Ia drugs (including quinidine, disopyramide and procainamide) even at low or subtherapeutic concentrations.[94]

Non-cardiac drugs

Many commonly prescribed non-cardiac drugs also have the potential to prolong the QT interval, with the consequent risk of provoking significant ventricular arrhythmias, particularly torsade de pointes. Regulatory bodies have ruled that the QT-interval-prolonging properties of every new chemical entity should be extensively investigated.[95] The incidence of drug-induced torsade de pointes in the population is largely unknown.[96] It is well recognised that the combination of a slow heart rate and hypokalaemia (both of which prolong the QT interval) increase the probability of the development of torsade de pointes when a

Table 5 The 10 drugs most commonly reported in association with torsade de pointes between 1983 and 1999 (based on adverse drug reaction reports to the WHO).

Drug	Reports of TdP (n)	Reports of fatal TdP (n)	Total reports of adverse reaction	TdP as % of total reports
Sotalol	130	1	2758	4.71
Cisapride	97	6	6489	1.49
Amiodarone	47	1	13,725	0.34
Erythromycin	44	2	24,776	0.18
Ibutilide	43	1	173	24.86
Terfenadine	41	1	10,047	0.41
Quinidine	33	2	7353	0.45
Clarithromycin	33	0	17,448	0.19
Haloperodol	21	6	15,431	0.14
Fluoxetine	20	1	70,929	0.03

TdP = torsade de pointes
Adapted from Darpö.[96]

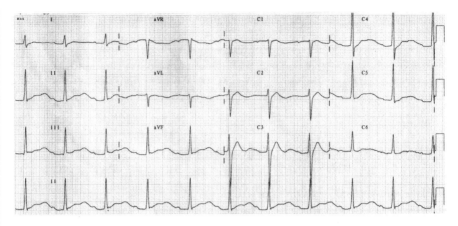

Fig. 33 Dramatic ST segment changes associated with profound hypokalaemia ([K+] 1.9 mmol/l). There are abnormally tall and abnormally wide U waves, well seen in II, III, aVF and V_3–V_6. The PR interval is prolonged (0.31 s). Note the strikingly wide Ta waves (best seen in II and III) indicating prolongation of atrial myocardial repolarisation.

QT-prolonging drug is used. Females have a greater propensity than males for the development of torsade de pointes.[94]

Table 5 lists the ten drugs most commonly reported in association with torsade de pointes, based on spontaneous adverse drug reaction reports reported to the World Health Organization (WHO) Drug Monitoring Centre between 1983 and 1999 (761 cases in all).[96]

More than 50 drugs have, so far, been shown to prolong the QT interval and, because of the continuously evolving data concerning drug-related QT interval changes, a static list can never be considered to be comprehensive. In this area, internet-based databases are invaluable.[97]

METABOLIC AND PHYSIOLOGICAL FACTORS

Hypokalaemia, hypocalcaemia, hypomagnesaemia, bradycardia and hypothermia all prolong the QT interval. QT prolongation can also occur in organic heart disease (congenital long QT, ischaemic heart disease, dilated cardiomyopathy, myocarditis, hypertrophic cardiomyopathy, congestive heart failure and Kawasaki syndrome).

Conversely, the QT interval is shortened by hyperkalaemia, hypercalcaemia, tachycardia, hyperthermia, increased sympathetic tone, acidosis, and digitalis.[98]

Figure 33 shows an example of the ECG changes in severe hypokalaemia (serum [K+] 1.9 mmol/l). There is very marked QT prolongation (0.79 s,; heart rate, 60 per min). There is equally dramatic prolongation of the Ta wave (well seen in II, III and aVF).

TORSADE DE POINTES

The main concern in relation to QT prolongation is the risk of the development of torsade de pointes. This arrhythmia was first described by Francois Dessertenne in 1966.[99] The varying morphology and amplitude of the QRS complexes gives rise to the typical 'twisting' appearance, the periods of ventricular arrhythmia are often self-limiting, brief and repetitive and the onset of the arrhythmia often follows a long–short sequence of RR intervals (Fig. 34).

Cellular mechanisms involved in torsade de pointes

The precise pathophysiology of this condition has not been fully worked out. Liu and Laurita,[100] using the arterially perfused canine left ventricular wedge

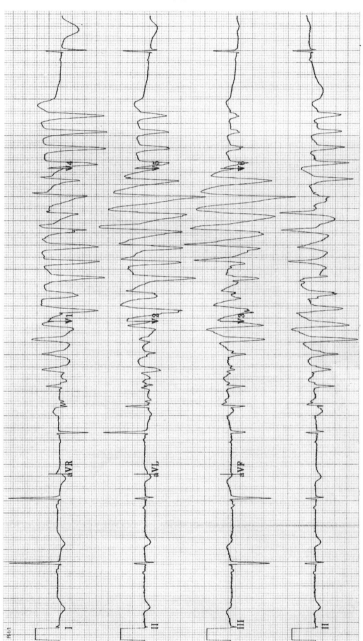

Fig. 34 Onset of torsade de pointes in a 54-year-old man with hypertension and ischaemic heart disease. He was receiving treatment with bendroflumethiazide, and had a low potassium level (3.3 mmol/l).

preparation with drug-induced models of LQT2 and LQT3, showed that 'under LQT2 and LQT3 conditions' the action potential duration (APD) of the M cells increased more than that of the epicardial cells with the result that the transmural dispersion of repolarisation (DOR) increased from a control value of 18 ms to 58 ms in LQT2 and to 115 ms in LQT3. After a pause, transmural APD and DOR increased compared with baseline values, under LQT2 and (to a greater extent) under LQT3 conditions, and discrete regions or 'islands' of prolonged APD with areas of unidirectional block were demonstrated. The pause associated with a short–long cycle length sequence also facilitated the formation of early after depolarisations.

REPOLARISATION CHANGES IN ISCHAEMIA AND INFARCTION

The earliest electrocardiographic manifestations of myocardial ischaemia are T-wave and ST-segment changes. Increased hyperacute T-wave amplitude with prominent symmetrical T waves in at least two contiguous leads is an early sign that may precede ST segment elevation.[101] The term 'contiguous leads' refers to leads considered to be adjacent to one another in the 3-dimensional arrangement of the 12-lead ECG. Thus any two or more adjacent leads in the groups (V_1–V_6), (II aVF and III) or (I and aVL), are held to be contiguous. It seems reasonable also to regard (aVF, II, V_6 and V_5) and (V_5, V_6, I and aVL) as being groupings appropriate to the use of the term 'contiguous' in relation, respectively, to inferolateral and anterolateral infarction or ischaemia.

There may be even earlier changes, which usually pass unnoticed. Kenigsberg et al.[102] have recently reported the observation that the Bazett-corrected QTc interval prolongs in 100% patients during early transmural ischaemia in patients undergoing balloon angioplasty. There was no significant change in the QRS duration. The authors suggested that the measurement of QTc prolongation might be used to detect early or intermittent transmural ischaemia. Somewhat disturbingly, the authors note that the uncorrected QT interval increased in only 80% or 77% patients (depending on which of two automatic interpretation programmes was used) and decreased in 20% or 23%. These latter patients had a significantly greater heart rate increment during balloon inflation. This, of course, raises the question of the reliability of the Bazett formula. Ischaemia-induced QTc prolongation was seen in 92% cases when the Fredericia formula was used and 93% with the Framingham formula.

ST ELEVATION MYOCARDIAL INFARCTION (STEMI)

STEMI is usually transmural and, most commonly, results from acute occlusion of a major epicardial coronary artery.[103] The greatest degree of ST elevation is seen in those leads facing the acutely ischaemic area. This basic fact is widely recognised by the ECG classification of acute STEMI as being anterior, inferior, anterolateral or inferolateral.

Use of ST segment vector in localisation of the site of block in STEMI
It is not widely appreciated that the identification of the direction of maximum ST elevation in the frontal plane leads is a useful guide to the site of the arterial occlusion, not only in relation to inferior infarction but also in relation to anterior infarction.[9]

Thus, acute inferior STEMI following occlusion of the right coronary artery gives maximum ST elevation in lead III with lesser ST elevation in aVF and less still in II (*i.e.* the frontal plane ST vector is directed at +120°), whereas acute inferior STEMI following occlusion of the circumflex coronary artery gives maximum ST elevation in lead II with lesser ST elevation in aVF and less still in III (frontal plane ST vector directed at +60°).[9]

In acute anterior STEMI, the direction of the maximal ST segment vector gives an important clue to the anatomical level of the occlusion within the anterior descending branch (LAD) of the left coronary artery. In using the ECG to localise the arterial block in relation to acute anterior STEMI, it is important

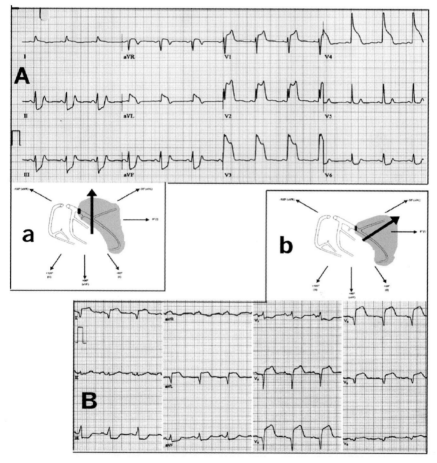

Fig. 35 Examples of the value of the frontal plane ST vector in the localisation of the site of occlusion of the left anterior descending artery in cases of anterior STEMI. In (A), the maximum limb lead ST shift is in aVF and III, the ST segment is negative in these leads and the ST vector is, therefore, directed superiorly at −90° (a). The ST segment elevation is directed towards the zone of maximum ischaemia and the appearances indicate an LAD lesion proximal to the first septal perforating branch (a). It is important to recognise that, in relation to acute anterior STEMI, ST elevation in aVR (even the modest degree seen here) is important because it indicates that the frontal plane ST vector is further to the left than −60°. In (B), the maximum limb lead ST segment shift is in aVL, giving a frontal plane ST vector of −30°. This suggests that the LAD occlusion is distal to the first septal perforating artery but proximal to the diagonal branch (b). Reproduced and modified, with permission, from Rowlands and Moore.[9]

to look for the greatest degree of ST shift (elevation or depression). The frontal plane vector of the maximum ST elevation is thus directed most closely either towards that frontal plane lead with the greatest degree of ST elevation or directly opposite to the frontal plane lead with the greatest degree of ST depression, using whichever lead has the greater ST shift. This concept effectively involves the use of twelve, rather than six limb leads (I, II, III, aVR, aVL and aVF as well as the standard six limb leads).[104] Engelen *et al.*[105] showed that, in the context of acute anterior myocardial infarction, the presence of ST elevation in aVR, usually of very small degree (in their series 0.2–1.8 mm), was very suggestive of a block proximal to the first septal perforator. This sign had a sensitivity of 43%, specificity of 86% and a positive predictive accuracy of 70%. In the same series, ST elevation in aVL was present in 83% of cases (though this finding was also present in 61% of more distal lesions). Examples are shown in Figure 35.

POSSIBLE CELLULAR MECHANISMS IN THE ECG CHANGES OF STEMI

Di Diego and Antzelevitch[106] have provided a valuable and revealing insight into some of the cellular mechanisms likely to be involved in the ECG changes of acute STEMI.

In the perfused canine right ventricular wedge preparation, they demonstrated two distinct mechanisms for the development of acute ST elevation in the transmural ECG following periods of induced ischaemia. They showed that, in transmural ischaemia, the striking electrophysiological change was

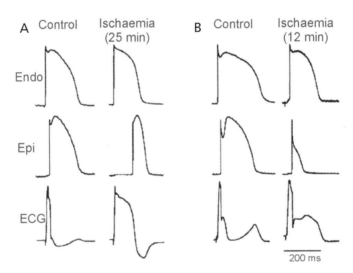

Fig. 36 Electrophysiological effects of ischaemia in the canine perfused right ventricular wedge model. Results from two different preparations. Each panel shows (from top to bottom) simultaneous transmembrane action potentials from endocardium (Endo), and epicardium (Epi) and the transmural ECG obtained along the same axis. (A) Recordings obtained under control conditions and after 25 min of ischaemia. (B) Recordings obtained under control conditions and after 12 min of ischaemia. The basic cycle length was 800 ms. Two distinctly different mechanisms involving (i) markedly delayed transmural conduction (A) and (ii) loss of the epicardial action potential dome (B) underlie the apparent ST-segment elevation encountered during acute ischaemia. Reproduced with permission of Elsevier Ltd from Di Diego and Antzelevitch,[106] © 2003 Elsevier Ltd.

delay in the onset of the epicardial action potential (Fig. 36A). This indicates major delay in transmural conduction from endocardium to epicardium. Thus, the apparent ST elevation (right-hand ECG trace in Fig. 36A) is actually caused by a marked prolongation of the R-wave duration (the R-wave duration extends from the time of origin of phase 0 of the action potential of the endocardial cells to the end of phase 0 of the action potential of the epicardial cells [Fig. 5]). In those preparations initially having a prominent notch in the right ventricular action potential (Fig. 36B), ischaemia-induced loss of the dome voltage occurs in epicardial cells but not in the endocardial cells, giving rise to true ST segment elevation. The prominent notch is associated with a voltage-gated potassium current (I_{to}). A prominent I_{to} current is commoner in males than in females.

INFARCTION ASSOCIATED WITH NON-SPECIFIC ST ELEVATION MYOCARDIAL INFARCTION CHANGES (NSTEMI)

The ECG changes in NSTEMI are not in themselves diagnostic. Non-specific ST depression and T wave changes occur in up to 50% of patients.[107] No specific pattern is recognisable and the pathophysiology of the group is unlikely to be homogeneous. Attempts to identify the source of ST depression in subendocardial ischaemia using animal models have shown no consistent relationship between the source of induced ischaemia (left anterior descending or circumflex arteries) and the location (within the 12-lead ECG) of the resulting ST depression.[108] This fits in with the limited ability to localise myocardial ischaemia in man from the distribution of ischaemic ST depression during exercise.[109]

As with acute STEMI, so with acute coronary syndromes such as unstable angina or NSTEMI, in the presence of a very proximal, critical narrowing of the left coronary system, the limb leads may give a clue to the site of the critical lesion. Figure 37 shows an ECG taken from a patient with acute, unstable angina during a spontaneous anginal episode at rest. The patient had had a successful angioplasty and stent insertion into a dominant right coronary artery 6 weeks earlier (at that time, visualisation of the left coronary system had been less than satisfactory). Wide-spread ST depression is seen (in I, II, aVL, aVF and V_4–V_6). The very highly significant finding, however, is the

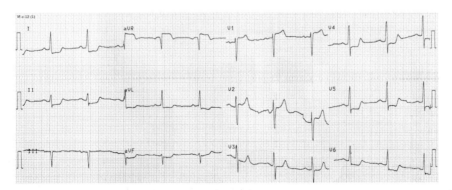

Fig. 37 The 12-lead ECG taken during a spontaneous episode of angina in a patient who had had successful stenting of his right coronary artery 6 weeks earlier. In addition to the diffuse ST depression, note the ST elevation in aVR.

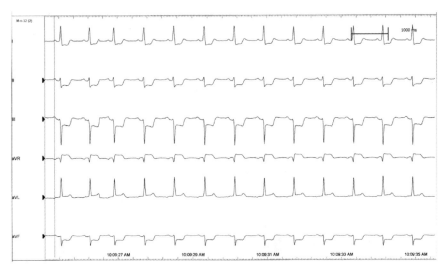

Fig. 38 Limb leads recorded from the same patient as in Figure 37, 2 days later at the onset of a procedure for repeat coronary angiography. Again, there is wide-spread ST depression but there was ST elevation in aVR. The patient had an entirely satisfactory right coronary artery with a critical stenosis at the origin of the left coronary artery.

presence of ST elevation in aVR. Figure 38 shows the limb leads from the same patient at the beginning of repeat angiography. Again, there is ST depression (this time in I, II, III and aVF) and, once more, there is ST elevation in aVR (and to a lesser extent in aVL). The patient proved to have a critical left main stem stenosis and subsequently had successful coronary artery bypass grafting. In the record shown in Figure 38, aVR was the only lead to show ST elevation. ST segment elevation in aVR suggests a very proximal lesion in the left coronary system, both in the situation of acute anterior STEMI and also in unstable angina/NSTEMI. In this latter situation, aVR may be the only lead showing ST elevation; all other leads may show ST depression or no ST shift.

UNIDENTIFIED ABNORMALITIES OF REPOLARISATION

Undoubtedly further, as yet undefined, repolarisation abnormalities await discovery and elucidation. Clinical practice is tantalising in so frequently providing a glimpse of the unknown. Figure 39 shows an example. This record was taken in 2007 from a patient who presented in 1993 with a cardiac arrest (in ventricular fibrillation). An ICD was implanted at that time and the device has given two appropriate shocks since then. The ECG has not changed significantly during the 14 years since initial presentation. No structural cardiac abnormality has been demonstrated and there is no family history of premature death. The exercise stress test, coronary angiogram, echocardiogram and electrophysiological studies had all given normal results. No biochemical or hormonal abnormality has been demonstrated and the patient is living a normal existence. The ECG shows no abnormalities of depolarisation but clearly shows repolarisation abnormalities. The obvious sign is the strikingly tall T waves in V_1–V_3 and the T waves are impressively symmetrical (angle of up-slope similar to angle of down-slope). The

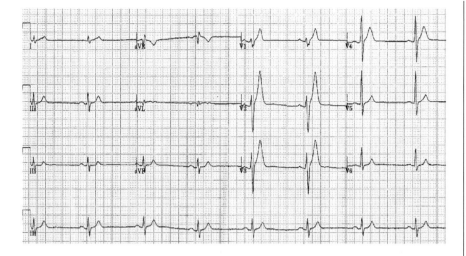

Fig. 39 The 12-lead ECG in a patient presenting with ventricular fibrillation. There is no abnormality in the form of the QRS complexes. The limb lead T waves show a minor abnormality in that, although the frontal plane QRS axis is virtually indeterminate, the frontal plane T wave axis is clearly determinate at +60°. The QT interval is normal at 360 ms and the QTc at 316 ms. However, there is virtually no ST segment in the right precordial leads (the T wave starts at the end of the S wave) and the T waves from V_1–V_3 are strikingly tall. This record, therefore, shows features often seen in the SQTS, even though the QT measurements are normal.

QT and QTc intervals are within normal limits at 360 ms and 316 ms, respectively (measured at a heart rate of 47 per min). The less obvious sign of repolarisation abnormality is in the limb leads. The frontal plane QRS axis is indeterminate (not an abnormality) but the T-wave axis is highly determinate at +60°. When repolarisation is normal, the T waves are concordant with the QRS complexes. Discordance (and, therefore, T-wave abnormality) occurs when either: (i) the angle between the frontal plane QRS and T wave axes exceeds ± 45°;[9] or (ii) the QRS axis is determinate and the T wave axis is not, or vice versa. It seems highly likely that this is a form of the short QT syndrome, albeit without a short QT! The tall, symmetrical T waves and absence of a detectable ST segment in all the precordial leads except V_6 strongly suggest SQTS or related condition, and the clinical history is in keeping with this. It may be that the criteria for the SQTS should be expanded to include the ratio of the T wave height to the QTc in the right precordial leads. No doubt further clarification of the heterogeneous nature[90] of the STQS will emerge.

ABNORMALITIES OF ATRIAL REPOLARISATION

The atrial repolarisation wave in the ECG (Ta wave) is discordant with the P wave, and typically appears as a small asymmetrical wave, opposite in polarity to the QRS complex and occurring at about the same time as the QRS complex. Abnormalities of atrial repolarisation are generally subtle, easily missed, and often obscured by the ensuing QRS complex except in situations where there is failure of, or delay in, atrioventricular conduction (Fig. 3) or when the Ta wave is increased in amplitude, for example during exercise (Fig. 4).

PROMINENT Ta WAVE

As noted earlier, the Ta wave increases both in depth and in duration during exercise. In the presence of normal sinus rhythm, with a P wave axis between 0° and 90°, the P wave is most commonly tallest in II and prominent (negative) Ta waves are, therefore, likely to be seen to best advantage in II, aVF, III (as well as in V_4–V_6). It is important not to mistake them for ST depression. The key is that the down-slope of the Ta wave clearly begins before the QRS (well seen in lead II of Fig. 4). The Ta wave is convex upwards in aVR (Fig. 4).

DEPRESSION OF THE PR SEGMENT

Depression of the PR segment is seen in pericarditis and in pericardial effusion.[110] In the context of acute inferior infarction, PQ segment depression has been shown to be an indicator of more extensive myocardial damage, extending to the posterior segments of the left ventricle.[111]

Depression of the R interval may occur as a result of a markedly prolonged Ta wave in severe hypokalaemia (Fig. 33).

Key points for clinical practice

- Depolarisation of myocardial cells is initiated by a sudden change in the relative permeabilities of the membrane to potassium and sodium ions. Within the ventricles, depolarisation spreads transmurally from endocardium to epicardium, both in terms of its initiation and its completion.

- Repolarisation begins in the endocardium at the peak of phase 0 of the action potential of the endocardial cells and finishes at the end of phase 3 of the action potential of the M cells, which are situated in the subendocardium. The process of completion of repolarisation, therefore, spreads from the epicardium towards the endocardium.

- In contrast to the dominantly radial (transmural) spread of depolarisation within the ventricles, spread in the atrial myocardium is dominantly longitudinal. In consequence, the Ta and P waves are discordant. The QRS and T waves are concordant because the direction of spread of completion of repolarisation is opposite to that of the completion of depolarisation.

- Repolarisation is a much more complex process than depolarisation.

- The ECG manifestations of repolarisation are highly informative in relation to clinical abnormalities.

- The demonstration of electrical heterogeneity of cell types at different levels within the ventricular wall has led to substantial progress in the understanding of the electrocardiographic manifestations of repolarisation both in the normal state and in association with clinically important abnormalities.

(continued on next page)

Key points for clinical practice *(continued)*

- It is important to recognise that variations in the ECG manifestations of repolarisation occur in healthy individuals, in the 'early repolarisation variant', and in the ECGs of athletes.

- ECG changes in the repolarisation phase are critical to the diagnosis of potentially fatal conditions such as Brugada syndrome, long QT syndrome and arrhythmogenic right ventricular cardiomyopathy.

- ECG changes of repolarisation are seen in association with electrolyte disturbances (especially in relation to K^+ and Ca^{2+}) and in association with a considerable number of drugs.

- Recent studies have thrown light on the mechanisms of ST elevation in relation to acute myocardial ischaemia and have highlighted the value of detailed assessment of the ST segment changes (particularly of the ST axis in the frontal plane) in localising the site of acute occlusion within the coronary arterial system.

ACKNOWLEDGEMENTS

The authors are grateful to Prof. C. Garratt for reading the manuscript and for his helpful comments. The authors also thank Dr Ronald Prineas (Wake Forest University Health Sciences, Suite 505, Piedmont Plaza Two, 2000 West First Street, Winston-Salem, NC 271904, USA) for very kindly making the highly specialised loupes available.

References

1. Hedén B, Ohlsson M, Holst H *et al.* Detection of frequently overlooked electrocardiographic lead reversals using artificial neural networks. *Am J Cardiol* 1996; **78**: 600–604.
2. Fozzard HA, Friedlander IR. Cellular electrophysiology. In: Macfarlane PW, Lawrie TDV. (eds) *Comprehensive Electrocardiology*. Oxford: Pergammon, Chapter 3, 1989.
3. McCullough JR, Chua WT, Rasmussen HH, Ten Eick RE, Singer DH. Two stable levels of diastolic potential at physiological K^+ concentrations in human ventricular myocardial cells. *Circ Res* 1980; **47**: 191–201.
4. Opie LH. *Heart Physiology: from cell to circulation*, 4th edn. New York: Lippincott Williams and Wilkins, 2004; p74.
5. Opie LH. *Heart Physiology: from cell to circulation*, 4th edn. New York: Lippincott Williams and Wilkins, 2004; p85.
6. Barr RC. Genesis of the electrocardiogram. In: Macfarlane PW, Lawrie TDV. (eds) *Comprehensive Electrocardiology*. Oxford: Pergammon, Chapter 5, 1989.
7. Spach MS, Barr RC, Benson DW *et al.* Body surface low-level potentials during ventricular repolarisation with analysis of the ST segment. Variability in normal subjects. *Circulation* 1979; **59**: 822–836.
8. Yan GX, Lankipalli RS, Burke JF *et al.* Ventricular repolarisation components on the electrocardiogram. Cellular basis and clinical significance. *J Am Coll Cardiol* 2003; **42**: 401–409.
9. Rowlands DJ, Moore PR. The limb leads and the frontal plane vectors; a poorly understood and underutilised resource. *Rec Adv Cardiol* 2007: **14**: 173–199.
10. Antzelevitch C, Sicouri S, Litovsky SH. Heterogeneity within the ventricular:

electrophysiology and pharmacology of epicardial, endocardial and M cells. *Circ Res* 1991; **69**: 1427–1449.

11. Sicouri S, Antzelevitch C. A subpopulation of cells with unique electrophysiological properties in the deep subepicardium of the canine ventricle. The M cell. *Circ Res* 1991; **68**: 1729–1741.

12. Yan GX, Shimizu W, Antzelevitch C. The characteristics and distribution of M cells in arterially perfused canine left ventricular wedge preparations. *Circulation* 1998; **88**: 1921–1927.

13. Antzelevitch C. Cellular basis for the repolarisation waves of the ECG. *Ann NY Acad Sci* 2006; **1080**: 268–281.

14. Yan GX, Antzelevitch C. Cellular basis for the normal T wave and the electrocardiographic manifestations of the long-QT syndrome. *Circulation* 1998; **98**: 1928–1936.

15. Antzelevitch C, Yan G-X, Shimizu W, Burashnikov A. Electrical heterogeneity, the ECG, and cardiac arrhythmias. In: Zipes DP, Jalife J. (eds) *Cardiac Electrophysiology: From Cell to Bedside*, 3rd edn. Philadelphia, PA: WB Saunders, 2000; p231.

16. Baker JM. *The unipolar electrocardiogram. A clinical interpretation.* New York: Appleton-Century-Crofts, 1952; p47.

17. Lepeschkin E. Physiologic basis of the U wave. In: Schlant RC, Hurst JW. (eds) *Advances in Electrocardiography*. New York: Grune and Stratton, 1972; 431.

18. Antzelevitch C, Nesterenko VV, Yan GX. The role of the M cells in acquired long QT syndrome, U waves and torsade de pointes. *J Electrocardiol* 1966; **28 (Suppl)**: 131–138.

19. Lepeshkin E. Genesis of the U wave. *Circulation* 1957; **15**: 77–81.

20. Gaita F, Giustetto C, Bianchi F *et al.* Short QT syndrome: a familial cause of sudden death. *Circulation* 2003; **109**: 30–35.

21. Hurst JW. Naming of the waves in the ECG, with a brief account of their genesis. *Circulation* 1998; **98**: 1937–1942.

22. Yan G-X, Antzelevitch C. Cellular basis for the electrocardiographic J wave. *Circulation* 1996; **93**: 372–379.

23. Di Diego JM, Antzelevitch C. High $[Ca^{2+}]$-induced electrical heterogeneity and extrasystolic activity in isolated canine ventricular epicardium: phase 2 reentry. *Circulation* 1994; **89**: 1839–1850.

24. Tranchesi J, Adelardi V, de Oliveira JM. Atrial repolarisation – its importance in clinical electrocardiography. *Circulation* 1960; **22**: 635–644.

25. Burashnikov A, Mannava S, Antzelevitch C. Transmembrane action potential heterogeneity in the canine isolated arterially perfused right atrium: effect of I_{Kr} and I_{Kur}/I_{to} block. *Am J Physiol* 2004; **286**: H2393–H2400.

26. Avanzino GL, Bianchi D, Calligaro A, Fisher M. Morphological and functional characteristics of the crista terminali in the rabbit right atrium. *J Physiol (Paris)* 1983; **78**: 848–853.

27. Gussak I, Antzelevitch C. Early repolarisation syndrome: clinical characteristics and possible cellular and ionic mechanisms. *J Electrocardiol* 2000; **33**: 299–309.

28. Mehta M, Jain AC, Mehta A. Early repolarisation. *Clin Cardiol* 1999; **22**: 59–65.

29. Boineau JP. The early repolarisation variant – an ECG enigma with both QRS and J-STT anomalies. *J Electrocardiol* 2007; **40**: 3.e1.

30. Boineau JP. The early repolarisation variant – normal or a marker of heart disease in certain subjects. *J Electrocardiol* 2007; **40**: 3.e11–3.e16.

31. Lux RL. Early repolarisation variant: interesting electrocardiographic anomaly or marker of arrhythmogenic risk? *J Electrocardiol* 2007; **40**: 4–5.

32. Liebman J. The early repolarisation syndrome is a variation of normal [Letter]. *J Electrocardiol* 2007; **40**: 392.

33. Bianco M, Bria S, Gianfelici A *et al.* Does early repolarisation in the athlete have analogies with the Brugada syndrome? *Eur Heart J* 2001; **22**: 504–510.

34. Serra-Grima R, Estorch M, Carrio I *et al.* Marked ventricular repolarisation abnormalities in highly trained athletes' electrocardiograms: clinical and prognostic implications. *J Am Coll Cardiol* 2000; **36**: 1310–1316.

35. Pelliccia A, Maron BJ, Culasso F *et al.* Clinical significance of abnormal electrocardiographic patterns in trained athletes. *Circulation* 2000; **102**: 278–284.

36. Brugada P, Brugada J. Right bundle branch block, persistent ST segment elevation and sudden cardiac death: a distinct clinical and electrocardiographic syndrome. A multicenter report. *J Am Coll Cardiol* 1992; **20**: 1391–1396.

37. Antzelevitch C, Brugada p, Brugada J *et al.* Brugada syndrome: 1992–2002. A historical perspective. *J Am Coll Cardiol* 2003; **41**: 1665–1671.

38. Mademanee K, Veerakul G, Mimmannit S *et al.* Arrhythmogenic marker for the sudden unexplained death syndrome in Thai men. *Circulation* 1997; **97**: 2595–2600.

39. Hermida JS, Lemoine JL, Aoun FB *et al.* Prevalence of the Brugada syndrome in an apparently healthy population. *Am J Cardiol* 2000; **86**: 91–94.

40. Monroe MH, Littman L. Two-year collection of the Brugada syndrome electrocardiogram pattern at a large teaching hospital. *Clin Cardiol* 2000; **23**: 849–851.

41. Surawicz B. Brugada syndrome: manifest, concealed, 'asymptomatic', suspected and simulated. *J Am Coll Cardiol* 2001; **38**: 775–777.

42. Wilde AAM, Antzelevitch C, Borggrefe M *et al.* Proposed diagnostic criteria for the Brugada syndrome. *Eur Heart J* 2002; **23**: 1648–1654.

43. Gussak I, Antzelevitch C, Bjerregaard P *et al.* The Brugada syndrome; clinical, electrophysiologic and genetic aspects. *J Am Coll Cardiol* 1999; **33**: 5–15.

44. Veltmann C, Schimpf R, Echternach C *et al.* A prospective study on spontaneous fluctuations between diagnostic and non-diagnostic ECGs in Brugada syndrome: implications for correct phenotyping and risk stratification. *Eur Heart J* 2006; **27**: 2544–2552.

45. Scheinman MM, Keung E. The year in clinical cardiac electrophysiology. *J Am Coll Cardiol* 2007; **49**: 2061–2069.

46. Antzelevitch C, Brugada P, Borggrefe M *et al.* Brugada syndrome. Report of the Second Consensus Conference. *Circulation* 2005; **111**: 659–670.

47. Brugada J, Brugada R, Antzelevitch C *et al.* Long-term follow-up of individuals with the electrocardiographic pattern of right bundle-branch block and ST elevation in precordial leads V1 to V3. *Circulation* 2002; **105**: 73–78.

48. Priori SG, Napolitano C, Gasparini M *et al.* Natural history of Brugada syndrome: insights for risk stratification and management. *Circulation* 2002; **105**: 1342–1347.

49. Viskin S. Inducible ventricular fibrillation in the Brugada syndrome; diagnostic and prognostic implications. *J Cardiovasc Electrophysiol* 2003; **14**: 458–460.

50. Junttila MJ, Raatikainen MJP, Karjalainen J *et al.* Prevalence and prognosis of subjects with Brugada-type ECG pattern in a young and middle-aged Finnish population. *Eur Heart J* 2004; **25**: 874–878.

51. Hermida J, Lemoine J, Aoun FB *et al.* Prevalence of the Brugada syndrome in an apparently healthy population. *Am J Cardiol* 2000; **86**: 91–94.

52. Eckardt L, Probst V, Jeroen SPP *et al.* Long-term prognosis of individuals with right precordial ST-segment-elevation Brugada syndrome. *Circulation* 2005; **111**: 257–263.

53. Priori SG, Napolitano C, Schwartz PJ. Genetics of cardiac arrhythmias. In: Splawski I, Shen J, Timothy KW. (eds) *Braunwald's Heart Disease*, 8th edn. Philadelphia, PA: Elsevier Saunders, 2007; p105.

54. Antzelevitch C. The Brugada syndrome: diagnostic criteria and cellular mechanisms [Editorial]. *Eur Heart J* 2001; **22**: 356–363.

55. Antzelevitch C. Cardiac repolarisation. The long and the short of it. *Europace Suppl* 2005; **7**: S3–S9.

56. Gemayel D, Pelliccia A, Thompson PD. Arrhythmogenic right ventricular cardiomyopathy. *J Am Coll Cardiol* 2001; **38**: 1773–1781.

57. Corrado D, Basso C, Thiene G *et al.* Spectrum of clinicopathologic manifestations of Arrhythmogenic right ventricular cardiomyopathy/dysplasia: a multicentre study. *J Am Coll Cardiol* 1997; **30**: 1512–1520.

58. Hess OM, McKenna W, Scultheiss H-P *et al.* Myocardial diseases. In: Camm AJ, Lüscher TF, Serruys PW. (eds) *The ESC Textbook of Cardiovascular Medicine*. Oxford: Blackwell, 2006; p487.

59. Marcus FI, Fontaine GH, Guiraudon G *et al.* Right ventricular dysplasia: a report of 24 adult cases. *Circulation* 1982; **65**: 384–398.

60. Nasir K, Bomma C, Tandri H *et al.* Electrocardiographic features of arrhythmogenic right. Ventricular dysplasia/cardiomyopathy according to disease severity: a need to

broaden diagnostic criteria. *Circulation* 2004; **110**; 1527–1534.

61. Marcus FI. Electrocardiographic features of inherited diseases that predispose to the development of cardiac arrhythmias, long QT syndrome, arrhythmogenic right ventricular cardiomyopathy/dysplasia, and Brugada syndrome. *J Electrocardiol* 2000; **33 (Suppl 1)**: 1–10.

62. Anan R, Takenaka T, Tei C. Epsilon waves in a patient with arrhythmogenic right ventricular cardiomyopathy. *Heart* 2002; **88**: 444.

63. Fontaine G, Guiraudon D, Frank R *et al*. Stimulation studies and epicardial mapping in ventricular tachycardia: study of mechanisms and selection for surgery. In: Kulbertus HE. (ed) *Re-entrant Arrhythmias: Mechanisms and Treatment*. Lancaster, PA: MTP, 1977; 334–350.

64. Zorio E, Arnau MA, Rueda J *et al*. The presence of epsilon waves in a patient with acute right ventricular infarction. *Pacing Clin Electrophysiol* 2005; **28**: 245–247.

65. Santucci PA, Morton JB, Picken MM *et al*. Electroanatomic mapping of the right ventricle in a patient with a giant epsilon wave, ventricular tachycardia, and cardiac sarcoidosis. *J Cardiovasc Electrophysiol* 2004; **15**: 1091–1094.

66. Gemayel C, Pelliccia A, Thompson PD. Arrhythmogenic right ventricular cardiomyopathy. *J Am Coll Cardiol* 2001; **38**: 1773–1781.

67. Aziz S, McMahon RFT, Garratt CJ. Sudden cardiac death in arrhythmogenic right ventricular dysplasia. *Circulation* 2000; **101**: 825–827.

68. Corrado D, Buja G, Basso C *et al*. Clinical diagnosis and management strategies in arrhythmogenic right ventricular cardiomyopathy. *J Electrocardiol* 2000; **33 (Suppl)**: 49–55.

69. Furushima H, Chinushi M, Okamura K *et al*. Comparison of conduction delay in the right ventricular outflow tract between Brugada syndrome and right ventricular cardiomyopathy: investigation of signal average ECG in the precordial leads. *Europace* 2007; **9**: eum128v 1–6.

70. Moss AJ. Long QT syndrome. *JAMA* 2003; **289**: 2041–2044.

71. Priori SG, Napolitano C, Schwartz PJ. Genetics of cardiac arrhythmias. In: Splawski I, Shen J, Timothy KW. (eds) *Braunwald's Heart Disease*, 8th edn. Philadelphia, PA: Elsevier Saunders, 2007; p102.

72. Splawski I, Shen J, Timothy KW *et al*. Spectrum of mutations in long-QT syndrome genes: KVLQT1, HERG, SCN5A, KCNE1, and KCNE2. *Circulation* 2000; **102**: 1178–1185.

73. Sauer AJ, Moss AJ, McNitt *et al*. Long QT syndrome in adults. *J Am Coll Cardiol* 2007; **49**: 329–337.

74. Lepesschkin E, Surawicz B. The measurement of the Q–T interval of the electrocardiogram. *Circulation* 1952; **6**: 378–388.

75. Goldenberg I, Moss AJ, Zareba W. QT interval: how to measure it and what is 'normal'. *J Cardiovasc Electrophysiol* 2006; **17**; 333–336.

76. Viskin S, Rosovski U, Sands AJ *et al*. Inaccurate electrocardiographic interpretation of long QT: the majority of physicians cannot recognise a long QT when they see one. *Heart Rhythm* 2005; **2**: 569–574.

77. Marek M. Errors and misconceptions in ECG measurement used for the detection of drug induced QT interval prolongation. *J Electrocardiol* 2004; **37 (Suppl)**: 25–33.

78. Bazett HC. An analysis of the time relations of electrocardiograms. *Heart* 1920; **7**: 353–370.

79. Macfarlane PW, Lawrie TDV. The normal electrocardiogram and vectorcardiogram. In: Macfarlane PW, Lawrie TDV. (eds) *Comprehensive Electrocardiology*. Oxford: Pergammon, 1989; p452.

80. Hodges M, Salerno D, Erlien D *et al*. Bazett's QT correction reviewed. Evidence that a linear correction for heart rate is better [Abstract]. *J Am Coll Cardiol* 1983; **Suppl 1**: 694.

81. Moss AJ. What duration of the QT interval should disqualify athletes from competitive sports? [Editorial]. *Eur Heart J* 2007; **28**: 2825–2826.

82. Corrado D, Pelliccia A, Bjornstad HH *et al*. Cardiovascular pre-participation screening of young competitive athletes for prevention of sudden cardiac death: proposal for a common European protocol. *Eur Heart J* 2005; **26**: 516–524.

83. Basavarajaiah S, Wilson M, Whyte G *et al*. Prevalence and significance of an isolated long QT interval in elite athletes. *Eur Heart J* 2007; **28**: 2944–2949.

84. Antzelevitch C. Heterogeneity of cellular repolarisation in LQTS: the role of M cells. *Eur Heart J Suppl* 2001; **3 (Suppl K)**: K2–K16.

85. Belardinlli L, Antzelevitch C. Assessing predictors of drug-induced torsade de pointes. *Trends Pharmacol Sci* 2003; **24**: 619–625.

86. Gussak I, Brugada P, Brugada J *et al*. Idiopathic short QT interval: a new clinical syndrome?

Cardiology 2000; **94**: 99–102.

87. Jervell A, Lange-Nielsen F. Congenital deaf-mutism, functional heart disease with prolongation of the QT interval and sudden death. *Am Heart J* 1957; **54**: 59–68.

88. Gaita F, Giustetto C, Bianchi F *et al*. Short QT syndrome: a familial cause of sudden death. *Circulation* 2003; **108**: 965–970.

89. Extramiana F, Antzelevitch C. Amplified transmural dispersion of repolarisation as the basis for arrhythmogenesis in a canine ventricular-wedge model of short-QT syndrome. *Circulation* 2004; **110**: 3661–3666.

90. Borggrefe M, Wolpert C, Antzelevitch C *et al*. Short QT syndrome genotype–phenotype correlations. *J Electrocardiol* 2005; **38**: 75–80.

91. Priori SG, Napolitano C, Schwartz PJ. Genetics of cardiac arrhythmias. In: Splawski I, Shen J, Timothy KW. (eds) *Braunwald's Heart Disease*, 8th edn. Philadelphia, PA: Elsevier Saunders, 2007; p108.

92. Brugada R, Hong K, Dumaine R *et al*. Sudden death associated with short-QT syndrome linked to mutations in HERG. *Circulation* 2004; **109**: 30–35.

93. Bellocq C, van Ginneken AGG, Bezzine CR *et al*. Mutation in the KCNQ1 gene leading to the short QT-interval syndrome. *Circulation* 2004; **109**: 2394–2397.

94. Yap YG, Camm AJ. Drug induced QT prolongation and torsade de pointes. *Heart* 2003; **89**: 1363–1372.

95. Kowey PR, Malik M. The QT interval as it relates to the safety of non-cardiac drugs. *Eur Heart J Suppl* 2007; **9 (Suppl G)**: G3–G8.

96. Darpö B. Spectrum of drugs prolonging QT interval and the incidence of torsade de pointes. *Eur Heart J Suppl* 2001; **3 (Suppl K)**: K70–K80.

97. University of Arizona, College of Pharmacy <http://www.qtdrugs.org/medical-pros/drug-lists/drug-lists.htm>.

98. Cheng TO. Digitalis administration: an underappreciated but common cause of short QT interval [Letter]. *Circulation* 2004; **109**: e159.

99. Dessertenne F. La tachycardre ventriculaire a deux foyers opposes variables. *Arch Mal Coeur Vaiss* 1966; **59**: 263–272.

100. Liu J, Laurita KR. The mechanism of pause-induced torsade de pointes in long QT syndrome. *J Cardiovasc Electrophysiol* 2005; **16**: 981–987.

101. Thygesen K, Alpert JS, White HD. Universal definition of myocardial infarction (ESC/ACCF/AHA/WHF Task Force for the Redefinition of Myocardial Infarction). *J Am Coll Cardiol* 2007; **50**: 2171–2195.

102. Kenigsberg DN, Khanal S, Kowalski M. Prolongation of the QTc interval is seen uniformly during early transmural ischemia. *J Am Coll Cardiol* 2007; **49**: 1299–1305.

103. Davis MJ. The pathophysiology of acute coronary syndromes. *Heart* 2000; **83**: 361–366.

104. Pahlm-Webb U, Pahlm O, Sadanandan S *et al*. A new method for using the direction of the ST-segment deviation to localise the site of acute coronary occlusion: the 24-view standard electrocardiogram. *Am J Med* 2002; **113**: 75–78.

105. Engelen DJ, Gorgels AP, Cheriex EC *et al*. Value of the electrocardiogram in localizing the occlusion site in the left anterior descending artery in acute anterior myocardial infarction. *J Am Coll Cardiol* 1999; **34**: 389–395.

106. Di Diego JM, Antzelevitch C. Cellular basis for ST-segment changes observed during ischemia. *J Electrocardiol* 2003; **36 (Suppl)**: 1–5.

107. Cannon CP, McCabe CH, Stone PH *et al*. The electrocardiogram predicts one-year outcome of patients with unstable angina and non-Q wave myocardial infarction: results of the TIMI III Registry ECG Ancillary Study. *J Am Coll Cardiol* 1997; **30**: 133–140.

108. Li D, Li CY, Yong AC *et al*. Source of electrocardiographic ST changes in subendocardial ischemia. *Circ Res* 1998; **82**: 957–970.

109. Mark DB, Hlatky MA, Lee KL. Localising coronary artery obstructions with the exercise treadmill test. *Ann Intern Med* 1987; **106**: 53–55.

110. Kudo Y, Yamasaki F, Doi Y *et al*. Clinical correlates of PR-segment depression in asymptomatic patients with pericardial effusion. *J Am Coll Cardiol* 2002; **39**: 2000–2004.

111. Nagahama Y, Sugiura T, Takehana K *et al*. PQ segment depression in acute Q wave inferior wall myocardial infarction. *Circulation* 1995; **91**: 641–644.

112. Pelliccia A, Paolo FM, Quattrini FM *et al*. Outcomes in athletes with marked ECG repolarisation abnormalities. *N Engl J Med* 2008; **358**: 152–161.

Wei C. Lau Kim A. Eagle

5

Evaluating the cardiac risk of non-cardiac surgery

The ageing patient population and advances in surgical and anaesthetic techniques have led to the performance of complex surgical procedures in greater number of patients with higher risk of cardiovascular disease.[1] The incidence of cardiac complications after non-cardiac surgery is approximately 0.5–1%.[2] Consequently, 200,000–400,000 people will suffer from peri-operative cardiac complications, and one in four or more of these patients will die.[3] Moreover, patients who survive a postoperative myocardial infarction (MI) are twice as likely to die in the following 2 years compared with patients with uneventful surgical procedures.[4] Thus, it is prudent for the practicing physician to perform a thoughtful evaluation of the surgical patient to provide an accurate pre-operative risk assessment, risk stratification, and risk modification that can then guide the strategies for optimum peri-operative risk reduction. This chapter outlines a systematic approach for cardiovascular risk assessment to guide peri-operative preventive therapies strategically to favour optimal outcome.

RISK OF PERI-OPERATIVE CARDIAC EVENTS DURING NON-CARDIAC SURGERY

Underlying significant coronary artery disease (CAD) is an important component in the pathophysiological processes of peri-operative MI. The risk of peri-operative MI is 0.1–0.6% in patients without a history of MI, 4.1–11% in

Wei C. Lau MD
Cardiovascular Center, University of Michigan Health Services, 1500 E. Medical Center Dr, Ann Arbor, MI 48109-5861, USA. E-mail: weiclau@med.umich.edu

Kim A. Eagle MD FACC (for correspondence)
Cardiovascular Center, University of Michigan Health Services, 1500 E. Medical Center Dr, Ann Arbor, MI 48109-5852, USA
E-mail: keagle@umich.edu

those with a 4–6-month history of prior MI, and 27–37% in patients who sustained MI within 3 months pre-operatively. Peri-operative MI is associated with > 50% mortality rates. A composite algorithm is thus provided in this chapter to improve the consensus-derived algorithm[5,6] recommended by the American College of Cardiology/American Heart Association (ACC/AHA) Task Force on Practice Guidelines,[5] and empiric risk indices,[7,8] such as the Revised Cardiac Risk Index (RCRI).[8]

PERI-OPERATIVE CARDIAC RISK ASSESSMENT

URGENCY OF THE SURGICAL PROCEDURE

Ascertaining the urgency of the surgery should be carefully assessed along with an initial history and physical examination in the evaluation of the surgical patients (Fig. 1). The urgency of surgery is dictated by patient- or surgery-specific factors and, in some instances, there may not be time for further cardiac assessment, as true emergency procedures are associated with an unavoidably higher morbidity and mortality. Recommendations should be provided for peri-operative medical management and surveillance in such instances. Selected patients felt to be at high risk for long-term coronary events may benefit from cardiac assessment after their recovery from surgery.

RECENT REVASCULARISATION AND CORONARY ARTERY DISEASE EVALUATION

A complete coronary revascularisation, in the form of coronary artery bypass grafting (CABG) in the previous 5 years or percutaneous transluminal coronary angioplasty in the previous 6 months to 5 years in a functionally active patient who is otherwise free of clinical symptoms of ischaemia, is associated with a low likelihood of peri-operative cardiac events.[9] Usually, such patients may proceed to surgery without further cardiac testing.

In those patients who have been evaluated in the past 2 years with either invasive or non-invasive techniques with favourable findings, no further cardiac work-up is generally necessary if they have been free of cardiac symptoms after the test. Patients with changing symptoms or signs of ischaemia should be considered for further evaluation.[5]

RISK ASSESSMENT FOR ADVERSE CARDIAC EVENTS

Evaluation of the surgical patient should begin with a thorough history and physical examination along with a 12-lead resting ECG in accordance with the ACC/AHA guideline recommendations.[5] If a patient has a major clinical predictor of adverse cardiac outcomes (Table 1) and is scheduled for elective surgery, a useful approach is to stratify further the patient using RCRI and, if indicated, to postpone surgery until the cardiac problem is adequately worked-up and optimally treated (Fig. 1). Patients with moderate or excellent functional capacity and one or more intermediate predictors of clinical risk can normally undergo low- and intermediate-risk surgery (Table 2) with low peri-operative cardiac risk. Patients with poor functional capacity or a combination

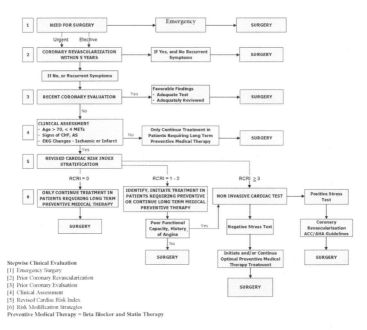

Fig. 1 Improved consensus-derived algorithm for cardiac risk assessment

Table 1 Clinical predictors of increased peri-operative cardiovascular risk

---

MAJOR

- Unstable or severe angina (Canadian Cardiovascular Society Class III or IV)
- Recent myocardial infarction (> 7 days but ≤ 30 days) with evidence of ischaemic risk by clinical symptoms or non-invasive testing
- Decompensated CHF
- Symptomatic arrhythmias (high-grade atrioventricular block, symptomatic ventricular arrhythmia with underlying heart disease, and supraventricular arrhythmias with uncontrolled ventricular rate)

INTERMEDIATE

- Mild angina (Canadian Cardiovascular Society Classes I and II)
- Prior myocardial infarction (history or ECG)
- Compensated or prior CHF
- Diabetes mellitus
- Renal insufficiency (creatinine = 2.0 mg/dl, ~175 μmol/l)

MINOR

- Advanced age
- Abnormal ECG (left ventricular hypertrophy, left bundle branch block, ST-T abnormalities)
- Rhythm other than sinus
- Low functional capacity
- History of stroke
- Uncontrolled systemic hypertension

CHF, congestive heart failure; ECG, electrocardiogram.
Adapted from *Guidelines for perioperative evaluation for noncardiac surgery.*[5]

Table 2 Surgery-specific cardiac risk (cardiac death and non-fatal MI)

HIGH (CARDIAC RISK > 5%)
• Emergency major operation, particularly in the elderly
• Aortic and other major vascular (endovascular or non-endovascular)
• Peripheral vascular
• Anticipated prolonged surgical procedures associated with large fluid shifts and/or blood loss
INTERMEDIATE (CARDIAC RISK < 5%)
• Intrathoracic
• Intraperitoneal
• Carotid endarterectomy
• Head and neck
• Orthopaedic
• Prostate
LOW (CARDIAC RISK < 1%)
• Endoscopic procedures
• Superficial procedures
• Cataract
• Breast

Adapted from *Guidelines for perioperative evaluation for noncardiac surgery.*[5]

of high-risk surgery, moderate functional capacity, and two or more intermediate clinical predictors of cardiac risk can be further assessed using RCRI stratification. In general, patients with minor or no clinical predictors of risk and with moderate or excellent functional capacity (> 4–6 metabolic equivalents [METs]) can safely undergo most types of non-cardiac surgery with low risk of cardiac complications.

Functional capacity

Various activities characterising functional capacity can be classified as excellent (METs > 7), moderate (METs 4–7), poor (METS < 4) or unknown (Table 3). Functional status is predictive of future cardiac events[10,11] and should be assessed in all pre-operative patients. Assessment of exercise tolerance in pre-operative risk stratification and precise prediction of in-hospital peri-operative risk is most applicable in patients who self-report worsening exercise-induced cardiopulmonary symptoms, patients who may benefit from non-invasive or invasive cardiac testing regardless of a scheduled surgical procedure, and patients with known coronary artery disease or with multiple risk factors and the ability to exercise. Patients with poor functional capacity facing intermediate- or high-risk surgery can generally be further stratified using the RCRI. Patients with moderate or excellent functional capacity and few or no clinical predictors of risk, or patients with a combination of intermediate predictors of cardiac risk, low- or intermediate-risk surgery, and preserved functional capacity, can usually proceed to elective surgery without undergoing further risk stratification or cardiac work-up.

Table 3 Functional capacity assessment from clinical history

EXCELLENT (> 7 METs)
- Carry 24 lb up eight steps
- Carry objects that weight 80 lb
- Outdoor work (shovel snow, spade soil)
- Recreation (ski, basketball, squash, handball, jog/walk 5 mph)

MODERATE (> 4 BUT < 7 METs)
- Have sexual intercourse without stopping
- Walk at 4 mph on level ground
- Outdoor work (garden, rake, weed)
- Recreation (roller-skate, dance, foxtrot)

POOR (<4 METs)
- Shower/dress without stopping, strip and make bed, dust, wash dishes
- Walk at 2.5 mph on level ground
- Outdoor work (clean windows)
- Recreation (play golf, bowl)

MET, metabolic equivalent.
Adapted from *Guidelines for perioperative evaluation for noncardiac surgery.*[5]

SURGERY-SPECIFIC RISK

The type of surgery also affects the pretest probability of cardiac complications (Table 2).[5] Emergency surgery is associated with a 4–5-fold increase in risk in comparison with elective surgery.[7] In addition, major vascular surgery or operations associated with large fluid shifts or blood loss have a 2–3-fold increased risk of cardiac complications. Risk classification of various surgical procedures should be considered along with the clinical predictors of risk and functional capacity in properly risk-stratifying patients before non-cardiac surgery.

THE REVISED CARDIAC RISK INDEX

Previous studies have compared several cardiac risk indices and the RCRI is favoured given its accuracy and simplicity.[8] The RCRI (Table 4) relies on the presence or absence of six identifiable predictive factors which include high-risk surgery, ischaemic heart disease, congestive heart failure, cerebrovascular disease, diabetes mellitus, and renal failure. Each of the RCRI predictors is assigned one point, when present. The risk of cardiac events (including MI, pulmonary oedema, ventricular fibrillation or primary cardiac arrest, and complete heart block) can then be predicted. Based on the presence of 0, 1, 2, 3, or more of these clinical predictors, the rate of major cardiac complications is estimated to be 0.4–0.5%, 0.9–1.3%, 4–6.6%, and 9–11%, respectively. Cardiac risk particularly increases with two or more predictors, and is greatest with three predictors or more. The clinical utility of the RCRI is to identify patients at higher risk for cardiac complications, and to determine whether they may

Table 4 Revised Cardiac Risk Index Clinical Markers

1 HIGH-RISK SURGICAL PROCEDURES
2 ISCHAEMIC HEART DISEASE
- History of myocardial infarction
- Current angina considered to be ischaemic
- Requiring sublingual nitroglycerin
- Positive exercise test
- Pathological Q-waves on ECG
- History of PTCA and/or CABG with current angina considered to be ischaemic

3 CONGESTIVE HEART FAILURE
- Left ventricular failure by physical examination
- History of paroxysmal nocturnal dyspnoea
- History of pulmonary oedema
- S3 gallop on cardiac auscultation
- Bilateral rales on pulmonary auscultation
- Pulmonary oedema on chest X-ray

4 CEREBROVASCULAR DISEASE
- History of transient ischaemic attack
- History of cerebrovascular accident

5 DIABETES MELLITUS
- Treatment with insulin

6 CHRONIC RENAL INSUFFICIENCY
- Serum creatinine > 2 mg/dl

Adapted from Lee et al.[8]

benefit from further risk stratification with non-invasive cardiac testing or initiation of pre-operative preventive medical management (Fig. 1).

NON-INVASIVE CARDIAC TESTING

Evidence discourages wide-spread application of pre-operative non-invasive cardiac testing for all patients. Rather, a selective approach based on clinical risk categorisation is both effective and cost-efficient. The selection of non-invasive cardiac stress tests for the occasional patient should anticipate that the patient will either meet guidelines for coronary revascularisation after coronary angiography or an adjustment in medical therapy, and no testing is recommended when it might delay surgical intervention for urgent or emergency conditions. Current thought recognises the potential benefit of occasional coronary revascularisation through identification of asymptomatic, but high-risk, patients (patients with left main, left main equivalent disease, or triple coronary vessel disease with poor left ventricular function). However, that evidence does not support aggressive attempts at identifying intermediate-risk patients with asymptomatic, but advanced, coronary artery disease where coronary revascularisation appears to offer little advantage over excellent medical therapy.[12,13] The ACC/AHA guidelines summarise recommendations for supplemental pre-operative evaluation in patients whose clinical history, physical examination, or exercise tolerance suggests they are intermediate- to high-risk regardless of planned major non-cardiac surgery.[5] Based on the RCRI score, medical therapy is appropriate to reduce peri-operative cardiovascular risk in selected intermediate (RCRI = 1–2) to high-risk (RCRI = 3) patients.[8] Patients with an RCRI of 3 should be considered for either pre-operative, non-invasive, cardiac testing or initiation of peri-operative medical therapy if there is either limited or no ischaemia during stress testing or if risks of coronary revascularisation are felt to exceed any potential benefit. An RCRI of 3 in patients with severe myocardial ischaemia suggestive of left main or three-vessel disease should lead to consideration of coronary revascularisation prior to non-cardiac surgery (Fig. 1). Non-invasive cardiac testing is most appropriate if it is anticipated that a patient will meet guidelines for initiation of important medical therapy or coronary angiography and coronary revascularisation in the event of a very positive test. Pharmacological cardiac stress tests should be used in patients with functional limitations which preclude exercise testing. Dobutamine stress echocardiography (DSE) and nuclear perfusion testing for purposes of identifying patients at risk for peri-operative myocardial infarction or death have excellent negative predictive values (near 100%) but poor positive predictive values (< 20%). Thus, a negative study is re-assuring but a positive study is still a relatively weak predictor of a 'hard' peri-operative cardiac event. Which higher risk patients are most likely to benefit from pre-operative non-invasive cardiac testing and treatment strategies to improve outcomes is not well defined.

PERI-OPERATIVE NON-INVASIVE CARDIAC TESTING

EXERCISE TESTING

Pre-operative cardiac exercise testing should be considered in the following situations:[5] (i) patients with intermediate pre-test probability of CAD; (ii) prognostic assessment of patients undergoing initial evaluation for suspected or proven CAD; (iii) evaluation of subjects with significant changes in clinical status; (iv) demonstration of proof of myocardial ischaemia before coronary revascularisation; (v) evaluation of adequacy of medical treatment; and (vi) prognostic assessment after an acute coronary syndrome. In patients with baseline ECG abnormalities and/or inability to exercise secondary to co-morbid conditions, pharmacological stress echocardiography or nuclear imaging are preferred.

PHARMACOLOGICAL STRESS TEST AND MYOCARDIAL PERFUSION IMAGING

The positive predictive value of pre-operative dipyridamole-thallium imaging for risk stratification has been consistently low, between 6–67%. On the other hand, pharmacological stress testing appears to have excellent negative predictive value (between 90–100%) making it more useful for reducing risk estimates when negative than for identifying very high risk when positive.

DOBUTAMINE STRESS ECHOCARDIOGRAPHY

There are limited studies comparing the prognostic accuracy of various non-invasive testing used for pre-operative cardiac risk assessment. The choices among non-invasive tests should thus be based on the need to assess valvular or ventricular function and on which test is most reliable and available locally. Dobutamine stress echocardiography (DSE) is attractive given that it may have better overall predictive performance,[14] as well as providing additional information about valvular and left ventricular dysfunction. A rapidly developing diagnostic modality is dobutamine stress magnetic resonance imaging, though sensitivity and specificity data are still pending at this time.[3]

PRE-OPERATIVE INVASIVE CARDIAC TESTING FOR RISK STRATIFICATION

Recommendations for peri-operative coronary angiography are similar to those for patients with suspected or known CAD in general and should conform to the ACC/AHA guidelines for coronary angiography.[5,15] This procedure should be considered for patients who have evidence for high risk of adverse outcome based on non-invasive test results, unstable angina, angina refractory to medical treatment, extensive ischaemia on non-invasive testing, or a non-diagnostic stress test in patients at high risk undergoing high-risk non-cardiac surgery. It should be considered on an individual basis for patients with limited to extensive ischaemia during non-invasive testing, for patients at intermediate risk undergoing high-risk surgery with non-diagnostic test results, for patients convalescing from MI who need urgent non-cardiac surgery, and for patients with peri-operative MI.[5,15] In general, patients who have a high clinical risk (RCRI > 3) and who have high-risk features on non-invasive cardiac testing should be considered for diagnostic cardiac catheterisation (Fig. 1).

PERI-OPERATIVE CORONARY REVASCULARISATION

Retrospective analyses of the Coronary Artery Surgery Study (CASS) registry, Bypass Angioplasty Revascularization Investigation (BARI),[16] and prospective study of patients enrolled in the Coronary Artery Revascularization Prophylaxis (CARP) trial[12] have shown that prophylactic coronary revascularisation with either CABG or percutaneous coronary intervention (PCI) before non-cardiac surgery provides no short- or mid-term benefit for patients without left main disease, or multivessel CAD in the presence of poor left ventricular systolic function. It is true that high-risk patients who have successfully undergone PCI or CABG prior to elective non-cardiac surgery experience fewer adverse peri-operative cardiovascular events compared to similar patients treated with medications alone. However, the mortality and morbidity associated with PCI or CABG appear to offset the potential benefit of coronary revascularisation prior to major non-cardiac surgery. Thus, evidence is lacking to support elective coronary revascularisation as a primary strategy in peri-operative risk reduction in intermediate-risk patients undergoing major non-cardiac surgery.

Recommendations for PCI prior to non-cardiac surgery are similar to those for patients with suspected or known CAD in general and should conform to the ACC/AHA guidelines for PCI.[17] While catheter-based percutaneous coronary revascularisation in the peri-operative setting is associated with lower procedural risk than CABG,[17] studies have shown that the placement of a stent in a coronary artery a short period of time prior to non-cardiac surgery may increase peri-operative risk of MI and cardiac death due to in-stent thrombosis.[3] This applies both to bare metal and to drug-eluting stents. In one report, patients could proceed to non-cardiac surgery as soon as 2 weeks or earlier after PCI, when only balloon angioplasty was employed.[18] On the other hand, a 6–8 week delay after PCI to allow for administration of dual antiplatelet therapy is preferable after bare metal coronary stent placement[19,20] and 3–6 months for a drug-eluting stent.[21] For patients who absolutely must undergo non-cardiac surgery early (first few days to 4 weeks) after PCI, balloon angioplasty appears to a reasonable alternative[18] since dual antiplatelet therapy is not required and acute thrombosis is rare after a few days. As with CABG, studies do not show that prophylactic PCI prior to non-cardiac surgery reduces the risk of peri-operative MI or cardiac death.

Currently, studies suggest that optimal medical therapy is the preferred strategy for the intermediate- to high-risk patient population with RCRI ≥ 2 without documented severe myocardial ischaemia.[12,13,22] Coronary revascularisation may be appropriate for selected patients when coronary angiography reveals left main disease and/or multivessel disease with depressed ejection fraction. A key decision is to determine whether the risk of peri-operative cardiac events is sufficiently low to proceed with surgery. For patients identified at high cardiac risk who are not candidates for coronary revascularisation, this may result in a decision to perform a less extensive non-cardiac procedure or attempt to modify cardiac risk by additional intra-operative and peri-operative medical therapies. For some high-risk patients who are considering elective surgery aimed at improving quality of life, a decision to postpone or cancel the operation may be the best strategy.

PHARMACOLOGICAL STRATEGY FOR PERI-OPERATIVE RISK MODIFICATION

Current peri-operative preventive medical therapy has the goal of reducing peri-operative adrenergic stimulation, peri-operative ischaemia, and inflammation which is triggered by adrenergic modulation, by using β-adrenergic antagonists or α_2-adrenergic agonists, HMG-CoA reductase inhibitors (statins), and aspirin during the peri-operative period.

ADRENERGIC MODULATION

β-Adrenergic antagonists

Two previous clinical trials have demonstrated the benefit of peri-operative β-blockers in reducing cardiac risk.[23,24] Mangano et al.[23] showed that patients undergoing vascular surgery who were randomly assigned to receive atenolol (versus placebo) had a reduced cardiac event rate over the first year or two after surgery. Poldermans et al.[24] studied 112 patients undergoing high-risk vascular procedures. Those with one or more clinical markers of risk and ischaemia demonstrated by DSE were randomly assigned to receive bisoprolol (titrated to a heart rate of 60 beats/min) or standard care before surgery. The incidence of death in the bisoprolol recipients was 3.4%, in contrast to 17% in the patients receiving standard care. There were no non-fatal MIs in the bisoprolol recipients, in contrast to a 17% incidence in the standard-care recipients. Overall, treatment with bisoprolol was associated with a 90% reduction in the composite end point of non-fatal MI and death. In a recent study, Poldermans *et al.*[13] demonstrated by using excellent β-blocker therapy with tight heart rate control below the ischaemic threshold of 60–65 beats/min in a total of 770 intermediate-risk pre-operative patients, that there was protection against major cardiac events after vascular surgery; non-invasive cardiac testing added little prognostic value among intermediate risk patients in this setting.[25]

Despite the promising results in retrospective and randomised control trials supporting the use of β-blockers for peri-operative cardiac risk, the prescribing of peri-operative β-blocker should be based on a thorough assessment of a patient's peri-operative RCRI ≥ 2, and not broad inclusion criteria, to yield a favourable risk-to-benefit ratio in patients who are at increased cardiac risk. Also, the effectiveness of metoprolol in peri-operative cardiac risk reduction has recently been challenged. Where metoprolol was shown to reduce peri-operative ischaemia and MI,[26,27] metoprolol may not be as effective as atenolol for peri-operative cardioprotection.[28–30]

For patients with mild-to-moderate reactive airway disease, it is advised to use the cardioselective β-blocker of choice, and titrate to a target resting heart rate of 60–65 beats/min. In intermediate- to high-risk patients without a long-term indication for β-blockers, the medications can be administered intravenously as a pre-operative medication on the day of surgery, with a targeted heart rate of 60–65 beats/min, and continued for > 7 days, preferably 30 days postoperatively. Intravenous preparations should be substituted for oral medication if patients are unable to take or absorb pills in the peri-operative period. Definitive indications for peri-operative β-blocker prophylaxis beyond higher risk patients undergoing vascular surgery awaits the result of the on-going Perioperative Ischemia Evaluation (POISE) trial.

A recent, expedited update on the ACC/AHA guideline focusing on recommendations for peri-operative β-blocker therapy[31] suggests using β-blockers for the following situations: (i) β-blockers should be continued in all high-risk patients previously receiving β-blocker therapy undergoing vascular surgery; (ii) β-blockers should be administered to all high-risk patients identified by myocardial ischaemia on pre-operative assessment undergoing vascular surgery; (iii) β-blockers are probably recommended for high-risk patients defined by multiple clinical predictors undergoing intermediate- or high-risk procedures; (iv) they may be considered for intermediate-risk patients defined by a single clinical predictor undergoing intermediate- or high-risk procedures; (v) β-blockers may be considered in low-risk patients defined by clinical predictors not receiving β-blocker therapy undergoing vascular surgery; and (vi) they should not be administered in pre-operative patients with absolute contra-indications to β-blocker. In addition, this focused update emphasised that current recommendations are limited by the fact that there are very few randomised controlled trials to answer several questions: What are the beneficial effects of different beta blocker agents? How should the medications be titrated? What is an optimal dosing regimen? What route of administration is optimal? What are the risks? As noted in the guideline update, the data favouring benefit of β-blockers for peri-operative risk reduction are most robust in patients undergoing vascular surgery where concomitant coronary artery disease is particularly common.

α_2-Adrenergic agonists

For intermediate to higher risk patients undergoing major non-cardiac surgery who are intolerant of β-blockers, evidence supports alternative prophylactic use of α_2-agonist for peri-operative cardiac risk reduction. This treatment should only be initiated in stable patients and should be titrated carefully to prevent significant hypotension and bradycardia.

HMG-CoA REDUCTASE INHIBITORS (STATINS)

Evidence supports the peri-operative prophylactic use of statins for reduction of peri-operative cardiac complications in patients with established atherosclerosis. Although the future role of statin prophylaxis in the reduction of peri-operative cardiac risk reduction awaits definitive clarification by the on-going European (DECREASE IV) trial, peri-operative statin therapy should currently be considered in intermediate- to high-risk patients undergoing major non-cardiac surgery to reduce peri-operative cardiac risk, and should be continued or initiated if the patient has known atherosclerotic vascular disease in any vascular territory.

CALCIUM CHANNEL BLOCKERS

There is no evidence supporting the use of calcium channel blockers for prophylaxis strategy to decrease peri-operative risk for major non-cardiac surgery.

ANGIOTENSIN-CONVERTING ENZYME (ACE) INHIBITORS

ACE inhibitors and angiotensin II receptor antagonists are frequently prescribed for the management of hypertension, congestive heart failure, chronic renal failure, and ischaemic heart disease. Evidence supports the discontinuation of ACE inhibitors and angiotensin receptor antagonists for 24 h prior to non-cardiac surgery owing to adverse circulatory effects after induction of anaesthesia in patients on a chronic ACE inhibitor regimen, and use of vasopressin agonists for refractory hypotension after induction of anaesthesia.

ORAL ANTITHROMBOTIC AGENTS

Recommendations regarding peri-operative use of aspirin and / or clopidogrel to reduce cardiac risk currently lacks clarity. Studies demonstrate a substantial increase in peri-operative bleeding and transfusion requirement in patients receiving dual antiplatelet therapy. Evidence supporting discontinuation of clopidogrel 5 days before surgery and the decision to hold aspirin 5–7 days prior to major surgery to minimise the risk of peri-operative bleeding and transfusion must be balanced with the potential increased risk of an acute coronary syndrome, especially in the high-risk patients with recent coronary stent implantation. If clinicians elect to withhold aspirin prior to surgery, it should be restarted as soon as possible postoperatively, especially following vascular graft procedures. Whether short-acting intravenous GPIIb/IIIa platelet receptor antagonists are useful in 'bridging' such patients through the peri-operative period has not been clarified.

OTHER STRATEGIES FOR REDUCING PERI-OPERATIVE RISK

ANAESTHETIC MANAGEMENT

Mortality is low with safe delivery of modern-day anaesthesia, especially in the low-risk patients undergoing low-risk surgery (Table 2). Inhalational anaesthetics have predictable circulatory and respiratory effects. All of the potent drugs decrease arterial pressure in a dose-related manner by systemic vasodilation, decreased cardiac output, and myocardial depression. Inhaled anaesthetics cause respiratory depression with diminished response to both hypercapnia and hypoxaemia, in a dose-related manner. In combination with neuromuscular blockade, inhalational anaesthetic agents cause marked reduction in functional residual capacity due to loss of diaphragmatic and intercostal muscle function, thereby decreasing thoracic volume. This decrease in lung volume leads to atelectasis in the dependent lung regions and, subsequently, may result in arterial hypoxaemia from ventilation perfusion mismatch leading to an increased risk of postoperative pulmonary complications.

Postoperative epidural analgesia > 24 h is beneficial in reducing the rate of postoperative MI (-3.8%; 95% CI, -7.4% to -0.2%; $P = 0.049$), with subgroup analysis favouring thoracic epidural analgesia compared with systemic analgesia. However, conflicting evidence limits the support for its broad recommendation as the technique of choice for major surgery.

MONITORING FOR PERI-OPERATIVE MYOCARDIAL INFARCTION

A protocol involving an ECG immediately after surgery and on the first and second postoperative days for the diagnosis of peri-operative MI provides the highest sensitivity, whereas routine measurements of serial cardiac biomarkers had higher false positive rates and did not increase the sensitivity.[32] Detection of elevated postoperative cardiac troponins I and troponin T have emerged as the most sensitive and specific biochemical markers of myocardial injury and infarction, and have been shown to be associated with increased risk of cardiac events. Current recommendations favour monitoring for signs of cardiac dysfunction in patients with prior evidence of CAD. In such patients undergoing surgical procedures associated with high cardiac risk, ECG at baseline, immediately after surgery and on the first 2 days postoperatively, should be obtained. Measurement of cardiac biomarkers should be reserved for patients at high risk and for those who demonstrate clinical, ECG, or haemodynamic evidence of cardiovascular dysfunction.

LONG-TERM RISK STRATIFICATION AND MANAGEMENT STRATEGIES

Postoperative patient care involves assessment and treatment of modifiable cardiac risk factors, including hypertension, hyperlipidaemia, smoking, obesity, hyperglycaemia, and physical inactivity. Patients who sustain a peri-operative MI or develop evidence of ischaemia should be carefully investigated, because they are at substantial cardiac risk over the subsequent 5–10 years. Non-invasive testing to assess left ventricular function and inducible ischaemia should be undertaken to identify patients who may benefit from revascularisation and/or optimisation of medical therapy. Postoperative heart failure and pulmonary oedema should be treated as for pulmonary oedema in the non-operative setting. An emergency ECG and a troponin level are helpful in the event of acute myocardial ischaemia.

SPECIFIC CARDIOVASCULAR CONDITIONS

VALVULAR HEART DISEASE

Special consideration has to be given in pre-operative risk assessment in patients with valvular heart disease. All patients undergoing non-cardiac surgery should be assessed for aortic valve stenosis by physical examination, and two-dimensional echocardiography for any suspicious murmur. Significant aortic stenosis carries a 5-fold increased risk of peri-operative mortality and non-fatal myocardial infarction compared with patients without aortic stenosis. The adjusted relative risks for adverse events is 5.2 for asymptomatic aortic valve gradients between 25–50 mmHg (moderate aortic valve stenosis), and 6.8 for gradient above 50 mmHg (severe aortic valve stenosis).[33,34] Thus, all patients undergoing non-cardiac surgery should be carefully evaluated for systolic murmurs accompanied with chest radiography electrocardiography and echocardiographic confirmation when aortic valve stenosis is suspected.

There is less known about peri-operative risks associated with mitral stenosis and mitral regurgitation in patients undergoing non-cardiac surgery. Clearly, a pre-operative history and physical examination, chest radiograph and/or electrocardiogram will usually provide clues to the diagnosis, which can be confirmed by echocardiography. Accurate diagnosis may help optimise intra-operative anaesthetic strategies, choice of pharmacological intervention and invasive monitoring, as well as postoperative medical management. Except for peri-operative antibiotic prophylaxis to prevent bacterial endocarditis, and the need for effective anticoagulation strategies, peri-operative complications in patients with prosthetic heart valves are probably similar to patients with comparable degrees of native valvular heart disease.

Severe aortic valve stenosis poses a higher risk in non-cardiac surgery. Patients with severe symptomatic aortic stenosis should undergo aortic valve replacement before non-cardiac surgery, if they are felt to be acceptable surgical candidates. In rare instances, balloon aortic valvuloplasty may be justified before elective non-cardiac surgery. A retrospective study suggested that selected patients with asymptomatic severe aortic stenosis could safely undergo non-cardiac surgery with careful haemodynamic monitoring.[35]

In patients with mild-to-moderate mitral stenosis, the heart rate should be controlled to ensure a sufficient diastolic filling period and to avoid pulmonary congestion. Patients with severe mitral stenosis likely benefit from balloon mitral valvuloplasty or surgical repair before high-risk surgery. Patients with aortic or mitral regurgitation benefit from volume control and after-load reduction. A slow heart rate increases diastolic filling per minute and can, theoretically, exacerbate left ventricular volume overload owing to aortic regurgitation. Faster heart rates are better tolerated in this particular condition.

In patients with a mechanical valve prosthesis, the prothrombin time should be reduced briefly to the low or subtherapeutic range for minor procedures such as dental work and superficial biopsies, and anticoagulation should be resumed immediately after the procedure. Patients at high risk of bleeding while taking oral anticoagulants and those at high risk of thrombotic complications when not taking them should receive peri-operative heparin 'bridging'. Patients between these two extremes should undergo individual assessment for the risk and benefit of reduced anticoagulation with warfarin versus peri-operative heparin initiation and brief interruption surrounding surgery. Patients with valvular heart disease require appropriate antibiotic prophylaxis for endocarditis.

ARRYTHMIAS AND CONDUCTION DEFECT

Ventricular and atrial arrhythmias are identified as predictors of peri-operative cardiac complications.[36] As such, identification of pre-operative arrhythmias warrants careful evaluation for the presence and severity of underlying ischaemic heart disease, cardiomyopathy, or other condition(s) that may contribute to peri-operative outcome. Generally, asymptomatic arrhythmias warrant observation only and maintenance of an optimal metabolic state. However, third-degree atrioventricular block can increase operative risk and necessitates pacing.[5]

CONGESTIVE HEART FAILURE AND LEFT VENTRICULAR DYSFUNCTION

Congestive heart failure (CHF) has been identified as a significant marker of cardiac risk for non-cardiac surgery.[37] Every effort should be made to identify the aetiology of CHF and, optimally, to control it pre-operatively. However, there are currently no evidence-based recommendations for optimal peri-operative strategy in patients with heart failure undergoing intermediate- to high-risk non-cardiac surgery other than making sure that such patients are on medications known to improve patients with heart failure in the long-term. Close monitoring of the volume status is needed to avoid peri-operative decompensation. Use of intravenous inotropic agents, vasodilators, or both, for a short duration in the peri-operative period may be useful to prevent and/or treat CHF.

HYPERTROPHIC CARDIOMYOPATHY

Patients with echocardiographically documented hypertrophic cardiomyopathy (HCM) are at risk for exacerbation of dynamic left ventricular outflow tract

(LVOT) obstruction. General anaesthesia or neuro-axial block can lead to peripheral vasodilation and sympathetic autonomic blockade that may decrease venous return and further exacerbate LVOT obstruction. Peri-operative cardiac risk reduction strategies should include avoidance of hypovolaemia, vasodilators, phosphodiesterase inhibitors, β-adrenergic agonists, and diligent attention to volume repletion and selected use of α-adrenergic agonists. Patients with hypertrophic cardiomyopathy are at significant risk for developing peri-operative hypotension, CHF, and arrhythmias and should be monitored closely.

CONGENITAL HEART DISEASE

Patients with left-to-right cardiac shunts with residual haemodynamic abnormalities after surgical repair have decreased cardiac output in response to stress.[38,39] Patients with a large left-to-right shunt but only a slight increase in pulmonary artery resistance should undergo cardiac repair before non-cardiac surgery. Patients with irreversible pulmonary artery hypertension have an extremely high risk associated with non-surgical procedures and should not undergo elective procedures unless there is absolutely no alternative.

Patients with prior repair of coarctation of the aorta have a significant risk of sudden death during follow-up.[40,41] These deaths are related to residual cardiac defects with CHF, rupture of a major vessel, dissecting aneurysm, or complications arising from severe atherosclerosis. Such patients also have a high incidence of residual hypertension. Therefore, these patients require careful pre-operative assessment and close haemodynamic monitoring during the intra-operative and postoperative periods. Patients with tetralogy of Fallot are also prone to sudden cardiac death. Monitoring and aggressive prevention and treatment of life-threatening arrhythmias such as ventricular tachycardia or atrioventricular block are needed for such patients in the peri-operative period. Surgery in patients with cyanotic congenital heart disease with right-to-left shunts poses several unique problems. Most cyanotic patients are polycythemic and, therefore, are prone to thrombotic complications. Use of diuretics should thus be avoided to decrease the tendency for thrombosis, particularly cerebral thrombosis in such patients. Patients with a haematocrit greater than 70% should be considered for plasmapheresis before non-cardiac surgery. Phlebotomy is not advisable in this circumstance, because this can decrease intravascular blood volume and thus increase cyanosis. Patients with a haematocrit between 55–65% should receive intravenous fluids starting the night before the surgery. Patients with congenital heart disease should also receive appropriate prophylaxis for bacterial endocarditis. With careful monitoring and precautions as outlined previously, patients with right-to-left shunts should be able to undergo non-cardiac surgery with relatively few complications.

Key points for clinical practice

- Coronary artery disease accounts for most deaths in patients undergoing non-cardiac surgery.

- Peri-operative myocardial infarction is associated with high mortality rates.

(continued)

Key points for clinical practice *(continued)*

- Risk of a peri-operative cardiac complication varies with the severity of the surgical procedure and with the Revised Cardiac Risk Index stratification.

- All information obtained from a systematic step-wise approach for pre-operative cardiac risk assessment for non-cardiac surgery should be used to decide whether the risk of peri-operative cardiac events is sufficiently low to proceed with surgery.

- Pre-operative, non-invasive cardiac testing should be based on a discrete clinical risk categorisation. The choices among non-invasive tests should be based on the need for valvular or ventricular function assessment and on which test is most reliable and available locally.

- In patients with strong suspicion of having, or being at risk for, coronary artery disease, β-blockers should be given in the peri-operative period starting at least 24 h before the procedure, titrated rapidly to a heart rate of 60 beats/min and continued postoperatively.

- Optimal postoperative patient care involves assessment and treatment of modifiable cardiac risk factors, including pain management, hypertension, hyperlipidaemia, smoking, obesity, hyperglycaemia, and physical inactivity.

- Patients who sustain a peri-operative myocardial infarction or develop evidence of ischaemia should be carefully investigated because they are at substantial cardiac risk over subsequent months and years.

References

1. Dudley JC, Brandenburg JA, Hartley LH, Harris S, Lee TH. Last-minute preoperative cardiology consultations: epidemiology and impact. *Am Heart J* 1996; **131**: 245–249.
2. Boersma E, Kertai MD, Schouten O *et al*. Perioperative cardiovascular mortality in noncardiac surgery: validation of the Lee cardiac risk index. *Am J Med* 2005; **118**: 1134–1141.
3. Schouten O, Bax JJ, Poldermans D. Assessment of cardiac risk before non-cardiac general surgery. *Heart* 2006; **92**: 1866–1872.
4. Landesberg G, Shatz V, Akopnik I *et al*. Association of cardiac troponin, CK-MB, and postoperative myocardial ischemia with long-term survival after major vascular surgery. *J Am Coll Cardiol* 2003; **42**: 1547–1554.
5. Eagle KA, Berger PB, Calkins H *et al*. ACC/AHA guideline update for perioperative cardiovascular evaluation for noncardiac surgery – executive summary: a report of the American College of Cardiology/American Heart Association Task Force on Practice Guidelines (Committee to Update the 1996 Guidelines on Perioperative Cardiovascular Evaluation for Noncardiac Surgery). *J Am Coll Cardiol* 2002; **39**: 542–553.
6. Palda VA. Detsky aortic valve stenosis. Perioperative assessment and management of risk from coronary artery disease. *Ann Intern Med* 1997; **127**: 313–328.
7. Goldman L, Caldera DL, Nussbaum SR *et al*. Multifactorial index of cardiac risk in noncardiac surgical procedures. *N Engl J Med* 1977; **297**: 845–850.
8. Lee TH, Marcantonio ER, Mangione CM *et al*. Derivation and prospective validation of a

simple index for prediction of cardiac risk of major noncardiac surgery. *Circulation* 1999; **100**: 1043–1049.

9. Mahar LJ, Steen PA, Tinker JH *et al.* Perioperative myocardial infarction in patients with coronary artery disease with and without aorta–coronary artery bypass grafts. *J Thorac Cardiovasc Surg* 1978; **76**: 533–537.

10. Weiner DA, Ryan TJ, McCabe CH *et al.* Prognostic importance of a clinical profile and exercise test in medically treated patients with coronary artery disease. *J Am Coll Cardiol* 1984; **3**: 772–779.

11. Weiner DA, Ryan TJ, Parsons L *et al.* Long-term prognostic value of exercise testing in men and women from the Coronary Artery Surgery Study (CASS) registry. *Am J Cardiol* 1995; **75**: 865–870.

12. McFalls EO, Ward HB, Moritz TE *et al.* Coronary-artery revascularization before elective major vascular surgery. *N Engl J Med* 2004; **351**: 2795–2804.

13. Poldermans D, Bax JJ, Schouten O *et al.* Should major vascular surgery be delayed because of preoperative cardiac testing in intermediate-risk patients receiving beta-blocker therapy with tight heart rate control? *J Am Coll Cardiol* 2006; **48**: 964–969.

14. Kertai MD, Boersma E, Sicari R *et al.* Which stress test is superior for perioperative cardiac risk stratification in patients undergoing major vascular surgery? *Eur J Vasc Endovasc Surg* 2002; **24**: 222–229.

15. Scanlon PJ, Faxon DP, Audet AM *et al.* ACC/AHA guidelines for coronary angiography. A report of the American College of Cardiology/American Heart Association Task Force on practice guidelines (Committee on Coronary Angiography). Developed in collaboration with the Society for Cardiac Angiography and Interventions. *J Am Coll Cardiol* 1999; **33**: 1756–1824.

16. Hassan SA, Hlatky MA, Boothroyd DB *et al.* Outcomes of noncardiac surgery after coronary bypass surgery or coronary angioplasty in the Bypass Angioplasty Revascularization Investigation (BARI). *Am J Med* 2001; **110**: 260–266.

17. Smith Jr SC, Dove JT, Jacobs AK *et al.* ACC/AHA guidelines for percutaneous coronary intervention (revision of the 1993 PTCA guidelines) – executive summary: a report of the American College of Cardiology/American Heart Association task force on practice guidelines (Committee to revise the 1993 guidelines for percutaneous transluminal coronary angioplasty) endorsed by the Society for Cardiac Angiography and Interventions. Circulation 2001; **103**: 3019–3041.

18. Brilakis ES, Orford JL, Fasseas P *et al.* Outcome of patients undergoing balloon angioplasty in the two months prior to noncardiac surgery. *Am J Cardiol* 2005; **96**: 512–514.

19. Kaluza GL, Joseph J, Lee JR, Raizner ME, Raizner AE. Catastrophic outcomes of noncardiac surgery soon after coronary stenting. *J Am Coll Cardiol* 2000; **35**: 1288–1294.

20. Wilson SH, Fasseas P, Orford JL *et al.* Clinical outcome of patients undergoing non-cardiac surgery in the two months following coronary stenting. *J Am Coll Cardiol* 2003; **42**: 234–240.

21. Babapulle MN, Joseph L, Belisle P, Brophy JM, Eisenberg MJ. A hierarchical Bayesian meta-analysis of randomised clinical trials of drug-eluting stents. *Lancet* 2004; **364**: 583–591.

22. Lindenauer PK, Pekow P, Wang K *et al.* Perioperative beta-blocker therapy and mortality after major noncardiac surgery. *N Engl J Med* 2005; **353**: 349–361.

23. Mangano DT, Layug EL, Wallace A, Tateo I. Effect of atenolol on mortality and cardiovascular morbidity after noncardiac surgery. Multicenter Study of Perioperative Ischemia Research Group. *N Engl J Med* 1996; **335**: 1713–1720.

24. Poldermans D, Boersma E, Bax JJ *et al.* The effect of bisoprolol on perioperative mortality and myocardial infarction in high-risk patients undergoing vascular surgery. Dutch Echocardiographic Cardiac Risk Evaluation Applying Stress Echocardiography Study Group. *N Engl J Med* 1999; **341**: 1789–1794.

25. Eagle KA, Lau WC. Any need for preoperative cardiac testing in intermediate-risk patients with tight beta-adrenergic blockade? *J Am Coll Cardiol* 2006; **48**: 970–972.

26. Pasternack PF, Grossi EA, Baumann FG *et al.* Beta blockade to decrease silent myocardial ischemia during peripheral vascular surgery. *Am J Surg* 1989; **158**: 113–116.

27. Pasternack PF, Imparato AM, Baumann FG *et al.* The hemodynamics of beta-blockade in

patients undergoing abdominal aortic aneurysm repair. *Circulation* 1987; **76**: III1–III7.

28. Redelmeier D, Scales D, Kopp A. Beta blockers for elective surgery in elderly patients: population based, retrospective cohort study. *BMJ* 2005; **331**: 932.

29. Brady AR, Gibbs JS, Greenhalgh RM, Powell JT, Sydes MR. Perioperative beta-blockade (POBBLE) for patients undergoing infrarenal vascular surgery: results of a randomized double-blind controlled trial. *J Vasc Surg* 2005; **41**: 602–609.

30. Yang H, Raymer K, Butler R, Parlow J, Roberts R. The effects of perioperative beta-blockade: results of the Metoprolol after Vascular Surgery (MaVS) study, a randomized controlled trial. *Am Heart J* 2006; **152**: 983–990.

31. Fleisher LA, Beckman JA, Brown KA *et al*. ACC/AHA 2006 guideline update for perioperative cardiovascular evaluation for noncardiac surgery: focused update on perioperative beta-blocker therapy – a report of the American College of Cardiology/American Heart Association Task Force on Practice Guidelines (writing committee to update the 2002 guidelines on perioperative cardiovascular evaluation for noncardiac surgery. *J Am Coll Cardiol* 2006; 47: In press.

32. Charlson ME, MacKenzie CR, Ales K *et al*. Surveillance for postoperative myocardial infarction after noncardiac operations. *Surg Gynecol Obstet* 1988; **167**: 407–414.

33. Kertai MD, Bountioukos M, Boersma E *et al*. Aortic stenosis: an underestimated risk factor for perioperative complications in patients undergoing noncardiac surgery. *Am J Med* 2004; **116**: 8–13.

34. Goldman L. Aortic stenosis in noncardiac surgery: underappreciated in more ways than one? *Am J Med* 2004; **116**: 60–62.

35. O'Keefe Jr JH, Shub C, Rettke SR. Risk of noncardiac surgical procedures in patients with aortic stenosis. *Mayo Clin Proc* 1989; **64**: 400–405.

36. Goldman L, Caldera DL, Southwick FS *et al*. Cardiac risk factors and complications in non-cardiac surgery. *Medicine (Baltimore)* 1978; **57**: 357–370.

37. Abrams HB, McLaughlin JR *et al*. Predicting cardiac complications in patients undergoing non-cardiac surgery. *J Gen Intern Med* 1986; **1**: 211–219.

38. Tikoff G, Keith TB, Nelson RM, Kuida H. Clinical and hemodynamic observations after surgical closure of large atrial septal defect complicated by heart failure. *Am J Cardiol* 1969; **23**: 810–817.

39. Lueker RD, Vogel JH, Blount Jr SG. Cardiovascular abnormalities following surgery for left-to-right shunts. Observations in atrial septal defects, ventricular septal defects, and patent ductus arteriosus. *Circulation* 1969; **40**: 785–801.

40. Maron BJ, Humphries JO, Rowe RD, Mellits ED. Prognosis of surgically corrected coarctation of the aorta. A 20-year postoperative appraisal. *Circulation* 1973; **47**: 119–126.

41. Simon AB, Zloto AE. Coarctation of the aorta. Longitudinal assessment of operated patients. *Circulation* 1974; **50**: 456–464.

Marc E. Shelton   Gregory J. Mishkel
Anna L. Moore   Amanda M. Pfeiffer

6

Late stent thrombosis: incidence, significance, outcomes, management

The advent of balloon angioplasty in the 1970s and the 1980s ushered in a host of minimally invasive therapeutic modalities aimed at treating coronary artery disease (CAD), currently referred to as percutaneous coronary interventions (PCI). Although commonly successful, balloon angioplasty was soon found to have significant limitations including the risk of abrupt closure (3–8% of cases), need for urgent coronary artery bypass surgery (3–5% of cases), and recurrence of symptoms from restenosis (approximately 30% of cases within 6–9 months of the procedure).[1] Years of development of other interventional techniques followed, but only coronary stenting consistently improved safety and late clinical outcomes compared with balloon angioplasty.

Historically, clinical outcome data comparing balloon angioplasty and bare metal stenting (BMS) in landmark trials (STRESS, BENESTENT, BENESTENT II, REST, SAVED, TOSCA) were limited to follow-up periods of less than 1 year. The mid-term clinical outcomes reported in these trials ranged between 0–9% for mortality, between 0.5–5% for ST segment elevation myocardial infarction (STEMI), and between 9–27% for repeat revascularisation.[2]

PCI treatment has recently evolved even further with the introduction of drug-eluting stents (DES) to address persistent and problematic restenosis. The randomised controlled trials of the Cypher® sirolimus-eluting stent (SES; Cordis Corporation/J&J, Miami Lakes, FL, USA) versus BMS (RAVEL, SIRIUS, E-SIRIUS, C-SIRIUS, SES SMART, DIABETES) showed a striking and clinically significant reduction in the need for target lesion revascularisation (TLR). Stent thrombosis was not identified as an issue with either stent platform during the first year of follow-up.[3] The randomised controlled trials of the TAXUS®

Marc E. Shelton MD (for correspondence)
Prairie Cardiovascular Consultants Ltd, 3700 Vanderbilt Circle, Springfield, IL 62711, USA
E-mail: mshelton@prairieheart.com

Gregory J. Mishkel MD, **Anna L. Moore** MPH, **Amanda M. Pfeiffer** BS, Prairie Education & Research Cooperative, Prairie Heart Institute of St John's Hospital, Springfield, Illinois, USA

paclitaxel-eluting stent (PES; Boston Scientific, Natick, MA, USA) versus BMS (TAXUS I, II, IV, VI) revealed similar results, with a significant reduction in clinically important events. Once again, stent thrombosis was not viewed as an issue with this DES platform.[4]

Given the impressive, consistent reductions in the need for repeat revascularisation demonstrated in the early studies, DES adoption in the US was rapid after the first US Food and Drug Administration (FDA) approval in 2003.[5] The use of DES in the US expanded from approximately 20% immediately following commercial release to nearly 80% by 2005. Although the carefully designed randomised controlled DES studies[6] suggested that ST rates in the control and treatment arms were similar out to 1 year, concern later surfaced about a possible slight increase in very late (beyond 1 year) thrombogenesis in DES.[7,8]

The early randomised clinical trials were underpowered to detect small potential differences in ST in the treatment groups and the initial follow-up period (1 year) after randomisation was insufficient to demonstrate differences in very late ST. Accordingly, the true frequency and clinical significance of this problem remains unclear in the 'real world' today.

LATE STENT THROMBOSIS IN THE BMS ERA

In the BMS era, the development of ST was primarily considered to be an acute event that occurred within the initial 30 days following stent implantation, although a few studies were published that reported ST beyond 30 days.

A study by Orford et al.[9] examined the frequency of early ST in BMS. A total of 4509 patients underwent successful stent implantation and were treated with dual anti-platelet therapy. Amongst these, ST occurred in 23 patients (0.51%) within 30 days following stent placement. A multivariate analysis was performed indicating that the number of stents placed was an independent correlate of ST (odds ratio, 1.80; $P < 0.001$). The frequencies of death and non-fatal myocardial infarction (MI) among the 23 patients were 48% and 39%, respectively.

A pooled analysis of six clinical trials performed by Cutlip et al.[10] further evaluated the incidence of ST. From a total cohort of 6186 patients (6219 vessels), clinical ST developed within 30 days in 53 patients (0.9%), 45 of which were documented angiographically. Six-month outcomes following clinical ST were very poor – death, 20.8%; STEMI, 15.1%; and non-STEMI, 41.5%. These studies and others highlight the dire outcomes associated with any stent thrombosis.

A separate, single-centre study[11] of 1855 consecutive stent recipients found that, during a 12-month follow-up period, 34 patients (1.8%) developed ST. Of those 34 patients, 22 developed ST within the first 15 days following their procedure, while 12 additional patients presented with ST between 33–270 days. A similar study was performed by Wang et al.[12] in a cohort of 1191 consecutive stent recipients; there were 11 (0.92%) early (first 30 days) STs reported, and 9 (0.76%) late (after 30 days) STs reported. The average time to late ST was 109 days (range, 39–211 days). Some of the proposed mechanisms for late ST in BMS were stenting across ostial segments, exposure to brachytherapy, vulnerable plaque disruption, diffuse in-stent restenosis, and incomplete neointimal healing.[13]

Together, these studies illustrate that the risk of ST was a recognised, published phenomenon prior to the arrival of DES. However, there is a paucity of data to evaluate the incidence of very late ST (beyond 1 year) following BMS implantation. It is unknown whether very late ST was truly an extremely rare event, or was simply underappreciated and under-reported, in the BMS era.[14]

LATE STENT THROMBOSIS IN THE DES ERA

Soon after the commercial release of DES in the US, several case reports described the clinical phenomenon of very late ST, which had not previously been appreciated with BMS.[15–18] McFadden et al.[16] sparked the concern of very late ST in DES with a report of 4 cases of angiographically confirmed ST (two with PES at 343 and 442 days, and two with SES at 335 and 375 days). Interestingly, these cases of ST all arose soon after anti-platelet therapy interruption. Kavouni et al.[17] subsequently described one case report of very late ST that occurred in a DES 17 months post-procedure, and Feres et al.[18] reported on two cases of very late ST in DES at approximately 12 and 40 months post-procedure. Again, these cases occurred after the discontinuation of anti-platelet therapy.

Ong et al.[19] reported long-term (at least 1 year) follow-up of a consecutive cohort of 2006 patients who received either SES (1017 patients) or PES (989 patients), and found 8 angiographically confirmed late (greater than 30 days after implant) ST events in 7 patients (two of whom died because of ST), with an incidence of 0.35%.

Joner et al.[20] reported from a registry of 40 autopsies (68 stents), in which 23 DES patients > 30 days following PCI were matched to 25 BMS patients. Late ST (> 30 days) was discovered in 14 of the DES patients. Both SES and PES showed greater delayed healing and poorer endothelialisation in comparison to BMS. Moreover, anti-platelet therapy had been withdrawn in 5 of the 14 patients. This study proposed that the cause of late ST was most likely 'multifactorial', in addition to the interruption of anti-platelet therapy.

BASKET-LATE was the first randomised trial that observed higher rates of late cardiac death and MI after DES than after BMS implantation, in part due to thrombotic events that occurred after the discontinuation of clopidogrel.[21] Following the release of the BASKET-LATE results, researchers began scrambling to analyse ST incidence and outcomes in DES, in an attempt to determine whether or not DES posed a greater risk of late and very late ST than BMS.

THE DES ST CONTROVERSY HEIGHTENS

EUROPEAN SOCIETY OF CARDIOLOGY 2006

At the 2006 European Society of Cardiology (ESC) congress, the Swedish Coronary Angiography and Angioplasty Registry (SCAAR) reported an increased in clinical events (death or MI) among DES patients (published later in *The New England Journal of Medicine* in 2007).[22] This landmark analysis evaluated events after the first 6 months following stent placement on 19,771 BMS and DES patients with 2.5 years of follow-up. The study revealed a significantly higher rate of death (relative risk [RR], 1.32; 95% confidence interval [CI], 1.11–1.57) and composite events (death or MI) in DES patients (RR, 1.20; 95% CI, 1.05–1.37) compared to BMS patients. Furthermore, Camenzind et al.[23] reported results from a meta-analysis indicating that the incidence of total mortality and Q-wave MI combined was 6.3% in SES patients versus 3.9% in BMS patients ($P = 0.03$). Together, the findings from these studies attracted the attention of the media and greatly heightened the concerns in the cardiovascular community about the safety of DES.

When Camenzind et al.[23] formally published their meta-analysis in *Circulation* in March 2007, the pooled data from the randomised clinical trials comparing SES or PES to BMS did show a trend toward increased death and Q-wave MI with DES. However, a response by Serruys and Daemen,[24] in the same volume of *Circulation*, explained that, in contrast to the data proposed at the ESC congress, the total death and MI (Q-wave and non-Q-wave) at 4 years was 11.4% in SES and 10.1% in BMS ($P = 0.40$). It was noted that the meta-analysis of Camenzind et al.[23] was derived from data at different follow-up time periods and non-Q-wave MI was not included in their clinical end-point, both details that were overlooked at the ESC meeting.

TCT 2006

Following the ESC meeting, information presented at the Transcatheter Cardiovascular Therapeutics (TCT) conference in October 2006 also suggested a possible increase of late ST in DES. Data from the Bern–Rotterdam registry (published later in *The Lancet* in 2007)[25] analysed 8146 DES patients, and reported a late ST rate of approximately 0.6% per year (between 30 days and 3 years). Stone et al.[26] presented results from a meta-analysis of RAVEL, SIRIUS, E-SIRIUS, and C-SIRIUS, and TAXUS-I, TAXUS-II, TAXUS-III, TAXUS-IV, and TAXUS-V, and suggested that while the ST rates were similar from 0–365 days, there was a slight but significant increase of very late ST in DES (> 1 year following PCI) when compared to BMS. Importantly, no significant increase in death or MI was found.

Together, the ESC and TCT 2006 meetings fuelled the concerns in the medical community regarding the safety of DES, and whether or not the

Table 1 Coronary stent thrombosis definitions differ between programmes

TAXUS® stent programme	Cypher® stent programme	
	≤ 30 days	≥ 30 days
Angiographic confirmation	Angiographic confirmation	Angiographic confirmation
OR	OR	AND
QWMI or NQWMI in target vessel territory	QWMI in target vessel territory	MI in target vessel
OR	OR	
Sudden, unexplained death (≤ 30 days)	Sudden, unexplained death	

benefits of decreased restenosis outweighed the increased risk of catastrophic clinical events. Additionally, it had become apparent that the lack of standardised ST definitions was hindering the effort to analyse the available data accurately. The protocol definitions of ST from different stent programmes varied widely (see Table 1) and were further perturbed by censoring patients from follow-up if they experienced a TLR event, even if ST occurred at a later date. Therefore, meta-analyses could not properly pool data, which made it very difficult to compare ST rates that were being reported from studies around the world.

US FDA CIRCULATORY SYSTEM DEVICES ADVISORY PANEL

By December 2006, the DES thrombosis controversy had been sensationalised in the media, produced a significant effect on the stock market, and served as grist for the medicolegal industrial mill. Clinicians were gripped with uncertainty about the safety of the everyday use of DES. In response to concern for the public health, the US FDA assembled a special Circulatory System Devices Panel to evaluate these alarming issues.[27] Experts from industry, academia, and community-based clinical practice presented detailed data on DES utilisation and outcomes. The FDA urged each presenter to analyse their data according to the standardised ST definitions that had been developed by the Academic Research Consortium (ARC).

After deliberation, the panel supported the 'on-label' use of DES and agreed that, although the incidence of ST appeared to be slightly increased in DES patients after 1 year, there was no evidence for a concomitant increase in death or MI when compared to BMS patients. Conversely, the panel agreed that the 'off-label' use of DES was associated with a higher risk of ST, MI, or death when compared to the 'on-label' use. The FDA recommended that DES labelling state that results from 'off-label' use of DES should not be expected to mirror the results found in pivotal trials. The FDA panel concluded that continued study of complex patients and lesions was needed to truly assess the risks/benefits of 'off-label' DES usage.

ACADEMIC RESEARCH CONSORTIUM

The ARC definitions were developed in an effort to standardise the identification of ST, and to provide consistency in analysing previous and future studies. In May 2007, Cutlip et al.[28] formally published the ARC definitions (summarised in Table 2). Clearly, identification of definite ST by angiographic or autopsy evidence of thrombus or occlusion is the most specific classification; however, the definite ST definition does not allow for the inclusion of events in the absence of physical evidence. The use of the probable ST definition captures patients with clinical events that most likely represent ST, but for whom hard evidence is not available. The probable ST classification yields a group that, unfortunately, is likely to be somewhat heterogeneous, since this group would include patients with true ST and some patients with new clinical events caused by disease either upstream or downstream from the old stent. Since progression of the underlying disease process can be expected in some number of cases, the amount of contamination of this group caused by

Table 2 Academic Research Consortium (ARC) definitions

Stent thrombosis	
Definite ST	Acute coronary syndrome (ACS)
	AND
	Angiographic evidence of thrombus/occlusion
	Autopsy evidence of thrombus/occlusion
Probable ST	Sudden, unexplained death within 30 days following stent placement
	OR
	Target vessel MI without angiographic confirmation of ST or other identified culprit lesion
Possible ST	Sudden, unexplained death >30 days following stent placement
Stent thrombosis timing	
Early ST	0–30 days
Acute ST	0–24 h after stent placement
Subacute ST	Between 24 h and 30 days following stent placement
Late ST	Between 30 days and 365 days following stent placement
Very late ST	> 365 days following stent placement

the inclusion of non-stent related complications is unknown. The possible ST category includes all sudden, unexplained deaths greater than 30 days post-stent placement. While some of the deaths in the possible ST group are due to ST, another portion of the deaths are likely to be from cardiac arrest from other causes. Due to the lack of specificity in the possible ST group, many authors have suggested that the definite + probable ST combined group is the most accurate representation of thrombotic events.[29,30]

The importance of using the ARC temporal classification follows the logic that the mechanisms of acute ST (0–24 h following PCI), subacute ST (1–30 days following PCI), late ST (between 1–12 months following PCI), or very late ST (more than 1 year following PCI), may be disparate. Contributors to ST are likely to include thrombosis, mechanical factors (such as residual stenosis, residual dissection flaps, and side-branch occlusions), incomplete endothelialisation, immunological reaction to metals and coatings, genetic factors, and compliance factors. Accordingly, time-to-occlusion data might yield clues that help clinicians with selection of treatment options in a given patient.

CURRENT ASSESSMENT OF ARC ST IN DES

META-ANALYSES

The ARC definitions have been accepted widely in recent studies of DES. An examination of the contemporary ARC-defined studies may give a better insight into the very late ST phenomenon in DES.

In a meta-analysis of 8 randomised trials involving 4545 patients, the 4-year incidence of ST was not significantly different between DES and BMS patients.[30] Using the newly developed ARC definitions, the cumulative incidence of definite + probable ST in the SES cohort was 1.5% compared to 1.7% in BMS ($P = 0.70$; 95% CI, 1.5 to 1.0) and 1.8% in the PES cohort compared to 1.4% in BMS ($P = 0.52$; 95% CI, 0.7 to 1.4). The incidence of very late (> 360 days) definite + probable ST events was 0.9% in SES versus 0.4% in BMS and 0.9% in PES versus 0.6% in BMS. Unfortunately, of the 68 (1.5%) definite + probable patients, 30.9% (21 patients) died and 83.8% (57 patients) suffered a MI.

Spaulding *et al.*[31] also performed a pooled analysis comparing data from 4 randomised trials that included 1748 SES and BMS patients. According to the ARC definitions, overall ST (definite + probable + possible) was observed in 30 (3.6%) cases in the SES group, compared to 28 (3.3%) cases in the BMS group ($P = 0.80$). There was a significantly lower occurrence of late overall ST in the SES group (0.3% versus 1.3%; $P = 0.03$). At 4 years, cumulative mortality between SES and BMS was similar: 6.7% versus 5.4%, respectively (HR, 1.24; 95% CI, 0.84–1.83; $P = 0.28$). The study concluded that SES did not increase the risk for death, MI, or ST.

Stettler *et al.*[32] conducted a meta-analysis comparing the safety and efficacy of DES versus BMS and found no significant difference in the risk of long-term definite ST. A total of 38 trials (18,023 patients) were included, with patients categorised into three different treatment groups (PES, SES, and BMS), followed out to 4 years. The cumulative incidences of overall mortality, cardiac mortality, definite ST, and combined death + MI were similar for the three treatment options. However, the risk of definite ST beyond 30 days was significantly higher for PES when compared to BMS (HR, 2.11; 95% CI, 1.19–4.23; $P = 0.017$) and when compared to SES (HR, 1.85; 95% CI, 1.02–3.85; $P = 0.041$). The estimated risks for MI were 0.81 (95% CI, 0.66–0.97; $P = 0.030$) for SES versus BMS, 1.00 (95% CI, 0.81–1.23; $P = 0.99$) for PES versus BMS, and 0.83 (95% CI, 0.71–1.00; $P = 0.045$) for SES versus PES. The estimated risks for TLR were 0.30 (95% CI, 0.24–0.37; $P < 0.0001$) for SES versus BMS, 0.42 (95% CI, 0.33–0.53; $P < 0.0001$) for PES versus BMS, and 0.70 (95% CI, 0.56–0.84; $P = 0.0021$) for SES versus PES. This large study indicated that the risk of definite ST may, in fact, be higher in DES than BMS after 1 year; however, the incidence of death between groups was similar, and the incidence of TLR in DES (SES in particular) was significantly reduced over 4 years of follow-up.

'REAL-WORLD' DATA

In July 2007, the Western Denmark Heart Registry published data on 12,395 consecutive patients (17,152 lesions) treated with DES (3548 patients) or BMS (8847 patients).[33] Jensen and colleagues compared rates of ST, MI, mortality, and TLR after stent implantation over a follow-up period of 15 months. Overall ST (definite + probable + possible ST) was observed in 190 (2.15%) patients in the BMS cohort compared to 64 (1.80%) patients in the DES cohort. The risk of overall ST among patients was similar between treatment options with a hazard ratio of 0.91 (95% CI, 0.67–1.24; $P = 0.57$). The risk of all-cause death over the follow-up period was also similar between groups (HR, 0.90;

95% CI, 0.75–1.09; $P = 0.29$). On the other hand, the risk of MI between 12–15 months was significantly greater in patients treated with DES (HR, 4.00; 95% CI, 2.06–7.79; $P < 0.001$).

Machecourt *et al.*[34] reported findings from the EVASTENT registry of 1731 patients undergoing revascularisation with SES. In this matched-cohort registry, each diabetic patient included in the study was paired with a non-diabetic patient. During the 1-year follow-up period, 35 (2.1%) patients died and 78 (4.5%) patients suffered a MACE. According to ARC classifications, 45 (2.6%) patients experienced ST at a 1-year rate of 2.4%. The ST rate in diabetic patients was significantly higher versus non-diabetics at 1 year (3.2% versus 1.7%; $P = 0.03$). Diabetics with multivessel disease suffered the highest ST rate of 4.3% compared to 0.8% of non-diabetics with single-vessel disease ($P < 0.001$). Early (≤ 30 days) ST was observed in 23 cases (16 in diabetics versus 7 in non-diabetics). In a multivariate analysis, independent predictors for ST were: renal failure, low left ventricular ejection fraction, lesions involving a bifurcation, long lesions, calcified lesions, history of stroke, and insulin-dependent diabetes.

At the Prairie Heart Institute at St John's Hospital, Springfield, IL, USA, we evaluated 5342 consecutive patients (representing 8067 lesions) who underwent placement of a first DES between May 2003 and December 2006.[35] The ARC definitions were applied to identify 50 definite, 13 probable, and 54 possible cases of ST. From the definite + probable group of 63 patients, there were 24 recorded early ST (between 0–30 days), 13 late ST (between 31–365 days), and 26 very late ST (> 365 days). Of the patients with definite late ST, 66.7% were taking dual anti-platelet therapy and 50% of the definite very late ST patients were known to be taking dual anti-platelet therapy during the time of ST. The cumulative 3-year event rate for definite + probable beyond 30 days was 1.5%, with a rate of 0.5% per year, which is comparable to rates found in other studies. From multivariate Cox regression, we identified predictors of ST: younger age, current smoker, prior PCI, 'off-label' stent use, bifurcation stenting, and total occlusion stenting.

LONG-TERM OUTCOMES OF DES

While the problem of late and very late ST has garnered considerable attention, the unanswered question remains – does the benefit of greatly reduced need for revascularisation with DES outweigh the risk of ST?

At the ESC congress in September 2007, data from Sweden on the long-term outcomes of DES versus BMS were comparable.[36] The updated SCAAR registry was presented with 4 years of follow-up; in contrast to the 2006 results, the data no longer showed an increased risk of mortality in DES patients compared to BMS patients. The cumulative risk of death or MI between treatment options was 1.01 (95% CI, 0.94–1.09) in the total cohort of 35,262 patients and 0.91 (95% CI, 0.82–1.01) in the single stent cohort of 18,937 patients. When patients were grouped according to year of implantation (2003, 2004 and 2005), a decreased risk of death or MI was found with each year of implantation (excluding the first 30 days following PCI in each group). The relative risks of death or MI with each year were 1.31 (95% CI, 1.12–1.53), 1.22 (95% CI, 1.05–1.43), and 0.93 (95% CI, 0.76–1.13), respectively. Better outcomes in the 2005 cohort could be due to increased awareness of the risk of late ST associated with DES by requiring longer duration of dual anti-platelet therapy, improved stenting techniques with higher balloon pressure and more accurately sized stents, and/or improved selection of patients for DES. In the total cohort of 41,775 stents (20,058 BMS and 21,717 DES), the cumulative risk of ST was 0.5% per year out to 4 years.

In October 2007, Tu et al.[37] published data from the Cardiac Care Network registry in Ontario, Canada. In the matched-cohort study of 3751 DES and BMS patients, the rate of TVR at 2 years was significantly lower in DES patients compared to BMS patients (7.4% versus 10.7%; $P < 0.0001$). The rates of death or MI at 6 months, 1 year, and 2 years were significantly lower in DES (4.8%; 6.1%; and 9.3%, respectively) compared to BMS (5.7%; 7.5%; and 10.5%, respectively; $P = 0.02$ for the distributions of the DES versus BMS Kaplan–Meier curves). This study concluded that DES were effective in reducing revascularisation rates, without significantly increasing the rate of death or MI.

The long-term outcomes of DES patients in our Prairie Data Registry to date have demonstrated cumulative, actuarialised 3-year results as follows: overall death rate of 12.4%, cardiac death rate of 5.5%, and a MI rate of 5.0% in an unselected population of 'real world' patients.[35]

SUMMARY OF PUBLISHED DATA

In aggregate, recent studies suggest that although there may be a slight increased risk of late ST in the DES population, the mortality risk is likely offset by the reduced need for TLR. The extensive evaluation of the DES safety data over the past 2 years has highlighted several important clinical factors that should be carefully considered in treatment strategies for patients today.

LESSONS LEARNED TO IMPROVE PATIENT CARE

THE IMPORTANCE OF DUAL-ANTIPLATELET THERAPY

Although many of the early case reports noted that ST occurred after cessation of dual anti-platelet therapy, the Duke Heart Center better quantified the substantially increased risk of ST in a study of DES patients in whom clopidogrel was discontinued between 6–12 months after initial PCI.[38] Further, continued clopidogrel use was a significant predictor of lower adjusted rates of death or MI (3.1% versus 7.2%; $P = 0.02$) at 24 months. The BMS group in the Duke study showed no differences in death or MI whether or not clopidogrel was continued for 6 or 12 months. Clinicians are lacking definite data to guide the continuation of dual anti-platelet therapy after 1 year. Accordingly, the AHA/ACC/SCAI/ACS/ADA Science Advisory recommended continuation of dual anti-platelet therapy following DES placement for at least 1 year, if not longer for those patients who are not at high risk of bleeding.[39] Prolonged dual anti-platelet therapy may be especially warranted in cases for which clinical (e.g. age, acute coronary syndrome, diabetes mellitus, low ejection fraction, current smoking, prior PCI, 'off-label' DES placement) and angiographic factors (e.g. bifurcation stenting, total occlusion stenting, overlapping stents) have been associated with increased risk for ST.[35,39]

Clinicians should carefully consider whether or not a patient is likely to comply with extended dual anti-platelet use. The impact of potential contributors to non-compliance on the overall, long-term outcome of patients was clearly delineated by Spertus *et al.*[40] in a review of the PREMIER Registry. Several risk factors for early cessation of thienopyridine therapy were identified, including: avoidance of healthcare because of cost, advanced age, lower education level, and lack of follow-up. This study concluded that almost 1 in 7 MI patients who received DES were no longer taking thienopyridine by 30 days, and those non-compliant patients were more likely to die within the next 11 months. Randomised clinical trial patients are more likely to receive close follow-up than are 'real world' patients, an important difference which may improve compliance with prescribed therapy. Interventionalists need to consider all of these issues when choosing a treatment plan for a given procedure. These issues should be addressed with the patient when procedural consent is obtained; if determined to be at high-risk for non-compliance, the patient might be more suited to conservative medical therapy or coronary artery bypass graft (CABG) than PCI.

ADDITIONAL PROCEDURAL CONSIDERATIONS

'OFF-LABEL' USE

Currently, the FDA 'on-label' indications for use of DES include short (< 28 mm), *de novo* lesions in native vessels between 2.5–3.5 mm in diameter for SES, or 2.5–3.75 mm in diameter for PES. These indications are similar to 'on-label' use of most current BMS. Clinical trials used to obtain FDA commercial labelling have historically excluded patients at high risk for cardiac events. In fact, typical large-centre PCI practice involves care for patients who commonly have higher risk features. Approximately 50–80% of PCI procedures in the 'real world' are 'off-label'.[37,43] Therefore, safety and efficacy data from the initial randomised trials may not extrapolate to the 'real world' experience. Not surprisingly, DES long-term safety and efficacy have been reported to be worse in 'off-label' procedures, although the absolute event rates have remained low.[35,42] This highlights the need for outcomes research in 'real world' practice over long periods of time to ensure detection of uncommon adverse events.

SAPHENOUS VEIN GRAFT

Saphenous vein graft (SVG) PCI remains an area of challenge for interventionalists. Lesions in SVGs have been generally excluded in early stent trials. Early reports of SES in SVG showed reduced TLR at 6 months versus BMS, but longer term follow-up of the same patients of up to 3 years later demonstrated that the early benefit was lost.[43] In fact, the RRISC trial suggested that the BMS group had lower mortality than the DES group after longer follow-up. The power of this conclusion is somewhat limited due to the small sample size in each group (38 SES patients; 37 BMS patients), but the observation highlighted the difficulty in projecting future outcomes based on early observations.

LARGE VESSELS

Early DES trials highlighted the benefit of DES over BMS with TLR in vessels ~3.0 mm in diameter or less. Large coronary arteries ($\geq$ 3.5 mm) have less risk of the need for TLR with BMS than small vessels. In fact, a recent study by Steinberg et al.[44] found that BMS and DES had equally favourable clinical outcomes and were similar at 1-year follow-up in large vessels. Accordingly, if further data confirm the findings of Steinburg and colleagues, BMS should be considered over DES in the large vessel subset, since BMS requires shorter-term dual anti-platelet therapy.

PERI-OPERATIVE MANAGEMENT OF PATIENTS WITH CORONARY STENTS

Since premature withdrawal of dual anti-platelet therapy is associated with significant increased risk of ST, peri-operative issues in a stent patient are very important clinically. Considerations about these issues are nicely reviewed in an article by Brilakis et al.[45] In summary, peri-operative care should be individualised for a given patient. Factors such as the urgency of the surgery, the severity of bleeding risks of the surgery, and the timing of surgery following stent implantation should be considered. In general, elective surgery should be delayed for 6 weeks following placement of a BMS, and ideally for 1 year following DES stenting. If a stent needs to be deployed in a patient who may need surgery in the foreseeable future, a BMS should be used since anti-platelet therapy can be interrupted after a shorter duration following implantation. If surgery is needed earlier after DES implantation, consideration should be given to continuing dual anti-platelet therapy if there is a low risk of bleeding. In a patient with higher risk of bleeding, duration of anti-platelet cessation should be individualised, and the interventional cardiologist should ideally be consulted to help with discussion making, if feasible. There are currently no approved 'bridging strategies' for patients who need to come off their clopidogrel and/or aspirin. Peri-operative ST has been observed as late as 35 months in our study[35] and is associated with a high morbidity and mortality. Primary PCI may be the preferred strategy for patients who develop peri-operative ST.

FUTURE STUDIES

Future studies of new stent coatings may lead to improved outcomes for our patients. Many early studies are underway including the use of stents with other anti-proliferative agents, anti-platelet coatings, anti-thrombin coatings, bio-absorbable stents, and novel peptide brief proliferative agents, such as cRGD.[46] Lessons learned from the early BMS/DES era should lead us to be objectively critical and circumspect about the initial claims. Randomised and 'real world' subsets will need to be followed, and early and late outcomes monitored before mass adoption of the new technologies.

Key points for clinical practice

- Stent thrombosis (ST) during 4 years of follow-up based on randomised clinical trials is approximately the same in bare metal stenting (BMS) and drug-eluting stent (DES) groups, although the time course is different with more late ST occurring in DES.

- Late ST is a rare, but clinically important, event occurring at a rate of approximately 0.5% per year after DES in the 'real world'.

- Late ST may be reduced somewhat by longer-term dual anti-platelet therapy; no benefit has been demonstrated conclusively to extending therapy beyond 1 year.

- At the present time, after 4 years of follow-up, there seems to be no significant difference in the end-point of death between the DES and BMS groups.

- There are multiple clinically determined risk factors for ST including age, acute coronary syndrome, diabetes mellitus, low ejection fraction, prior brachytherapy, reduced renal function, and tobacco use.

- There are multiple angiographic risk factors for ST including long lesions, multiple overlapping stents, ostial stenting, bifurcation stenting, small vessels, and sub-optimal stent results.

- Patient compliance issues are clinically relevant to long-term outcomes and, therefore, must be considered when making choices of therapy.

- Peri-operative management of anti-platelet agents in patients with stents is important. Cessation of anti-platelet agent use in the peri-operative period should be individualised and based on patient and surgical considerations.

- In patients for whom percutaneous coronary intervention is needed and future near-term surgery is planned, BMS should be considered over DES.

- Insurers, governmental bodies, and pharmaceutical companies should ensure that issues such as drug cost do not cause patients to discontinue thienopyridine therapy prematurely, which could lead to rare, but potentially catastrophic, secondary cardiovascular complications.

References

1. Detre K, Holubkof R, Kelsey S et al. PTCA in 1985 to 1986 and 1977 to 1981. The National Heart, Lung, and Blood Institute Registry. N Engl J Med 1988; **318**: 265–270.
2. Braunwald's Heart Disease, 7th edn 2005. Table 52-3,1375.
3. Baim D. Grossman's Cardiac Catheterization, Angiography, and Intervention, 7th edn. Table 24.13,519.
4. Baim D. Grossman's Cardiac Catheterization, Angiography, and Intervention, 7th edn. Table 24.14,521.
5. Rao SV, Shaw RE, Brindis RG et al. Patterns and outcomes of drug-eluting coronary stent use in clinical practice. Am Heart J 2006; **152**: 321–326.

6. Holmes DR, Leon MB, Moses JW *et al.* Analysis of 1-year clinical outcomes in the SIRIUS trial: a randomized trial of a sirolimus-eluting stent versus a standard stent in patients at high risk for coronary restenosis. *Circulation* 2004; **109**: 634–640.

7. Muni NI, Gross TP. Problems with drug-eluting coronary stents – The FDA perspective. *N Engl J Med* 2004; **351**: 1593–1595.

8. Moreno R, Fernandez C, Hernandez R *et al.* Drug-eluting stent thrombosis – Results from a pooled analysis including 10 randomized studies. *J Am Coll Cardiol* 2005; **45**: 954–959.

9. Orford J, Lennon R, Melby S *et al.* Frequency and correlates of coronary stent thrombosis in the modern era. *J Am Coll Cardiol* 2002; **40**: 1567–1572.

10. Cutlip DE, Baim DS, Ho KKL *et al.* Stent thrombosis in the modern era: a pooled analysis of multicenter coronary stent clinical trials. *Circulation* 2001; **103**: 1967–1971.

11. Heller LI, Shemwell KC, Hug K. Late stent thrombosis in the absence of prior intracoronary brachytherapy. *Cathet Cardiovasc Intervent* 2001; **54**: 5323–5328.

12. Wang F, Stouffer GA, Waxman S, Uretsky B. Late coronary stent thrombosis: early vs. late stent thrombosis in the stent era. *Cathet Cardiovasc Intervent* 2002; **55**: 142–147.

13. Farb A, Burke AP, Kolodgie FD, Virmani R. Pathological mechanisms of fatal late coronary stent thrombosis in humans. *Circulation* 2003; **108**: 1701–1706.

14. Casserly IP, Goldstein JA, Lasala JM. Interventional rounds – Late stent thrombosis in the nonbrachytherapy population: a real phenomenon? *Cathet Cardiovasc Intervent* 2002; **59**: 504–508.

15. Virmani R, Guagliumi G, Farb A *et al.* Localized hypersensitivity and late coronary thrombosis secondary to a sirolimus-eluting stent – Should we be cautious? *Circulation* 2004; **109**: 701–705.

16. McFadden EP, Stabile E, Regar E *et al.* Late thrombosis in drug-eluting coronary stents after discontinuation of antiplatelet therapy. *Lancet* 2004; **364**: 1519–1521.

17. Karvouni E, Korovesis S, Katritsis DG. Very late thrombosis after implantation of sirolimus eluting stent. *Heart* 2005; **91**: e45.

18. Feres F, Costa Jr JR, Abizaid A. Very late thrombosis after drug-eluting stents. *Cathet Cardiovasc Intervent* 2006; **68**: 83–88.

19. Ong ATL, McFadden EP, Regar E *et al.* Late angiographic stent thrombosis (LAST) events with drug-eluting stents. *J Am Coll Cardiol* 2005; **45**: 2088–2092.

20. Joner M, Finn A, Farb A *et al.* Pathology of drug-eluting stents in humans. *J Am Coll Cardiol* 2006; **48**: 193–202.

21. Pfisterer M, Brunner-La Rocca HP, Buser PT *et al.* and BASKET-LATE Investigators. Late clinical events after clopidogrel discontinuation may limit the benefit of drug-eluting stents: an observational study of drug-eluting versus bare-metal stents. *J Am Coll Cardiol* 2006; **48**: 2584–2591.

22. Lagerqvist B, James SK, Stenestrand U *et al.*; for the SCAAR Study Group. Long-term outcomes with drug-eluting stents versus bare-metal stents in Sweden. *N Engl J Med* 2007; **356**: 1009–1019.

23. Camenzind E, Steg PG, Wijns W. Stent thrombosis late after implantation of first-generation drug-eluting stents: a cause for concern. *Circulation* 2007; **115**: 1440–1455.

24. Serruys PW, Daemen J. Late stent thrombosis: a nuisance in both bare metal and drug-eluting stents. *Circulation* 2007; **115**: 1433–1439.

25. Daemen J, Wenaweser P, Tsuchida K *et al.* Early and late coronary stent thrombosis of sirolimus-eluting and paclitaxel-eluting stents in routine clinical practice: data from a large two-institutional cohort study. *Lancet* 2007; **369**: 667–678.

26. Stone *et al.* DES evidence-based medicine perspectives on emerging safety concerns, real world outcomes, and use recommendations. Presented at Transcatheter Cardiovascular Therapeutics, Washington, DC, October 2006.

27. Summary from the Circulatory System Devices Panel Meeting. Available at: <http://www.fda.gov/cdrh/panel/summary/circ-120706.html>.

28. Cutlip DE, Windecker S, Mehran R *et al.*; on behalf of the Academic Research Consortium. Clinical end points in coronary stent trials: a case for standardized definitions. *Circulation* 2007; **115**: 2344–2351.

29. Holmes DR, Kereiakes DJ, Laskey WK *et al.* Thrombosis and drug-eluting stents: an objective appraisal. *J Am Coll Cardiol* 2007; **50**: 109–118.

30. Mauri L, Hsieh W, Massaro JM *et al*. Drug-eluting stent thrombosis results from a pooled analysis including 10 randomized studies. *J Am Coll Cardiol* 2005; **45**: 954–959.

31. Spaulding C, Daemen J, Boersma E, Cutlip D, Serruys P. A pooled analysis of data comparing sirolimus-eluting stents with bare-metal stents. *N Engl J Med* 2007; **356**: 989–997.

32. Stettler C, Wandel S, Allemann S *et al*. Outcomes associated with drug-eluting and bare-metal stents: a collaborative network meta-analysis. *Lancet* 2007; **370**: 937–948.

33. Jensen LO, Maeng M, Kaltoft A *et al*. Stent thrombosis, myocardial infarction, and death after drug-eluting and bare-metal stent coronary interventions. *J Am Coll Cardiol* 2007; **50**: 463–470.

34. Machecourt J, Danchin N, Lablanche JM *et al*.; for the EVASTENT Investigators. Risk factors for stent thrombosis after implantation of sirolimus-eluting stents in diabetic and nondiabetic patients. *J Am Coll Cardiol* 2007; **50**: 501–508.

35. Mishkel GJ, Moore, AL, Pfeiffer AM, Markwell SJ, Shelton ME. Predictors of stent thrombosis following implantation of a drug-eluting stent. Presented at the European Society of Cardiology Congress, Vienna, Austria, September 2007.

36. James S, Carlsson J, Lindbäck J *et al*. Long term outcome with drug eluting stents vs. bare metal stents in Sweden – One additional year of follow-up. Presented at European Society of Cardiology Congress, September 2007.

37. Tu JV, Bowen J, Chiu M *et al*. Effectiveness and safety of drug-eluting stents in Ontario. *N Engl J Med* 2007; **357**: 1393–1402.

38. Eisenstein EL, Anstrom KJ, Kong DJ *et al*. Clopidogrel use and long-term clinical outcomes after drug-eluting stent implantation. *JAMA* 2007; **297**: 159–168.

39. Grines CL, Bonow RO, Casey DE *et al*. Prevention of premature discontinuation of dual antiplatelet therapy in patients with coronary artery stents: a science advisory from the American Heart Association, American College of Cardiology, Society for Cardiovascular Angiography and Interventions, American College of Surgeons, and American Dental Association, with representation from the American College of Physicians. *Circulation* 2007; **115**: 813–818.

40. Spertus JA, Kettelkamp R, Vance C *et al*. Prevalence, predictors, and outcomes of premature discontinuation of thienopyridine therapy after drug-eluting stent placement: results from the PREMIER registry. *Circulation* 2006; **113**: 2803–2809.

41. Win HK, Caldera AE, Maresh K *et al*. Clinical outcomes and stent thrombosis following off-label use of drug-eluting stents. *JAMA* 2007; **297**: 2028–2030.

42. Beohar N, Davidson CH, Kip KE *et al*. Outcomes and complications associated with off-label and untested use of drug-eluting stents. *JAMA* 2007; **297**: 1992–2000.

43. Vermeersch P, Agostoni P, Verheye S *et al*. Increased late mortality after sirolimus-eluting stents versus bare-metal stents in diseased saphenous vein grafts: Results from the DELAYED-RRISC trial. *J Am Coll Cardiol* 2007; **50**: 261–267.

44. Steinberg DH, Mishra S, Javaid A *et al*. Comparison of effectiveness of bare-metal stents versus drug-eluting stents in large ($\geq$ 3.5 mm) coronary arteries. *Am J Cardiol* 2007; **99**: 599–602.

45. Brilakis ES, Baerjee S, Berger PB. Perioperative management of patients with coronary stents. *J Am Coll Cardiol* 2007; **49**: 2145–2150.

46. Dixon SR, Grines CL, O'Neill WW. The year in interventional cardiology. *J Am Coll Cardiol* 2007; **50**: 269–285.

Philippe Gabriel Steg Isabelle Boutron

7

How far are clinical trial data reliable guides to the optimal treatment of acute myocardial infarction?

In the past 20 years, giant strides have been made in the treatment of acute myocardial infarction (MI). With the advent of reperfusion therapy (intravenous thrombolysis and primary percutaneous coronary intervention) as well as with improvements in the in-hospital management, the acute outcomes of patients presenting alive to the hospital with ST segment elevation acute myocardial infarction (STEMI) have markedly improved. Recent data from the Global Registry of Acute Coronary syndromEs (GRACE) have shown that the in-hospital mortality and complications of acute STEMI have continued to dwindle as recently as the past 7 years.[1] One of the key factors in establishing the value of the new therapies which have changed the outcomes of MI has been the emergence of large, co-operative, randomised, clinical trials (RCTs). Starting with the ISIS trials, the GISSI, TIMI and GUSTO 1 studies, a series of very large, usually international, multicentre, randomised trials addressed simple and clear questions, with the appropriate power to provide unambiguous demonstration of success or failure, using clinically relevant 'hard' end-points, such as mortality (for most of the original studies).

This was consistent with the philosophy put forward a few years earlier by Yusuf, Collins and Peto, of the need for large-scale, simple RCTs[2] and took advantage of the fact that the relatively high short-term mortality of acute myocardial infarction provided a frequent, simple, unambiguous, and solid end-point for trials – mortality. This also provided a strong impetus for changing clinical care once a trial demonstrated a reduction in mortality.

Philippe Gabriel Steg MD FESC FACC FCCP
Professor, INSERM U-698 et Université Paris VII – Denis Diderot, Hôpital Bichat-Claude Bernard; Assistance Publique, Hôpitaux de Paris, Paris, France
For correspondence: Professor Philippe Gabriel Steg, Centre Hospitalier Bichat-Claude Bernard, 46 rue Henri Huchard, 75018 Paris, France. E-mail: gabriel.steg@bch.aphp.fr

Isabelle Boutron MD PhD
INSERM U738, Paris, France; Université Paris VII – Denis Diderot, UFR de Médecine, Paris, France; AP-HP, Hôpital Bichat, Département d'Epidémiologie, Biostatistique et Recherche Clinique, Paris, France

Therefore, RCTs have been an essential tool in establishing the value of new therapies for acute MI in a convincing and unequivocal fashion. The clear-cut results from these trials, whether negative or positive, have been incorporated into clinical guidelines, in which the strength of the evidence and the strength of the recommendation are graded to help practitioners understand the value (or lack thereof) of new therapies and to embrace rapidly the effective ones. However, over time, a number of issues has emerged regarding the external validity (or generalisability) of RCT results. External validity is crucial because, if the trial results only apply to a very select group of patients but not to the broader patient population with a given condition, then the results may not be generally applicable and the treatment may not be approved by regulators or embraced by practitioners. However, the assessment and reporting of the external validity of trials is usually very limited. Given that the treatment of acute myocardial infarction has been one of the fields in which RCTs have led to the greatest advances, it is also one in which the importance of these issues have been exemplified. The issue of external validity has been recently reviewed extensively by Rothwell.[3] A large number of factors can affect external validity, and these can be summarised under the broad categories discussed below.

ISSUES WITH SELECTION OF END-POINTS FOR CLINICAL TRIALS IN ACUTE MYOCARDIAL INFARCTION

As mortality began to improve, the size of the studies required to demonstrate further improvement started to become extremely large, commonly exceeding 10,000 or 20,000 patients. In order to avoid requiring such large sample sizes, investigators have resorted to using surrogate end-points or composite end-points, the latter often involving the combination of mortality, stroke and re-infarction.

The use of surrogate end-points as a substitute for mortality and other important clinical end-points has been well documented to be potentially misleading.[3–5] A famous example in the setting of myocardial infarction is the fact that anti-arrhythmic drugs produced a reduction in ventricular arrhythmias after myocardial infarction, yet were associated with an increased mortality.[6]

To avoid this pitfall, another solution is to use clinical end-points but to combine them into 'composite' end-points, which are likely to be more frequent than death alone and which, therefore, provide more statistical power for a smaller size population. However, even when the components of composite end-points are genuine clinical end-points, the use of composite end-points is fraught with problems. Using composite end-points increases the power of a trial to detect differences between study arms and, therefore, reduces the sample size requirements for the trial. In addition, it can be said that composite end-points may best capture the overall impact of therapeutic interventions. Yet the interpretation of composite end-points can be very difficult, as discussed below. These issues have been extensively reviewed.[7–10]

1. The various components of the composite end-points may be of differing value to the patient and physician; this is particularly true when a

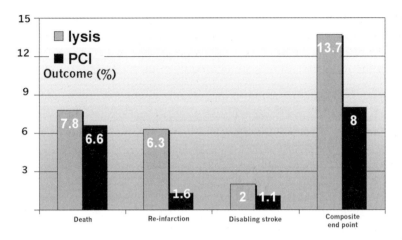

Fig. 1 Thirty-day outcome in the DANAMI-2 randomised trial comparing primary PCI and intravenous thrombolysis for STEMI. The reduction in the composite end-point is largely (although not exclusively) driven by a reduction in the end-point of re-infarction.

composite end-point includes fatal and non-fatal events. Often, it is the component of least importance which is the most frequent and for which treatment benefit will be greatest.[10] Conversely, the number of events in the component of greatest importance (such as death) will often be small. It is, therefore, essential that the impact of the therapy tested on each of the components of the composite end-point be reported separately in detail.

2. The magnitude of the benefit, and even the direction of the benefit, may vary between the components of the composite. Sometimes, the benefit is largely driven by one of the components of the composite. An example is the DANAMI-2 trial comparing primary percutaneous coronary intervention and intravenous thrombolysis for STEMI. The trial demonstrated an unambiguous reduction in the primary composite end-point of death, re-infarction and disabling stroke, from 13.7% to 8% with percutaneous coronary intervention over thrombolysis ($P = 0.001$).[11] However, among the various components of the composite end-point, it is apparent that the reduction was largely (although not exclusively) driven by a reduction in re-infarction (Fig. 1).

3. Given that some of the most important end-points (such as mortality) may be less frequent, the uncertainty around the estimates will be greater and there may be lack of consistency between fatal and non-fatal events. It remains unclear how a reduction of a composite end-point is to be interpreted when it is associated with a non-significant trend towards increased mortality. It may very well be due to chance. An example is the CLARITY trial comparing clopidogrel to placebo as an adjunct to thrombolysis and aspirin for ST-segment elevation acute myocardial infarction.[12] The primary end-point in that study was the composite of an occluded infarct artery on the coronary angiogram done before hospital discharge and death or myocardial infarction if occurring before the angiogram. The trial demonstrated a clear 31% reduction in the primary endpoint (Table 1), but this was driven by a 36% reduction in occlusion of

Table 1 An example of inconsistency between components of a composite end-point. Primary composite end-point of the CLARITY trial and its components

	Clopidogrel (n = 1752)	Placebo (n = 1739)	Odds ratio (95% CI)	P-value
Principal end-point (%)				
TIMI 0/1 flow, MI or death	15.0	21.7	0.64 (0.53–0.76)	< 0.001
Individual components of the primary end-point (%)				
TIMI 0/1 flow	11.7	18.4	0.59 (0.48–0.72)	< 0.001
Re-infarction	2.5	3.6	0.70 (0.47–1.04)	0.08
Death	2.6	2.2	1.17 (0.75–1.82)	0.49

Clopidogrel treatment was associated with a clear reduction in the risk of occurrence of two of the three components of the primary end-point, but with a trend towards an increase in death (although confidence intervals are very wide, given the low mortality). Adapted from Sabatine et al.[12]

the infarct artery and a 31% reduction in re-infarction. In contrast, there was an 18% non-significant increase in death (OR, 1.17; 95% CI, 0.75–1.82). Because the death rates were low, a likely explanation was chance. In fact, when focusing on cardiovascular mortality, there was a trend towards a modest (3%) reduction with clopidogrel. Fortunately, a simultaneous report from a very large Chinese RCT of over 45,000 patients (the COMMIT trial)[13] was able to demonstrate a 7% reduction in hospital mortality with clopidogrel over placebo as an adjunct to standard therapy (including aspirin) in ST-segment elevation acute myocardial infarction, thereby providing strong re-assurance that the benefit observed in CLARITY in terms of patency and re-infarction was not offset by a small increase in mortality.

Even if all components of the composite end-point demonstrate directionally consistent benefit, it may be misleading to claim a reduction in the composite if the latter is almost exclusively driven by one of the components.

TRIAL SETTING

The country, type of healthcare system, type of recruitment setting, as well as selection of participating centres or physicians all can affect the outcome of a randomised trial. An example is the GUSTO-IV ACS trial in which results obtained in North America with prolonged abciximab infusion in acute coronary syndromes appeared beneficial whereas results from Europe and the rest of the world suggested no benefit, or even harm, from treatment.[14] Apart from the well-known limitations of subset analyses,[15] there are numerous potential mechanisms by which such variations can be explained (Table 2).

The influence of participating centres' volume of care and physicians' expertise is particularly important for trials assessing percutaneous coronary interventions. In fact, there is abundant evidence that hospitals with a larger volume of activity tend to have better outcomes and that the expertise of

Table 2 Mechanisms of variations in trial outcomes in acute coronary syndromes

- Random variation in *post-hoc* subset analyses
- Variations between study centres
- Variations in baseline demographics
- Variations in adjunctive therapy
- Variations in use and timing of revascularisation
- Variations in staffing of sites
- Variations in the ascertainment and adjudication of events
- Unmeasured socio-economic factors
- Variations in genetic susceptibility to atherosclerosis or thrombosis

interventionalists and other care providers is also a determinant for outcomes.[16–19] The organisation of the hospital (*e.g.* presence on-site of a cardiologist, activation of the catheterisation laboratory by emergency physician or prehospital personnel) also has an impact on outcomes.[20,21] However, in published randomised trials, data related to the number and expertise of the centres and operators involved in the trial are frequently lacking.

Another example, which is particularly relevant in the case of myocardial infarction, is the trial setting. Nearly all RCTs performed in acute myocardial infarction have addressed patients hospitalised with acute myocardial infarction. However, it is established that at least half of the deaths related to acute myocardial infarction occur before the patient actually reaches the hospital. In the early minutes and hours after the onset of symptoms, the risk of ventricular tachyarrhythmia and sudden death is maximal. Therefore, hospital presenters are in fact 'survivors' or the prehospital phase and it is clear that the improvement in hospital outcomes of acute myocardial infarction seen in the last two decades is not paralleled by a similar improvement in prehospital outcomes. In fact, prehospital death rates have undergone a much smaller decline than in-hospital death rates.[22]

TRIAL SELECTION PROCESS AND CHARACTERISTICS OF PARTICIPANTS

It is common for RCTs in acute myocardial infarction to recruit only a minority of the patients screened and the latter number is often not reported, particularly in trials performed in acute settings such as acute myocardial infarction. The selection process is actually a key factor in determining the external validity of a trial. RCTs usually enrol a highly selected patient population which may not be fully representative of the patients with the same condition encountered in routine practice. This is particularly true in respect of trials performed in the setting of acute myocardial infarction. Many of these trials have studied potent antithrombotic therapies, such as thrombolytic agents. In order to reduce the risk of the adverse effects of these therapies, such as bleeding (particularly intracerebral haemorrhage), patients deemed to be at high risk of bleeding are often routinely excluded from enrolment. In addition to these exclusion criteria, others such as absence of co-morbidities, an age limit, potential compliance to therapies and other factors are also used to select

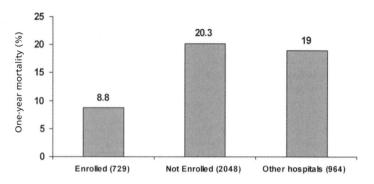

Fig. 2 One-year mortality in acute myocardial infarction patients enrolled in the ASSENT 2 trial, not enrolled in the trial but admitted to hospitals participating in the trial and in patients hospitalised in hospitals not participating in the trial.

trial participants. The net result is that the 'excluded group' often represents a very substantial fraction, and sometimes even the majority, of the patients screened. Yet, clearly, in routine practice, there is a host of data to demonstrate that patients who are excluded from participation in RCTs have worse outcomes than those of trial participants (Fig. 2).[23]

This is not the only problem with the representativeness of participants in RCTs. Not only do excluded patients fare worse than trial participants, but even trial participants fare worse than trial-eligible patients from routine practice. This is key because we usually assume that patients who are akin to trial participants have similar outcomes and will derive similar benefit from therapies to that observed in trial participants. In an analysis of participants with STEMI in the GRACE registry of acute coronary syndromes, enrolled at the approximate time of three large-scale international RCTs in STEMI (GUSTO V, DANAMI-2 and ASSENT-3), we categorised the registry patients into three groups: (i) patients who actually participated in a RCT during the study; (ii) patients who were eligible for any of the RCTs; and (iii) patients who were ineligible.[24] Base-line risk was markedly different for these three categories of patients, being lowest for actual trial participants, intermediate for trial-eligible patients and worst for trial-ineligible patients. The hospital outcomes for these three groups, particularly mortality, were then examined. The first finding, somewhat expected, is that trial-ineligible patients had the worst outcome. This is consistent with previous findings from several other studies. However, another important finding was that the trial-eligible patient population also had worse outcomes (an approximate doubling in mortality) compared to trial participants (Fig. 3) and this difference persisted after adjustment for base-line risk. This is crucial because a common assumption is that we can extend the outcomes observed in RCT participants to patients whom we encounter in clinical practice who have features similar to those of the trial participants. This analysis demonstrated that this was not the case. It does not necessarily imply that the directional effects of the therapy tested in RCTs would be different in routine practice, but rather that the overall outcomes are far better in trial participants than they are in 'the real world'. The problem of representativeness of trial participants is true not only for

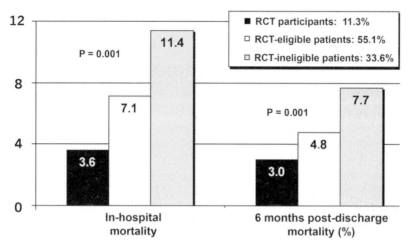

Fig. 3 In-hospital and 6-month post-discharge mortality in 8469 STEMI patients from the GRACE international registry of acute coronary syndromes, according to participation and eligibility in any of the three following randomised trials: GUSTO-V, DANAMI-2 and ASSENT-3.

efficacy but also for safety end-points. In another analysis from GRACE pertaining to non-ST segment elevation acute coronary syndromes,[25] similar differences were seen not only for 'efficacy' end-points (such as death), but also for bleeding (Fig. 4). Therefore, the assessment of external validity of a trial needs to account for both of these. It is not uncommon for a factor to influence both efficacy and safety in the same direction: for example, age is likely to be higher in patients who are excluded from participation in RCTs, yet is a strong risk factor for both death and bleeding. A more difficult situation would arise

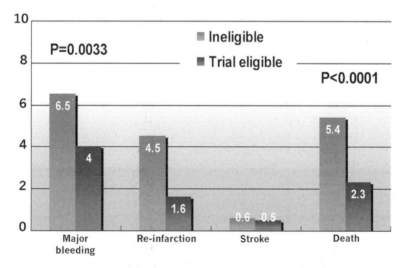

Fig. 4 In-hospital outcomes for non-ST segment elevation acute coronary syndromes in the GRACE registry according to eligibility for the randomised trials testing intravenous glycoprotein IIb/IIIa receptor blockers. Efficacy and safety outcomes, particularly bleeding, were consistently worse in ineligible patients compared to patients eligible for participation in the trial.

if a correlate of trial exclusion affected differentially efficacy and safety. Fortunately, this is a rare occurrence.

DIFFERENCES BETWEEN TRIAL PROTOCOL AND ROUTINE PRACTICE

Even when the patients enrolled and the hospitals participating in RCTs are truly representative of the real world, the external validity of the trial may still be limited by additional factors, such as differences between trial protocol and routine practice. These may affect the trial intervention, the timing of treatment, the use of co-therapies and changes in practice since the trial was performed. In addition, these differences may be geographically weighed: in other words, a trial performed in a given geographical setting may not have relevance for treatment of patients in another setting in which patient characteristics, management, healthcare and use of co-therapies may markedly differ. In the PURSUIT trial (testing eptifibatide versus placebo for non-ST elevation acute coronary syndromes), outcomes appeared to differ markedly according to the geographic distribution of centres: in centres from Latin America, treatment effect appeared neutral, whereas it was beneficial in centres from North America.[26] However, these geographical differences in outcomes were also associated with marked geographical differences in baseline characteristics and management, particularly a much lower use of revascularisation procedures in Latin America compared with North America, factors which significantly influence outcomes in this setting. Another example is the DANAMI-2 trial, alluded to earlier.[11] In that trial, angioplasty and intravenous thrombolysis were compared in the treatment of acute STEMI. However, patients treated by percutaneous coronary intervention also received dual antiplatelet therapy with clopidogrel in addition to aspirin, whereas patients treated by thrombolysis only received aspirin. This is because, at the time, there was no evidence of the efficacy or safety of clopidogrel added to aspirin as an adjunct to thrombolysis, whereas there was strong evidence of the need for clopidogrel added to aspirin to prevent subacute stent thrombosis. Yet, since that trial was performed, two large RCTs have demonstrated that clopidogrel as an adjunct to aspirin and thrombolysis has a major benefit in terms of reduction of mortality (with a 7% reduction in hospital mortality with 75 mg/day, but no loading dose in the COMMIT trial) and re-infarction.[12,13] In the CLARITY trial, use of clopidogrel (300 mg loading dose and 75 mg/day thereafter) was associated with an 18% reduction of the odds of death, re-infarction or stroke. Therefore, had clopidogrel been used in the thrombolysis arm of DANAMI-2, there would presumably have been less contrast between the two study arms. Yet, in today's practice, the combination of clopidogrel with aspirin is indeed used for all types of STEMI patients, given its benefits.

IS EXTERNAL VALIDITY SUFFICIENTLY CONSIDERED IN THE PLANNING, CONDUCTING AND REPORTING OF RCTS?

During recent years, increasing emphasis has been placed on the internal validity of RCTs (*i.e.* the extent to which systematic errors or bias are avoided): (i) regulatory agencies have proposed recommendations for the planning, conduct and analysis of RCTs; (ii) quality tools have been developed to evaluate internal validity of RCTs included in meta-analyses and in systematic reviews;[26] and (iii) the CONSORT published recommendations endorsed by editors to improve the reporting of published RCTs.[27] All these initiatives have improved the quality of trials. However, external validity (*i.e.* applicability of trials' results) is neglected. For example, most recommendations for cardiovascular risk management are based on internally valid RCTs, but less than one-third are based on high-quality evidence applicable to the populations, treatments, and outcomes specified in guideline recommendations.[28] External validity is not clearly taken into account in systematic reviews and meta-analyses and there is no validated tool for assessing the external validity of RCTs. This is problematical as lack of external validity is frequently put forward as the reason why interventions found to be effective in clinical trials are underused in clinical practice.[3]

THE WAY FORWARD

In order to improve the yield from RCTs for clinicians and patients alike, a number of steps are essential. It is necessary to:

1. Define a simple and clinically relevant question to study, and to address clinically relevant end-points, rather than waste resources in studies on surrogate markers of outcomes or on issues which are likely to represent only marginal advancement in medical knowledge.

2. Define a simple strategy for patient selection which captures a patient population as representative as possible of the patients encountered in everyday practice, with a limited number of exclusion criteria. The representativeness of the enrolled population should be assessed by means of a screening log which permits computation of the ratio of numbers enrolled to numbers screened.

3. Provide comprehensive reports of the trial selection process, management and outcomes (both for efficacy and adverse outcomes), following the internationally accepted sets of guidelines, such as the CONSORT statement.[28] The CONSORT group recently developed an extension of the CONSORT Statement for trials assessing non-pharmacological treatments. These guidelines clearly emphasise the need to report systematically physicians' expertise and centres' volume of care as well as all components of the intervention administered.[29,30]

4. Complement the results of RCTs with analyses of the management practices and outcomes of patients in everyday practice, as can be assessed from large-scale, representative registries. The goal of these analyses is not to replicate the assessment of efficacy or safety of the therapies or strategies tested in trials but rather to understand their relevance. A simple example is that of trials demonstrating the efficacy and safety of an antithrombotic treatment in a selected population capped for age. It then becomes important to know, from representative contemporary sources, what are the risks of bleeding in relation to age, co-morbidities and the use of co-therapies in patients from routine practice, as opposed to the highly selected trial population. This will help clarify the bleeding risk in patients who would receive the new therapy, which is highly likely to be higher than that of trial participants.

John G. Webb

8

Percutaneous aortic valve replacement

Aortic stenosis, when symptomatic, is associated with progressive deterioration and limited survival. Medical management has little to offer and balloon valvuloplasty can provide only limited benefit in terms of palliation. In contrast, surgical aortic valve replacement (AVR) is associated with symptomatic improvement and improved survival in appropriate patients.[1] However, surgical AVR requires general anaesthetic, thoracotomy, cardiotomy, aortotomy and cardiopulmonary bypass. Whilst well-tolerated, low-risk and effective in many patients, this is not the case in others.

Surgical risk is increased by advanced age as well as other co-morbidities, such as cerebrovascular, aortic, pulmonary, renal, hepatic and left ventricular disease as well as more subjective issues such as debility and frailty. Patients with aortic stenosis are most often elderly; a recent US community survey documented a prevalence of 4.6% in patients over the age of 75 years.[2] Many patients with co-morbidities, such as advanced age, are understandably reluctant to undergo conventional surgery and many physicians are reluctant to advise it.[2,3] Percutaneous AVR may offer a less invasive alternative with the potential for reduced morbidity and mortality in selected patients.[4]

PERCUTANEOUS VALVES

Two types of valves have been utilised in the great majority of the clinical experience to date. The prototypic balloon-expandable Cribier-Edwards™ valve (Edwards Lifesciences Inc.; Irvine, CA, USA) consisted of a stainless steel slotted tubular stent measuring approximately 15 mm in length. Equine pericardial leaflets were sewn to the stent frame and a synthetic fabric cuff covered the ventricular end of the stent so as to provide a seal around the

John G. Webb MD
McLeod Professor of Heart Valve Interventions, University of British Columbia; Director Cardiac Catheterization, Division of Cardiology, St Paul's Hospital, 1081 Burrard Street, Vancouver, BC, Canada V6Z 1Y6. E-mail: webb@providencehealth.bc.ca

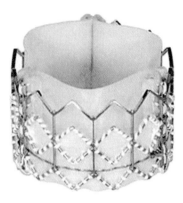

Fig. 1 The balloon-expandable Edwards SAPIEN transcatheter valve. The valve is constructed of a stainless steel frame with bovine pericardial leaflets and a fabric sealing cuff.

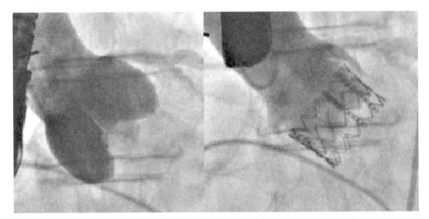

Fig. 2 Aortic angiogram before (left) and after (right) percutaneous valve implantation. Note that there is no aortic regurgitation following valve implantation as evidence by the absence of contrast within the left ventricle demonstrating a functioning prosthetic valve.

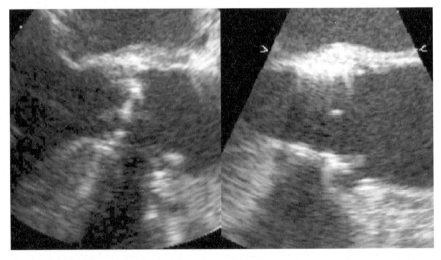

Fig. 3 Echocardiogram before (left) and after (right) percutaneous valve implantation.

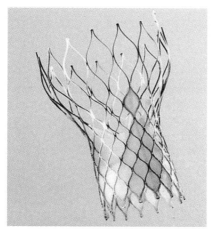

Fig. 4 The self-expanding CoreValve transcatheter valve. The valve is constructed of a nitinol alloy frame with porcine pericardial leaflets and a porcine pericardial sealing cuff.

valve.[5,6] The Edwards SAPIEN™ valve (Fig. 1) has replaced this first generation device, incorporating more durable bovine pericardial leaflets and a larger sealing cuff.[7] The stent is crimped onto a balloon catheter which is inflated then expanded within the native valve (Figs 2 and 3).

The self-expanding CoreValve™ device (CoreValve Inc.; Irvine, CA, USA) consists of a nitinol alloy stent measuring approximately 50 mm in length (Fig. 4). The stent is constrained within a long delivery sheath which is advanced to lie within the native aortic valve. As the sheath is withdrawn, the stent expands to assume its predetermined shape. The lower portion of the relatively long stent is positioned within the aortic annulus displacing and excluding the native leaflets. The middle portion contains the valve leaflets and is tapered to avoid contact with the coronary ostia. The upper portion extends above the coronary arteries and extends outwards to anchor the prosthesis against the ascending aorta.[8] Leaflets are pericardial with a pericardial sealing cuff.

Newer valves under development or in very early trials include the Sadra, 3F, Direct Flow and Paniagua valves among others.[9] These largely represent attempts to improve deliverability, positioning and the ability to reposition the valve if initial deployment is suboptimal.

As percutaneous AVR evolves, simple balloon valvuloplasty catheters have been replaced by integrated valve delivery systems. The Edwards system incorporates a specially constructed balloon catheter and deflectable catheter. The steerable catheter and relatively short stent facilitate manipulation through tortuous vessels and the stenotic valve.[6] A newer delivery system (RetroFlex II) improves deliverability further. The current Edwards delivery system has a profile of 22–24 French in diameter, depending on valve size, although a further reduction in delivery profile is anticipated. The CoreValve delivery system has been progressively reduced from 24 French to 18 French.[10]

ACCESS FOR PERCUTANEOUS AVR

Initial procedures were performed using femoral venous access.[5,11,12] Catheterisation of the right ventricle was followed by transeptal puncture of

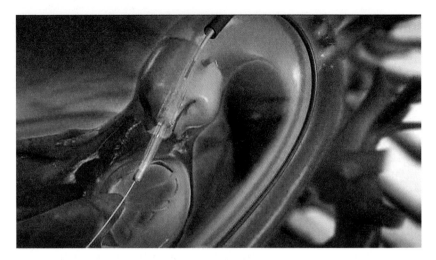

Fig. 5 A percutaneous valve crimped onto balloon catheter is advanced from the femoral artery, through the aorta and positioned within the stenotic native aortic valve.

the interatrial septum allowing antegrade access to the left heart and aortic valve. Subsequently, a transarterial procedure (Figs 5 and 6) utilising a steerable delivery catheter was developed in our centre and gained favour due to a lower rate of complications and greater reproducibility.[6,7] Although favoured over the transvenous approach, a major limitation of the femoral arterial approach is the large diameter of current valves and delivery catheters, particularly in the presence of iliofemoral arterial disease. Additional issues relate to manipulation of the prosthesis through tortuous aortic anatomy and through the stenotic native aortic valve. Various surgical approaches including cutdown and arteriotomy or temporary conduit access to the iliac or subclavian arteries have been utilised. However, the approach currently favoured when femoral access is problematic involves an intercostal incision

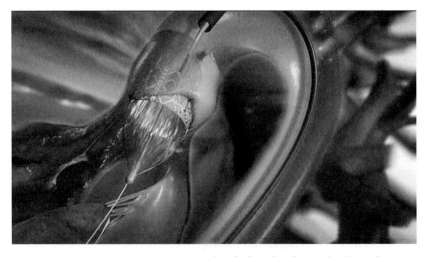

Fig. 6 The stent is expanded displacing and excluding the diseased native valve. Following balloon deflation the bioprosthetic leaflets will function in place of the native valve.

and direct left ventricular puncture with catheter introduction through the apical free wall of the left ventricle.[13-15] Currently, the femoral arterial approach is favoured with the left ventricular approach reserved for patients in whom femoral arterial access is suboptimal.[16]

PROCEDURAL OUTCOMES

Initial procedures utilising the transvenous procedure were problematic, although feasibility and potential benefit were dramatically demonstrated.[5,12] Subsequently, with the transarterial procedure, increased experience and procedural enhancements, in our experience the rate of successful implantation rose to 96%.[7] In our first human transarterial experience, intraprocedural mortality was low at 2%. Mortality at 30 days was initially 16%, falling to 8% with increased experience and comparing favourably to a logistic EuroSCORE predicted surgical mortality of 28% in high-risk patients declined surgery owing to co-morbidities.[7] Outcomes have continued to improve further in this single centre Vancouver experience.[16] Subsequently, favourable experience with the transarterial procedure has been duplicated in several other centres in Europe and the US. As of late 2007, over 300 transarterial procedures have been performed utilising the Cribier Edwards and Edwards SAPIEN valves. Preliminary unpublished data from the REVIVE II and REVIVAL II European, Canadian and US transarterial registries document a 12.5% mortality at 30 days in high-risk patients.

A similar story has unfolded with the self-expanding CoreValve device. Initial procedures in India demonstrated procedural success, but poor clinical outcomes. Subsequently, Grube in Germany reported a single centre experience in which implantation was successful in 88% of 25 patients with an in-hospital mortality of 20%.[8,17] A more recent multicentre report described 86 cases performed using the newer lower profile delivery systems.[10] Implantation was successful in 88% of patients. Periprocedural complications were primarily driven by stroke in 10% and tamponade in 7% with a 30-day mortality of 12%.[10] As of late 2007, the total number of CoreValve procedures exceeds 300. Preliminary, unpublished analysis of 175 patients treated with the lower profile device reportedly shows an increase in procedural success to 92% and a 30-day mortality of 15%, comparing favourably to a logistic EuroSCORE estimate of 24%.

VALVE FUNCTION

Percutaneous valves have two advantages over surgically implanted valves. The lack of a sewing ring allows for a larger orifice area for a given valve size. *In vitro* testing routinely demonstrates favourable haemodynamics with current percutaneous valves. In addition, expansion of the aortic annulus by balloon dilation and subsequent implantation of an oversized stent allows for implantation of a larger valve. In our experience, percutaneous AVR is associated with minimal or no discernible gradient at the time of catheterisation. In our initial 50-patient experience, echocardiography reported an increase in valve area from 0.6 cm^2 to 1.7 cm^2 (Fig. 7). Preliminary unpublished data from the combined European, Canadian and US high-risk transarterial Edwards Lifesciences registries documents a mean gradient

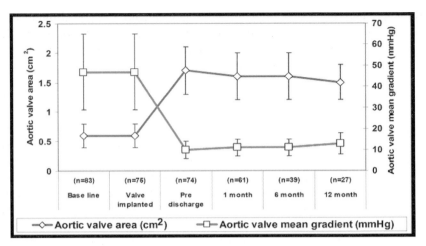

Fig. 7 Aortic valve area and mean gradient as assessed by echo following transarterial balloon expandable aortic valve implantation in 83 patients (Vancouver registry).

falling from 45 mmHg to 11 mmHg and valve area increasing from 0.6 cm^2 to 1.6 cm^2. Similarly, preliminary unpublished data from the recent global CoreValve experience with the newer devices valve documents an area increase in aortic valve area from 0.6 cm^2 to 1.6 cm^2.

Aortic regurgitation may be valvular (through the valve) or paravalvular (around the valve). Valvular regurgitation is commonly present in patients with aortic stenosis. Following percutaneous AVR, valvular regurgitation is generally absent or mild. However, ineffective sealing of the prosthesis within the aortic annulus allows for paravalvular regurgitation. Regurgitant leaks between the prosthesis and the native annulus are commonly present after valve implantation. Mild regurgitation may be apparent only as the auscultatory finding of a diastolic murmur, identical to that seen with native valvular regurgitation or echocardiographic regurgitant colour flow most commonly seen posteriorly adjacent to the mitral valve. More severe paravalvular regurgitation may result in heart failure or cardiogenic shock. Haemolysis has not been reported. Although severe leaks were common in the initial experience, concerns have been reduced primarily as a consequence of improved implantation techniques. Follow-up suggests that paravalvular leaks remain stable or decrease with time. Worsening regurgitation has not been reported. For the most part, some degree of valvular regurgitation prior to valve implantation is exchanged for a similar or lesser degree of paravalvular regurgitation after implantation. In general, the clinical benefit of relieving aortic stenosis greatly outweighs the consequences of paravalvular regurgitation. While this is true in older patients with co-morbidities currently considered candidates for percutaneous AVR, in future this may be a more important concern in younger, more active patients.

CORONARY ARTERY ISSUES

Coronary artery disease is common in patients with aortic stenosis. In our initial experience in percutaneous AVR in patients at high risk for surgery, significant coronary disease was present in 74% with prior bypass in 42%. Angioplasty is sometimes performed to reduce the likelihood of ischaemic ventricular dysfunction and haemodynamic instability at the time of the implant procedure. More often this is not necessary and coronary disease is relatively well tolerated following AVR.

Valve implantation does have the potential to provoke coronary obstruction. The major concern reported to date is obstruction of the left main coronary artery when the diseased native leaflet is displaced into the sinus of Valsalva by the implantable prosthesis.[6] It appears this is mainly a concern when the native valve is unusually bulky and in close proximity to the coronary ostium. The problem appears infrequent but has, on occasion, required angioplasty or bypass and has resulted in mortality. Currently, screening with echocardiography and aortic root angiography appears useful to exclude patients at risk for this problem.[7,18]

The stent component of percutaneous valves may extend to, or even above, the level of the coronary ostia. Generally, the open cells of the stent do not impair coronary perfusion. Intubation with angiographic catheters above, or through, the cells of the valved stent is still possible if clinically indicated.

STROKE

Stroke is a potentially devastating complication of surgical AVR and a major concern of patients. Similarly, stroke is a possible complication of percutaneous AVR. Reported rates of stroke with percutaneous AVR vary from 3–9% in high-risk elderly patients undergoing this procedure to date.[6–8,10,15,19] The most likely pathogenesis is embolisation of calcific debris from the native aortic valve or atheroma from the ascending aorta.[18] It seems reasonable to anticipate, and hope, that stroke rates will fall with increased experience, improved equipment and lower risk patients.

LATE OUTCOMES

Early experience demonstrated an acute improvement in left ventricular systolic function following successful percutaneous AVR.[12] Longer term follow-up confirmed improved left ventricular function was sustained at one year and was more dramatic in patients with more severe baseline ventricular dysfunction. Similarly, functional mitral insufficiency is reduced acutely with additional benefit at one year. Longer term follow-up has confirmed improvement in functional class is significant and sustained.[7]

VALVE DURABILITY

Percutaneous valves must not only function at the time of implantation but they must continue to function for a reasonable period of time to have clinical value. Poor durability of some early surgical valves was not initially apparent until catastrophic failure occurred. The majority of currently available surgical valves have been extensively tested and long-term durability has been documented. *In vitro* accelerated testing of currently available percutaneous valves suggests durability comparable to surgical bioprostheses, exceeding 10 years. However, *in vitro* testing may not duplicate the durability of a valve that has been constrained in a sheath, expanded with a balloon, expanded inadequately, excessively or asymmetrically or is compressible. Structural valve failure has not been reported to date; however, late follow-up in significant numbers of patients is only available to 2 years[16] with only anecdotal, unpublished reports of durability to 4 years. Eventually, structural valve failure can be expected to occur with all bioprostheses. Although very preliminary, early experience suggests that implantation of a second prosthesis within an earlier degenerated prosthesis is feasible and may extend the therapeutic reach of a percutaneous procedure.[20]

WHO IS A CANDIDATE?

According to American Heart Association/American College of Cardiology guidelines, severe aortic stenosis in combination with symptoms or left ventricular dysfunction is a class I indication for surgical valve replacement.[1] It seems reasonable to apply similar minimum requirements for considering percutaneous AVR. However, experience with percutaneous AVR is still limited, implications not entirely known and long-term follow-up lacking. Conversely, experience with conventional surgery is extensive, implications better defined and late outcome is known. Patients who are good candidates for conventional surgery should have this procedure. The temptation to offer a less invasive but less well investigated alternative in patients well suited to conventional surgery should be resisted pending greater experience.

Current information supports the use of percutaneous AVR in selected patients at particularly high risk with conventional surgery. What exactly constitutes 'high risk' is difficult to define and the term 'non-operable' is inherently controversial. A surgical consensus opinion that 30-day mortality exceeds 20% has been utilised by some groups. In an attempt to provide objective criteria, various models of surgical risk have been developed and calculators are readily available on-line. A logistic EuroSCORE estimate of > 20% (<www.euroscore.org>) or a STS estimate of > 10% (<www.sts.org>) have been suggested as appropriate thresholds. Unfortunately, both models fail to take into account many co-morbidities common with open heart surgery; for example, severe mitral or tricuspid regurgitation, porcelain aorta and hepatic failure. Moreover, surgical risks include not only mortality, but also morbidity. It appears likely that, in future, the potential for reduced morbidity with a percutaneous procedure may be a major factor in determining candidacy.

There are few absolute contra-indications to percutaneous AVR, meaning that the majority of patients with severe aortic stenosis are technically suitable candidates. Specific exclusions to percutaneous AVR are few. Current prosthetic valves are available in limited sizes appropriate for most, but not all, annulus diameters. The CoreValve device is unique in requiring points of fixation both in the annulus and the supracoronary aorta, which may exclude patients with a dilated ascending aorta. A very bulky aortic valve leaflet in close proximity to a coronary ostium may raise concerns about coronary obstruction. Current valves require annular disease and calcification for fixation and isolated regurgitation may not allow secure prosthesis seating. Perhaps the most common exclusion relates to inadequate arterial access.

Femoral or iliac arteries significantly smaller than current delivery catheters, particularly in the presence of severe calcification or tortuousity increase the risk of vascular injury during a transarterial implantation procedure.

TRAINING

Percutaneous AVR is relatively complex procedure with considerable potential for adverse outcomes. The literature clearly demonstrates a steep learning curve and improving outcomes with experience. In our initial human transarterial experience in high-risk, non-surgical candidates, outcomes improved dramatically and continue to improve.[6,7] Formal training appears important to minimise this learning curve. Formal educational programmes sponsored by the industry are evolving. Currently, these include formal instruction, case review, live case observation on on-site proctoring for initial cases. Virtual reality medical simulators have been developed for at least one device and appear helpful (Medical Simulation Inc.; Denver, CO, USA).

WHAT IS NEEDED TO START A PERCUTANEOUS AVR PROGRAMME?

This procedure crosses the traditional boundaries between cardiology and cardiac surgery. A combined programmatic approach is probably optimal for appropriate patient selection and management. To date, the procedure has been performed by interventional cardiologists, although cardiac surgeons with endovascular skills may also be able to perform the procedure. Vascular access assessment and management may require the skills of radiologists and vascular surgeons. Echocardiography is important in patient selection, annulus measurement and transoesophageal echocardiographic guidance and post-procedural assessment. Anaesthetic management is complex and best managed by anaesthetists with a special interest in the field. Elderly patients with co-morbidities may require geriatric, social work and specialised nursing management. Regional centres of expertise may be desirable to facilitate the development of expertise and good outcomes.

CURRENT AVAILABILITY

Both the Edwards SAPIEN and the CoreValve devices are available in limited European and Canadian centres under various clinical, compassionate and registry protocols. Both devices have now received CE mark approval in Europe, paving the way for commercialisation. A few other prototype devices have been implanted in small numbers of patients in single-site evaluations. In the US and Canada, a randomised clinical evaluation – the PARTNER (Placement of AoRTic TraNscathetER Valves) Trial – is currently underway.

SUMMARY

Percutaneous aortic valve implantation has evolved into a reproducible procedure with outcomes that compare favourably with conventional surgery in selected, high-risk patients. Outcomes are improving; however, experience remains limited.

Charles Ilsley Richard Grocott-Mason

9

Setting up a primary percutaneous coronary intervention service – the Harefield experience

The management of acute myocardial infarction has advanced dramatically and has continued to evolve over the past 40 years. Randomised controlled trial proven treatment strategies have led to marked improvements in mortality and quality of life, driven in large part by early reperfusion and by advances in medical therapy (aspirin, β-adrenergic blockers, heparin and ACE inhibitors).[1,2] ST segment elevation myocardial infarction (STEMI) is almost invariably caused by thrombotic occlusion of an epicardial artery due a ruptured atherosclerotic plaque (Fig. 1). The benefits of re-opening that blockage are offset by the risks of the intervention. From the late 1980s, rapid thrombolysis has been the treatment of first choice and, following the publication of the Coronary Heart Disease National Service framework in March 2000 (<http://www.dh.gov.uk/en/Publicationsandstatistics/Publications/PublicationsPolicyAndGuidance/DH_4094275>), substantial effort has been put into reducing delays in the treatment of patients with acute STEMI. A mandatory national database was set up (MINAP), with 'door-to-needle' times included as a measure of an acute trust's performance. Thrombolysis, despite the use of a variety of lytic agents and combination therapies, and even though driven by UK Government targets to be delivered within 30 min of presentation, only successfully re-opens up to 70% of arteries and, dependent largely on age and time to treatment, is associated with a hospital mortality of 11% (4% in under 60-year-olds to 35% in patients over 80 years of age). There are wide variations in the management and outcomes[3] and, since thrombolysis often fails to provide clinical or actual reperfusion, re-infarction is not infrequent (the unstable plaque is not healed) and a majority of patients undergo revascularisation at a later date. The clinical benefits of emergency

Charles Ilsley FRCP FRACP (for correspondence)
Director of Cardiology, Harefield Hospital, Hill End Road, Harefield, Middlesex UB9 6JH, UK
E-mail: c.ilsley@rbht.nhs.uk

Richard Grocott-Mason MD FRCP
Consultant Cardiologist, Hillingdon Hospital, Pield Heath Road, Uxbridge, Middlesex UB8 3NN, UK

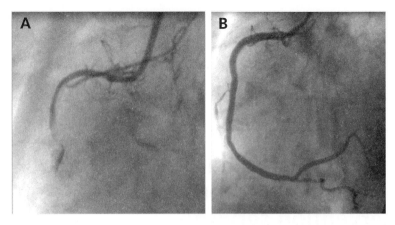

Fig. 1 (A) Single frame of a dominant right coronary showing mid-vessel occlusion in a patient presenting with pain and inferior ST elevation. (B) The vessel has been opened with a stent restoring antegrade flow and the ECG change and chest pain resolved.

'rescue' percutaneous coronary intervention (PCI) after failed thrombolysis are controversial. Even after clinically successful thrombolysis in patients without complications, early access to a non-invasive risk stratification test, such as a nuclear perfusion scan or dobutamine stress echocardiogram, is limited and patients often wait many days for transfer to a tertiary centre for such investigations and for subsequent angiography and revascularisation.

By 2003, a large body of evidence had demonstrated primary percutaneous coronary intervention (PPCI) to be a more effective treatment for STEMI, both for patients admitted directly to an intervention centre and also for those transferred from a district general hospital without PPCI facilities, especially if the procedure can be performed efficiently.[4–6] Patients treated with PPCI have a lower hospital mortality of around 5%, shorter hospital admission, better long-term survival, and fewer non-fatal re-infarctions and haemorrhagic strokes, compared with thrombolysis. In the longer term, left ventricular function is better and less heart failure ensues. Usually, the primary intervention is definitive. Moreover, many studies suggest that the overall cost of such treatment is lower, despite the initial relatively high cost of the index admission.[7] In addition, the information gained about the overall burden of coronary disease improves patient risk stratification and reduces delays to any further necessary revascularisation.

There has been debate in the literature about the importance of 'door-to-balloon' times in STEMI, but it is illogical to think anything other than that the quicker the artery is opened the smaller will be the infarct and the better the outcome.[8] It seems easier to administer an i.v. bolus of a thrombolytic agent rapidly rather than to organise the opening and staffing of a cardiac catheter laboratory with the appropriate expertise; however, the establishment of successful PPCI network programmes in Denmark, Czech Republic and southern Poland has shown that it is possible. We felt strongly that if a PPCI programme could be delivered in other parts of Europe, there was no reason why we could not do so locally. Our challenge was how to provide such optimal care in the NHS. We established the first 24-h primary angioplasty service in London at Harefield Hospital in March 2004, initially limited to the London Borough of Hillingdon, but subsequently expanded to cover a wider area of North West London and Hertfordshire. This article summarises the reasons for the change, the processes involved, the problems encountered, the results, and the lessons learned.

INTRODUCTION OF 24-h PPCI AT HAREFIELD HOSPITAL

The real world of STEMI treatment in 2003 is illustrated by an audit of 113 consecutive patients treated for STEMI at Hillingdon Hospital, a 400-bed district general hospital in West London serving a local population of about 270,000. In the study cohort, 88% had immediate reperfusion therapy (99 lysis; 1 PPCI); overall, nearly two-thirds of patients ($n = 71$) had coronary angiography and half had undergone revascularisation, the majority by angioplasty. One in four patients had pre-discharge coronary angiography either as an emergency (failed thrombolysis or re-infarction), or prior to discharge (for on-going angina or because they were thought to be at high risk of recurrent events in the short-term). There had been long delays for treatment, with some patients waiting in-hospital for up to 3 weeks for transfer. Those investigated as an out-patient had longer delays of up to 9 months for revascularisation (mean time from presentation to elective angiogram 171 days, and to elective angioplasty 276 days).

Harefield Hospital is a specialty cardiothoracic centre on the fringe of North-West London and, prior to 2004, its lack of an accident and emergency department (A&E) had precluded emergency admission of patients with STEMI. Consequently, they were taken to Hillingdon Hospital for thrombolysis. Although the lack of an A&E department was considered a formidable obstacle, there were three very important drivers for change: (i) the growing body of evidence that PPCI was clinically and cost effective (the most important feature of the latter being the saving in bed-days); (ii) the coming together of a district general hospital, tertiary centre and Primary Care Trust (PCT) in wanting the best care for their patients; and (iii) the ability and willingness of the London Ambulance Service (LAS) both to diagnose and to triage patients with chest pain. From the perspective of the tertiary centre, it seemed hugely sensible to treat patients in the early stages of infarction when the results would be favourable rather than to target the smaller, much sicker cohort of 'rescue' angioplasty (after failed thrombolysis). This latter group would, inevitably, have less satisfactory outcomes and prolonged (and, therefore, more expensive) hospital stays.

Integrating different organisations within the NHS was far from easy and required full collaboration and discussion with all disciplines involved even though there was already a very close working relationship between Harefield and Hillingdon Hospitals. Harefield Hospital had a 24-h on-call service covering the cardiac catheter laboratories but, since the vast majority of emergency patients received were inter-hospital transfers, there was sufficient time to call the catheter laboratory staff in from home prior to the patient's arrival. Generally, patients were transferred to a ward for assessment and then to the catheter laboratory. All this took considerable time. To establish the new service, three principles were considered important – the provision of rapid

PPCI, 24/7 availability and absence of any age limit at diagnosis. To minimise delays, the ideal service model was direct admission from home to Harefield Hospital by the LAS, with inter-hospital transfer (IHT) from Hillingdon Hospital A&E Department for patients initially presenting there. Protocols for the LAS, Hillingdon Hospital A&E Department and Harefield Hospital had to be considered and integrated. Service improvements, operational changes and training were implemented. We envisaged a hybrid system because, though many patients are brought from home by ambulance, at least a third self present to an A&E department. Equally, the diagnosis may not be clear on initial ECGs and may become apparent after the patient has been admitted to the local hospital.

LONDON AMBULANCE SERVICE

It was decided that, in order to deliver rapid PCI, the diagnosis of STEMI had to be made in the patient's home prior to direct transfer to Harefield Hospital, bypassing the traditional A&E department. In many ways, the debate preceding the acceptance of this policy was somewhat analogous to the debate, prevalent in the 1990s, about whether thrombolysis should be delivered in the A&E department or the coronary care unit (CCU). This policy clearly put the onus on the paramedic crew to make a correct diagnosis and the combination of enthusiastic crews, good training in ECG interpretation and the provision of 12-lead ECG machines as standard, laid the foundations of the service. With the Clinical Practice Manager, London Ambulance Service NHS Trust (Mark Whitbread) we established simple and achievable criteria for STEMI management (Table 1).

The policy was established that patients resuscitated from a cardiac arrest out of hospital would still taken directly to Harefield Hospital as long as the presumptive diagnosis was STEMI, they were breathing spontaneously and haemodynamically stable. Similarly, if a patient had a VF arrest en route to Harefield Hospital, the journey would continue as long as haemodynamic stability had been achieved. Unconscious or haemodynamically unstable patients would be taken to the nearest A&E department for further assessment and treatment.

LAS paramedic crews proved to be very capable in assessing symptoms, performing and interpreting a 12-lead ECG, diagnosing STEMI and, therefore, in deciding to which hospital the patient should be taken. This has been a particularly important change from the earlier principle of taking the patient to the nearest NHS A&E department. Following implementation of the new

Table 1 Eligibility/ineligibility criteria for PPCI

Eligible patients (no age limit)	Ineligible patients
Central chest pain ≤ 9 h	Haemodynamic instability
ST elevation* ≥ 2 contiguous leads	LBBB**
	Cardiac arrest – unconscious

*ST elevation ≥ 1 mm in inferior leads; ≥ 2 mm in chest leads.
**Crews were encouraged to bring patients with typical symptoms plus LBBB.

policy, patients who have a STEMI at Heathrow airport, for example, are picked up by the LAS, driven past the door of Hillingdon Hospital (about 3 miles) and taken to Harefield Hospital (about 11 miles away). As the distances and transfer times from patient pick-up to arrival at hospital are potentially short, we deliberately rejected telemetry of the ECG for review since any delay introduced by this process would be both medically and operationally inefficient.

The paramedics have, from the start, been highly enthusiastic about the programme, and this has been a major factor in its success. When the ambulance crew diagnose a STEMI, they take the patient to Harefield Hospital. The crew telephone Harefield switchboard, giving an estimated arrival time, using a dedicated telephone line, a call that at any time of day or night initiates the calling in to the hospital of the catheter laboratory team (including the on-call consultant cardiologist). Audit has shown mean time from the LAS call to arrival at the catheter laboratory to be 15 min and the mean time from first contact with the patient to arrival at Harefield Hospital to be 40 min. The crew, greeted at the door by a registrar and SHO, bring the patient directly to the catheter laboratory, discuss the ECGs and the case and usually watch the diagnostic angiogram and the procedure. For the paramedic teams, this immediate feedback and the positive stimulus of seeing a patient's blocked artery opened, within half-an-hour of arrival at the hospital is clearly much more rewarding than just delivering the patient to an A&E department. This feature has been vital to the sustainability of the PPCI programme. All members of the clinical team see the benefits, and can appreciate the importance of their own contribution. When the paramedics do not think the initial ECGs are diagnostic, or if the patient is very unstable, they have the option to take the patient to the nearest A&E department for assessment and stabilisation.

HILLINGDON HOSPITAL A&E DEPARTMENT

For patients who present themselves to Hillingdon Hospital A&E Department, are already in hospital, or are brought by LAS after non-diagnostic initial ECG, the referral process is a little more complicated than that of direct admission (Table 2). It had already been established as Hillingdon Hospital policy that patients presenting to A&E with chest pain should be triaged with an ECG within 10 min, because of the focus on delivering thrombolysis within 30 min. To implement the new regimen, the chest pain protocol was changed so that anyone eligible for thrombolysis would be referred for PPCI. Once a diagnosis of STEMI was suspected, patients would be treated with 300 mg aspirin and 600 mg clopidogrel and given a bolus of intravenous heparin. The A&E doctor, instead of administering thrombolysis would ring the on-call cardiology registrar at Harefield Hospital and refer the patient for PPCI. In cases of diagnostic difficulty, the ECGs might be faxed for review before the patient was accepted.

The inter-hospital transfer of patients raises different issues for the LAS. Once a patient has been brought by them to a hospital, or has presented to a hospital, the clinical responsibility for that patient lies with the hospital. It was, therefore, necessary to ensure that patient transfer to Harefield Hospital could be achieved rapidly and safely. In order to achieve the rapidity of transfer required, the 'critical transfer pathway' was used. This means that LAS treats

Table 2 Inter-hospital transfer protocol for PPCI from Hillingdon Hospital to Harefield Hospital

Immediate assessment
- Confirm diagnosis of AMI
- General haemodynamic assessment
- Assessment of pre-morbid state

Decision on PCI
- Made by A&E SHO usually as per thrombolysis
- Consent patient – not specifically for PCI but for transfer and angiography/PCI in general
- A&E SHO phones cardiology SpR at Harefield
- ECGs may be faxed for review and discussion
- Patient accepted

Mechanism of transfer
- Critical transfer ambulance called
- Transfer direct to Harefield catheter laboratory
- Harefield switchboard alerts catheter laboratory team

Immediate treatment
- Aspirin 300 mg p.o.
- Clopidogrel 300–600 mg p.o.
- Heparin 70–100 U/kg i.v.
- Morphine 2.5–10 mg + Maxalon 10 mg i.v.

Who accompanies patient?
- At first, a senior cardiac nurse or CCU nurse escorted the patient; after a few months experience, paramedic crews transferred patients without nurse escort

the call with the priority of a '999' call, rather than an 'urgent' inter-hospital transfer (which ambulance control treats less urgently).

'Sick patients' transferred between hospitals are usually accompanied by a nurse or doctor, because, for example, not all ambulance crews are able to administer resuscitation drugs. For an NHS Trust, this was naturally a difficult problem because of the infrequent and unpredictable timing of transfers. It was important that there was always enough cover for the wards/A&E (there being no financial scope for any additional staff). The senior cardiac nurse (previously the driving force behind the delivery of thrombolysis) took the lead in patient transfers. When a patient needed transfer between 9 am and 5 pm she would be called urgently and, whenever possible, would accompany the patient during the transfer. Out-of-hours, the transfer nurse would be one of the more senior CCU nurses. Once direct admission from LAS to Harefield Hospital had been established as the norm, however, the numbers involved in IHT have fallen, making it more difficult to justify having any 'spare' staff to provide this cover. As the ambulance service has become more confident, we have felt able to transfer patients from Hillingdon A&E Department to Harefield without an escort provided the paramedic crew are happy with this.

HAREFIELD HOSPITAL – DIRECT ADMISSION TO THE CATHETER LABORATORY FOR ANGIOGRAPHY

We decided that rapid provision for PPCI could only be achieved by direct admission to angiography. Since this was a hospital without an A&E department, many structural changes had to be planned and achieved, and we had to assume some diagnostic inaccuracy by the paramedics so that, inevitably, some patients with non-cardiac causes would be brought to Harefield Hospital (which only has cardiac and transplant physicians). The hospital, therefore, had to change its practice in order to be able to accept sick patients at very short notice. This required 'every cog in the wheel to change' – switchboard procedures, the admission process, bed allocation, nursing procedures, on-call arrangements and staffing levels. Although there had always been an existing 24-h service for inter-hospital transfers, some direct admissions for PPCI could now be expected to arrive with less than 10-min notice. It was established that the on-call catheter laboratory teams, including consultants, would be available immediately, with a target door-to-balloon time (arrival to successful revascularisation or demonstration that reperfusion had occurred) of 30 min. It was agreed that, for the first month of the service, all patients would be transferred to Harefield via Hillingdon A&E Department, in order for the process to be evaluated, paramedics to check their diagnostic skill and new admission protocols tested at Harefield Hospital. It was apparent very quickly that prompt angioplasty was deliverable.

Following the alert from the LAS, which gave the patient's age, sex and time of arrival, the protocol stated that the ambulance would be met by the duty registrar and SHO (both resident) and the catheter laboratory nurse. The LAS crew would have informed the patient during transit of what would happen; no patient in the first couple of years refused treatment. The registrar would check the patient's history and ECG en route to the catheter laboratory (on the ground floor and about 150 m from reception). Cases of doubt (in respect, for example, of age, diagnosis or co-morbid disease) are discussed with the consultant cardiologist who will usually arrive with or just after the ambulance. The catheter nurse, radiographer and physiology technician are non-resident but have to be in place and able to have the patient ready for the procedure within 30 min of the call. In practice, it has nearly always proved possible to open the laboratory, even at night, in 15–20 min and some staff choose to be in residence. In the event that two patients arrive at the same time, a ward area is available at all times to take the second patient, pending the subsequent availability of the catheter laboratory. This happened in 9 (4%) of the first 200 admissions. Staffing levels have been adjusted to take account of the unpredictable nature of such admissions and with the flow of patients now exceeding 40 per month, many individuals choose to live in when on-call. Salaries and on-call payments have been renegotiated to reflect this valuable service.

The initial prediction was that the first year would see about 100 patients treated at the heart attack centre. No increase in beds was envisaged though we felt that bed management might be the biggest challenge for our nurses and in relation to the general work. Only rarely did it prove necessary to activate programme closure (with the LAS diverting patients to the district general hospital for routine thrombolysis). From the first month, demand exceeded predictions and demand has grown year on year. A patient care plan was developed with the main tension being the question of length of stay (LOS) – providing a comprehensive service at Harefield Hospital against repatriating the patient at day 1 thereby reducing the pressure on precious tertiary centre beds. We did not have a clear discharge protocol at the outset of the service but we developed excellent lines of communication with Hillingdon Hospital. In 2005, the service was extended to outer NW Thames and more recently to SW Herts.

EVALUATION OF CHANGE ISSUES ENCOUNTERED IN ESTABLISHING PPCI

Every organisation involved in the PPCI pathway has had to undergo changes in thought processes or practice. Overall, the process has been remarkably smooth, which is a real testament to the motivation and enthusiasm of everyone involved.

There have been a number of benefits for Hillingdon Hospital with the introduction of the primary PCI service, chief, amongst others, being a reduction in costs and better access of other patient groups to consultant cardiologists. In the first year, the expenditure on thrombolytic drugs was more than £48,000 less than in the previous year. The mean LOS for STEMI patients has been reduced from 8.1 days to 3.7 days. In this group alone, this equates to a saving of more than 500 bed-days per year. Over the time period from the thrombolysis era to now, the hospital has reduced the number of acute medical beds by 60. In an age when there is a priority not to keep patients in A&E for more than 4 h, such a bed reduction can only be achieved with maximum efficiency in treatments. The days of having patients feeling well and waiting for up to 2 weeks for transfer for an in-patient coronary angiogram are, or should be, over. Patients with acute coronary syndromes generally have better access to urgent in-patient coronary angiography, as there has been a significant reduction in the number of patients waiting, and the waiting times. There has also been an increase in the access of acute patients with other cardiac problems to the cardiologists and the acute cardiac wards. In addition to the overwhelming benefit of the programme in improving treatment for acute STEMI patients, all other patients admitted with a primary cardiac diagnosis now come under the care of the cardiology team within 24 h and this has been achieved without any increase in the compliment of cardiologists.

There were some initial difficulties to be overcome in A&E and CCU. One of the A&E consultants was resistant to the introduction of PPCI, partly because the prevailing door-to-needle times were very good. Much effort had been expended into achieving this target, and it was a key indicator for A&E performance. Even careful planning fails to foresee every problem and concerns were voiced about the safety of transferring patients when one of the first patients died in the ambulance just on arrival at Harefield Hospital. The service was suspended for a week whilst everyone was reconvinced that the procedures were adequate and that the process was safe. The CCU nurses were reluctant to lose STEMI patients and their management with thrombolysis, as this represented their biggest patient group. Initially, there were concerns that there might be a reduction in CCU beds, staff cuts and a loss of their skills. However, the staff involved were able to understand the need for change, by reviewing the evidence for PPCI. Involving this key staff group in transferring patients to Harefield Hospital and then in watching the PPCI being performed rapidly and efficiently convinced them of the merits of the treatment. They themselves also developed new experience and the skills involved in transferring patients with a paramedic crew and in occasionally having to resuscitate patients en route. Inevitably there has been a change in patient profile on CCU and fewer nurses are now needed for the same number of beds, Patients with non-ST elevation acute coronary syndromes and other acute cardiac patients now have better access to CCU. In addition, the number of high-dependency medical patients has increased, although this has sometimes caused difficulties with the staffing numbers and skill mix of nurses.

The local PCT was very forward thinking and co-operative in the introduction of the PPCI programme. The CHD Local Implementation Group (set up after the NSF) were convinced by the case for PPCI and were very supportive to its introduction as a pilot study. The results of the pilot phase were reviewed at 6 months and, when the benefits were clearly demonstrated, they were happy to continue to fund the PPCI programme. The real-world data from the local audit, showing the proportion of STEMI patients who went on to have intervention and the delays involved, was an important argument in their decision. The group was also helpful in re-investing some of the cost savings outlined above into other areas of cardiology at Hillingdon Hospital, especially heart failure.

In the catheter laboratory, especially in relation to patients arriving within a couple of hours of the onset of symptoms, PPCI can be technically quite easy and the extra data provided by the angiogram assist in estimating a patient's risk. However, one has to be conscious of alternative diagnoses that can mimic or cause myocardial infarction (Table 3) though a non-STEMI diagnosis can prevent risky thrombolysis that such patients would have had otherwise. There is no age restriction but the very elderly, especially those with co-morbidities not necessarily fully evaluated in just a few minutes, do not always receive intervention. A sizeable minority of patients demonstrate a significant thrombus burden and others, probably because the procedure releases toxic radicals or thrombus into the distal vessels, demonstrate the phenomenon of 'no-reflow' (open artery, no flow). The unheralded arrival of potentially ill

Table 3 Diagnoses of patients presenting within the Harefield PPCI programme that did not need coronary intervention

Myocardial infarction not due to coronary thrombosis
Aortic dissection
Coronary artery dissection
Coronary embolism (from left atrium or through PFO)
Coronary spasm with drug abuse
Normal (near normal) coronary arteries
Patients who did not have myocardial infarction
Chest pain with LBBB
Chest pain, normal coronary arteries
Ruptured sinus of Valsalva
Coronary spasm
Myocarditis
Pericarditis, including cardiac tamponade
Cocaine abuse

patients increased our utilisation of ITU beds and forced us to implement CCU nurse training to bring intra-aortic balloon counter-pulsation, and CPAP management to our ward. By 2007, all but 2 of 40 cardiology beds at Harefield Hospital are now monitored beds, many operating at Level 2. There is little actual pressure on the cardiac surgeons directly, but the need for surgical back-up, especially in some rarer presentations like aortic dissection, is self-evident.

Patients and their relatives have made it clear that they are extremely impressed by the speed of treatment that includes assessment by a consultant cardiologist rather than only by non-specialised junior A&E doctors.

EARLY RESULTS OF PPCI AT HAREFIELD HOSPITAL

The PPCI programme began in March 2004 and we were able to deliver the programme goal of treatment delivery to all STEMI patients within 60 min of arrival at Harefield Hospital. Of patients admitted according to the PPCI protocol, 81% (290 of 358) underwent angioplasty, with nearly all of those having stent implantation. Twenty-five patients (7%) had normal coronary angiographic findings and 8% had coronary disease that either did not require intervention or needed elective urgent coronary bypass surgery. The various conditions encountered are presented in Table 3. Patients delivered directly by the LAS seemed to fare somewhat better than those who came via the A&E department at Hillingdon Hospital or elsewhere. Door-to-balloon times in the

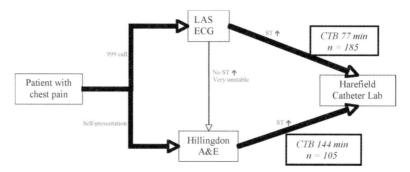

Fig. 2 Schematic diagram of pathway for patients with STEMI getting to the catheter laboratory for primary PCI. LAS, London Ambulance Service; STarrow, ST segment elevation on 12-lead ECG; CTB, median call-to-balloon time.

Table 4 Treatment times in Harefield PPCI programme. Historic thrombolysis data at Hillingdon (n = 183 patients) compared with the first 290 patients admitted to Harefield with confirmed myocardial infarction. Also shown, 30-day mortality for all three groups

	Thrombolysis (n = 183)	Inter-hospital transfer (n = 105)	Direct LAS (n = 185)
Symptom to needle/balloon	135 (85–225)	230 (175–394)	152 (102–255)
Call to needle/balloon	58 (49–73)	144 (124–184)	77 (68–90)
FPC to needle/balloon	46 (39–30)	131 (110–167)	68 (59–77)
First door to needle/balloon	18 (12–30)	97 (81–130)	24 (16–30)
30-day mortality	9.0%	7.8%	2.8%

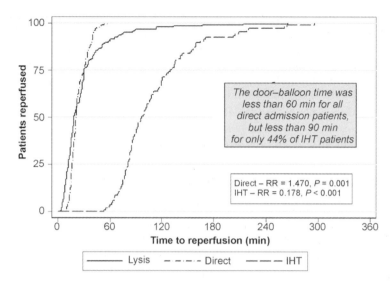

Fig. 3 Comparison of performance in treatment delivery represented in a Kaplan–Meier curve. The Hillingdon Hospital 2004 door-to-needle times are compared to direct LAS admissions and inter-hospital transfers (IHT). Direct LAS delivered PPCI provides a complete treatment strategy even faster than intravenous thrombolysis.

first 290 patients showed a mean of 27 min in all admissions, night and day; however, transferring a patient via A&E, even between well-informed and motivated departments, introduced a delay in treatment of at least 1 h (Figs 2 and 3). Our observational data show the lowest mortality to be in those patients admitted directly by the LAS from home (Table 4). The oldest patient treated was a 94-year-old woman, the youngest an 18-year-old man. The performance of the LAS was judged to be excellent, as it rarely delivered a patient with a normal ECG and no patients with serious non-cardiac illnesses were brought inappropriately to the specialist centre.

By mid-2007, about 45 patients a month were being referred, 60% of whom arrive outside of normal working hours. The impact on hospital stay has been dramatic. In relation to those patients with confirmed myocardial infarction, average stay has been reduced from 8.3 days to 3.7 days, releasing hundreds of bed-days (Fig. 4). The impact on Hillingdon Hospital has been even more

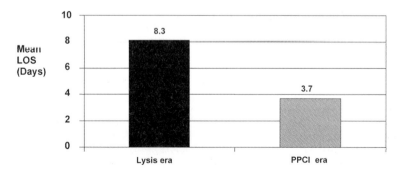

Fig. 4 Reduction in mean hospital length of stay (LOS) between thrombolysis era (2003) and the primary angioplasty era (2006).

pronounced with routine A&E targets improved beyond recognition. It is clear that the STEMI patients have been providing a significant burden to A&E.

All patients receive aspirin, clopidogrel and ReoPro® before angioplasty and by discharge most are on a cocktail (usually low dose) of ACE inhibitor, β–adrenergic blocker and statin. Ventricular function is assessed by echocardiography. Rehabilitation is discussed and all patients are offered programmed care either at Harefield or Hillingdon. All patients receive either a formal out-patient review, or telephone consultation if more appropriate, at about a month (also 6 months and annually thereafter) to check on patient information, clinical out-come and drug therapy.

DISCUSSION

Setting up a PPCI programme is not easy and PPCI is not to everyone's taste not least because consultants generally do not like to be working in the middle of the night only to have to report for duty as usual the following morning. Equally, patients, usually keen to be treated at their local hospital, have seen the advantage of rapid response and transfer and are almost uniformly in favour of travelling a little further to get the expertise and benefits of the PPCI team. That expertise requires elements including committed leadership, innovation, flexibility and team work, backed by senior management support, a commitment to explicit door-to-balloon times and data feedback to monitor progress. The key decision was to involve all interested parties (PCT, DGH, LAS and Harefield Hospital) at an early stage and to agree simple selection and treatment strategies. In both hospitals, all grades of staff were convinced of the quality-of-care benefits and these views were re-inforced by the obvious benefits individual patients demonstrated on a daily basis. At present perhaps only tertiary centres like Harefield can expect to have enough paramedical staff to run an effective on-call rota and together with the number of interventionists (on-call 1 in 5 at Harefield). Personnel issues may be the rate-limiting step for wide implementation of PPCI.

The CAPTIM and PRAGUE2 studies argue for equal or better results with 'early' thrombolysis.[5] However, the patients in these studies were treated at heart attack centres and 40% of those thrombolysed had early cross-over to PPCI; this does not match UK practice where patients predominantly do not have recourse to immediate PPCI. Good thrombolysis[9] is better than delayed (bad for outcomes) angioplasty as at some point the time taken to transfer and perform PPCI can be so delayed as even to lead to worse results.[10–12] The best available evidence suggests that PPCI loses its superiority over thrombolysis if door-to-balloon times exceed door-to-needle times by 60–90 min.[13,14] Time from the onset of infarction also matters but it is often difficult to be sure of when the clock starts. The patient history can be unreliable in this respect, and many patients present several hours after the onset of symptoms. When patients present very early, it may be difficult initially to establish a diagnosis of myocardial infarction. The population density and geography around Harefield allows of short ambulances journey times (half-hour or less), so our algorithm may not translate to such regions as Norfolk, Cornwall and Wales where preliminary thrombolytic therapy may well be more suitable strategies. What is clear, from such trials as CAPTIM and PRAGUE2, is that all patients with PPCI, even those potentially travelling large distances should be admitted to a heart attack centre to assess response to therapy and co-morbidity. On the other hand, patients with delayed pain-to-treatment times (greater than 3 or 4 h) may not benefit from PPCI as much as those subject to intervention somewhat earlier in the time course of their infarction. Our own results, whilst not randomised, support this concept with a lower mortality outcome of only 3% versus the 8% risk in the group 'delayed' by additional medical contact.

The role of the ambulance service is not to be understated; indeed, since 2006, nine infarct treatment centres, of which Harefield is one, cover the whole of London. Paramedics have the capacity to recognise myocardial infarction immediately and provide life-support during transfer. Without this triage, patients might not receive timely PPCI, whilst lack of confidence and over-triage could flood the heart attack centre with a host of patients who do not have myocardial infarction. Mis-triage (building delays which prevent either intervention) could be worse still. The evidence of our first 3 years of operations is that the LAS performs well with 83% of activations leading to immediate angiography. Our data, unrandomised and anecdotal, strongly support direct transfer of STEMI patients to a heart attack centre and with door-to-balloon times of less than 30 min, ambulance journeys of up to 60 min may be acceptable. Ambulance control rooms may not be able to cope with the dislocation such prolonged journeys involve even though STEMI transfer represents a mere fraction of the ambulance workload. Our experience, shared by others, demonstrates that despite the presence of committed and knowledgeable staff, an initial visit to an A&E department delays PPCI by about 1 h.

Myocardial infarction in the presence of either LBBB or ST depression carries a higher mortality risk than STEMI but these are more subtle clinical diagnoses that do not easily translate to LAS triage (though such possibilities are, nonetheless, under discussion for implementation London-wide in the foreseeable future). Acute myocardial infarction in patients with previous infarction, angioplasty or coronary bypass surgery can be challenging. Whilst it is clear that patients of all ages should be managed at a heart attack centre, the very elderly may not benefit even though they are at the highest risk – benefit may not be consistent across all age groups. A further question to be addressed is whether other severe coronary lesions, unrelated to the infarct vessel, should be treated during the index PPCI procedure. Such an approach would probably increase the potential risk but might reduce future risks. Clearly more trials are indicated.

CONCLUSIONS

A 'one-size-fits-all' strategy is neither practical nor advocated by these authors.[15] Thrombolysis should not be replaced by PPCI if the latter cannot be delivered within a couple of hours of first professional contact. Decisions on a national strategy seem blighted by lack of priority, funding and leadership. Ambulance services vary considerably, operational efficiency is under threat with ambulances travelling out of area (more ambulances equate to higher cost) and even in the LAS there are fears that the ambulances could be de-skilled with less paramedic crews. Local needs should be assessed and an optimal strategy designed for each region according to local geography and established facilities. The establishment of a PPCI service may be expensive if there is no infrastructure in place; PPCI does require more people and equipment than thrombolysis but, even though increased costs are of concern, it does lead to a more efficient, ultimately cheaper, evidence-based system that treats patients especially those at highest risk. The strategies of primary prevention of coronary disease may be reducing the prevalence of STEMI in under 75-year-olds, but acute coronary syndromes remain very common and eventually will be triaged much as STEMI is now. Improving outcomes for individuals with STEMI is an important health target and patients and the NHS can only benefit from increased implementation of PPCI programmes. The future for heart attack centres looks bright.

Key points for clinical practice

- European and US guidelines state: if immediately available, primary percutaneous coronary intervention (PPCI) should be performed in patients with ST segment elevation myocardial infarction (STEMI) or myocardial infarction with new or presumed new left bundle block who can undergo percutaneous coronary intervention of the infarct artery within 12 h of symptom onset.

- There is now a London-wide PPCI network. A 24-h service should be available to all patients in the UK.

- The treatment of acute myocardial infarction is time dependent and direct admission by ambulance to a heart attack centre will give best results. Even if ambulance journeys are long, patients will be delivered to specialist teams equipped with the resources to assess and treat each individual's needs.

- Timely PPCI can be achieved without an unacceptable increase in resources. Reperfusion strategies, PPCI or thrombolysis, should be dictated by local circumstances.

- Good thrombolysis is better than bad (late) angioplasty.

- Service change can be implemented quite easily in the NHS when all staff are motivated by improved patient outcomes.

- Innovations in service delivery should be monitored and adapted according to results and experience.

References

1. Rogers WJ, Canto JG, Lambrew CT, Tieffenbrunn AJ, Shoultz DA, Frederick PD. Temporal trends in the treatment of over 1.5 million patients with myocardial infarction in the US from 1990 through 1999: the National Registry of Myocardial Infarction 1, 2, and 3. *J Am Coll Cardiol* 2000; **36**: 2056–2063.
2. Task Force on the Management of Acute Myocardial Infarction of the European Society of Cardiology. Acute myocardial infarction: pre-hospital and in-hospital management.

Eur Heart J 1996; **17**: 43-63.

3. Birkhead JS, Weston C, Lowe D. Impact of specialty of admitting physician and type of hospital on care and outcome for myocardial infarction in England and Wales during 2004–5: observational study. *BMJ* 2006; **332**: 1306–1311.

4. Smith D, Channer K. Primary angioplasty should be first line treatment for acute myocardial infarction. *BMJ* 2004; **328**: 1254–1257.

5. Dalby M, Bouzamondo A, Lechat P, Montalescot G. Transfer for primary angioplasty versus immediate thrombolysis in acute myocardial infarction: a meta-analysis. *Circulation* 2003; **108**: 1809–1814.

6. Keeley EC, Boura JA, Grines CL. Primary angioplasty versus intravenous thrombolytic therapy for acute myocardial infarction: a quantitative review of 23 randomised trials. *Lancet* 2003; **361**: 13–20.

7. Vergel YB, Palmer S, Asseburg C *et al*. Is primary angioplasty cost effective in the UK? Results of a comprehensive decision analysis. *Heart* 2007; **93**: 1238–1243.

8. Hillis LD, Lange RA. Myocardial infarction and the open-artery hypothesis [Editorial]. *N Engl J Med* 2006; **355**: 2475–2477.

9. Verheugt F. Reperfusion therapy starts in the ambulance. *Circulation* 2006; **113**: 2377–2379.

10. De Luca G, Suryapranata H, Ottervanga VP, Antman EM. Time delay to treatment and mortality in primary angioplasty for acute myocardial infarction: every minute counts. *Circulation* 2004; **109**: 1023–1025.

11. Nallamothu BK, Bates ER. Percutaneous coronary intervention versus fibrinolyic therapy in acute myocardial infarction: is timing (almost) everything. *Am J Cardiol* 2003; **92**: 824–826.

12. Nallamothu BK, Fox KAA, Kennelly M *et al*. (on behalf of the GRACE investigators). Relationship of treatment delays and mortality in patients undergoing fibrinolysis and primary percutaneous coronary intervention. The Global Registry of Acute Coronary Events. *Heart* 2007; **93**: 1552–1555.

13. Terkelsen CJ, Lassen JF, Norgaard BL *et al*. Reduction of treatment delay in patients with ST-elevation myocardial infarction: impact of pre-hospital diagnosis and direct referral to primary percutaneous coronary intervention. *Eur Heart J* 2005; **26**: 770–777.

14. Asseburg C, Vergel YB, Palmer S *et al*. Assessing the effectiveness of primary angioplasty compared with thrombolysis and its relationship to time delay: a Bayesian evidence synthesis. *Heart* 2007; **93**: 1244–1250.

15. Faxon DP. Development of systems of care for ST-elevation myocardial infarction patients. Current state of ST-elevation myocardial infarction care. *Circulation* 2007; **116**: e29–e32.

Niall G. Keenan Dudley J. Pennell

10

Cardiovascular magnetic resonance of the atheromatous plaque: achievements, anticipated developments, clinical application

Atherosclerosis is the predominant cause of death and disability in the developed world today. Vessel wall imaging by cardiovascular magnetic resonance (CMR) is a relatively new and exciting technique for imaging atherosclerosis. It is used to identify atherosclerotic plaque, to characterise it (particularly in terms of vulnerability to rupture), and assess for plaque progression or regression, particularly in response to treatment. Much of the work that is described here involves the carotid arteries, but CMR can now image the coronary artery vessel wall.

Investigations for coronary artery disease (CAD) either indicate the functional importance of flow-limiting coronary stenoses (*e.g.* exercise electrocardiography [ECG]), or involve luminography for direct visualisation (*e.g.* coronary angiography). The presence of luminal stenoses implies thickening of the arterial wall, so a diagnosis of atherosclerosis is made, although the atherosclerosis itself remains invisible. Arterial wall imaging by CMR aims to make the atherosclerosis visible.

RATIONALE FOR VESSEL WALL IMAGING

It is well established that atherogenesis begins many years, even decades, before arterial stenoses develop, as the famous study of GIs in Vietnam demonstrated.[1] The first steps of the process, such as fatty streak formation, were identified in these young soldiers at post-mortem, at a stage when they could not be identified *in vivo* by coronary angiography. When an

Niall G. Keenan BM BCh MRCP (for correspondence)
Research Fellow, Cardiovascular Magnetic Resonance Unit, Royal Brompton Hospital, Sydney Street, London SW3 6NP, UK
E-mail: niall_keenan@hotmail.com

Dudley J. Pennell MD FRCP FESC FACC
Director Cardiovascular Magnetic Resonance Unit, Royal Brompton Hospital, Sydney Street, London SW3 6NP and Professor, Imperial College, London UK

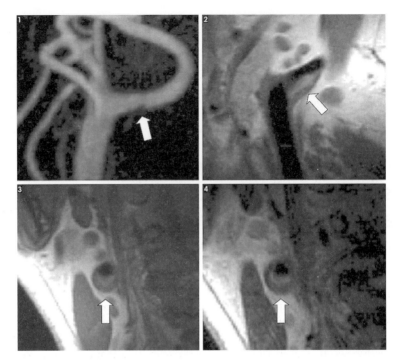

Fig. 1 Glagov remodelling *in vivo*. (1) MR angiogram. Targeted maximal intensity projection (MIP) of the right carotid artery bifurcation showing a 20–30% stenosis of the proximal right internal carotid artery. (2) A T1-weighted dark blood image longitudinal to the carotid bifurcation shows the plaque to be much larger than it appeared on the angiogram. (3,4) T1- and T2-weighted images perpendicular to the internal carotid artery show a large eccentric atherosclerotic plaque. The true degree of stenosis is 70%. In (4), the fibrous cap can be differentiated as an area of high signal adjacent to the lumen.

atherosclerotic plaque forms in the arterial wall and then begins to increase in size, it does not immediately start to intrude on and narrow the arterial lumen. In fact, the artery adapts, or 'remodels' outwards to make room for the plaque. In 1987, Glagov and colleagues[2] demonstrated this phenomenon in a series of left main stem coronary arteries at post mortem. They showed that in mild-to-moderate atherosclerosis, the lumen area increased with the amount of plaque present, so the greater the area of plaque, the greater the lumen area. The artery had remodelled outwards. However, in more severe disease, as plaques became larger, the lumen did then decrease in area. The point when the plaque began to intrude on the lumen occurred when about 40% of the vessel cross-section was occupied with plaque. The clear implication of this work was that many patients with 'normal' angiograms on luminography had atherosclerosis in the arterial wall (Fig. 1).[3]

WHICH PLAQUES RUPTURE?

This 'silent' atherosclerosis of the arterial wall became of greater interest when it was appreciated that a high proportion of myocardial infarctions were caused by the rupture of shallow, non-flow limiting plaques that might well be ignored on coronary angiography. It had generally been thought that atherosclerotic plaques grew by stages until, eventually, they occluded the arterial lumen. The paradigm was that angiography could identify patients 'at risk' of events by identifying high-grade stenoses. However, a case series of patients with myocardial infarction who had had a previous angiogram and were then re-studied at the time of the infarction showed that in 78% of the patients the culprit lesion was less than 70% stenosed at the time of the previous angiogram, in many cases much less than 70%.[4] This revealed further limitations of luminography.

CARDIOVASCULAR MAGNETIC RESONANCE

Cardiovascular magnetic resonance (CMR) is the term used for magnetic resonance imaging (MRI) applied to the heart and vasculature. MRI is a non-invasive imaging modality that acquires images using high-powered magnets and radiofrequency waves. Ionising radiation is not used, there are no known adverse direct effects. MR contrast media have an excellent safety profile compared with iodinated X-ray contrast media, although a small risk of nephrogenic systemic fibrosis exists with the older-generation, linear MR contrast agents in patients with severe renal failure.

The scanner is usually a 'doughnut' shape. This comprises a supercooled cylindrical electromagnet and a radiofrequency transmitter and receiver, known as 'coils'. The transmitter coil is built into the bore of the magnet. The receiver coil is placed as close as possible to the patient, either built into the table they lie on, or laid upon the region of interest.

The physics of image formation is complex.[5] In essence, when a patient lies in the bore of the magnet, all the protons in the body (mainly in water molecules) align with the magnetic field. When the transmitter coil is turned on, it releases a pulse of radiofrequency energy that knocks the protons out of alignment. The protons return to alignment with the strong magnetic field; as they do so, they release a small amount of radiofrequency energy. This is referred to as the 'echo', and it is picked up by the receiver coil. The more water in a tissue, the more protons, and the greater the echo. This is the basis of how MRI is used to characterise tissue.

In order to work out where in the tissue the signal is coming from, various techniques are used, generically referred to as 'spatial encoding'. For example, the magnetic field strength differs slightly from one end of the magnet to the other, so that different parts of the tissue produce an echo at slightly different radiofrequencies.

Different types of radiofrequency pulses are used to image different aspects of tissue. These are referred to as 'sequences'. For example, some sequences are designed to show fat as bright, whereas others show fat as dark. There are many sequences of which two well-known examples are spin echo and gradient echo.

CMR was first described for vessel wall imaging in 1982. Attempts to characterise atheromatous plaque by CMR began with *ex vivo* studies of specimens of iliac artery;[6] within a short time, the first clinical studies were performed.[7] Over the last 25 years, development has been rapid, following advances in MRI scanner, hardware and software technology. The majority of

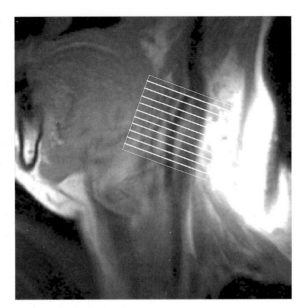

Fig. 2 T1-weighted fast spin echo CMR image. Longitudinal section through the carotid bifurcation, indicating the slice positions for vessel wall imaging in the carotid bifurcation. A typical pilot image used to acquire a series of images such as those shown in Figure 4.

this work has concentrated on the carotid arteries as they are large, relatively immobile, and near the surface (Figs 2–4). The aortic wall has also been studied. More recent work has examined the coronary artery wall.

Plaque imaging has been extensively validated. This was done initially by imaging *ex vivo* arteries, and comparing images with histology (Fig. 5).

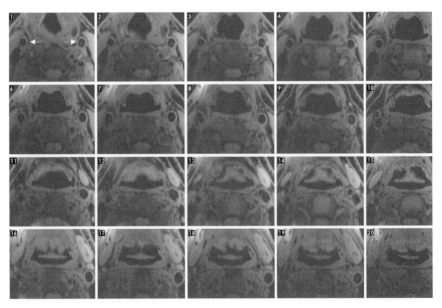

Fig. 3 T1-weighted fast spin echo CMR images. A series of 20 contiguous slices through the carotid bifurcations bilaterally. The carotid arteries are arrowed in image 1.

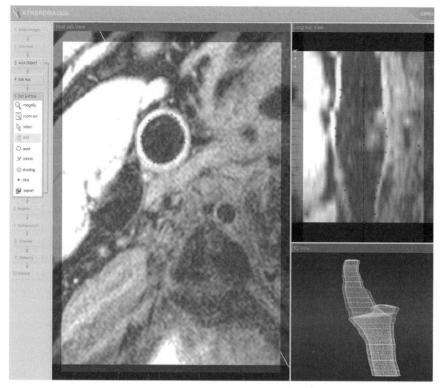

Fig. 4 The user interface of a semi-automated software solution used to model the carotid arterial wall at the bifurcation (AtheromaTools, a plug in of CMRTools, CVIS Ltd, London, UK). This sort of analysis is essential for quantitative work, such as studies of plaque regression.

However, the majority of this work has involved imaging patients' carotid arteries before carotid endarterectomy, and then comparing the images with histological images of the excised plaque. Many studies of this type have been performed, and they have refined the accuracy of carotid CMR for characterising plaque morphology and composition.

PLAQUE CHARACTERISATION BY CMR

The understanding that plaque composition is as important as plaque size in causing clinical events led to efforts to characterise plaque. A large plaque with a thick fibrous cap and a small lipid core is stable and highly unlikely to rupture and cause vessel occlusion. Conversely, a smaller plaque with a thin fibrous cap, a large lipid core and areas of dense neovascularisation and inflammation is more unstable. MRI is an ideal tool for plaque imaging because its high degree of soft tissue contrast means that lipid and fibrous tissue can be distinguished.

Initial studies used only one MRI 'weighting'. For example, using only T2-weighted imaging, Serfaty and colleagues[8] were able to classify *ex vivo* plaque according to the American Heart Association (AHA) classification with a sensitivity of 67–90% and a specificity of 85–100%.

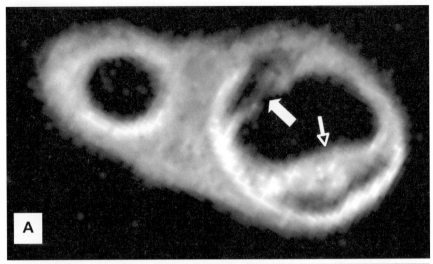

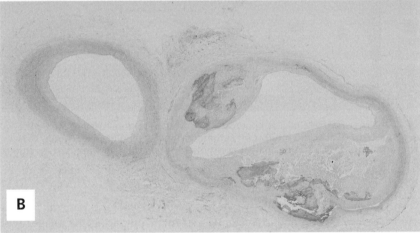

Fig. 5 *Ex vivo* correlation of carotid plaque histology with CMR. (A) High-resolution, T1-weighted, fast spin echo CMR of an *ex vivo* carotid artery – transverse section immediately above the carotid bifurcation, external carotid artery to the left and internal carotid artery to the right. Two plaques are present, one with a thin/ruptured fibrous cap (large arrow), the other with a thick fibrous cap (small arrow). (B) Matched hematoxylin and eosin (H&E) histological section.

The first attempt to characterise plaque *in vivo* was performed in 1996. Toussaint and co-workers[9] demonstrated an excellent correlation between *in vivo* and *ex vivo* T2 relaxation times for areas of fibrous cap and lipid core in carotid plaque of 6 patients undergoing endarterectomy, showing that the *ex vivo* work was clinically applicable.

The ability of CMR to discriminate between tissue components was not fully utilised as only one contrast weighting (T2) was used. Imaging the same tissue several times with different contrast weightings, and then combining the information enables a much greater degree of tissue characterisation to be performed. This process is called multicontrast, or 'multispectral' imaging.

Table 1 Signal characteristics of different tissues by CMR

Sequence weighting	Signal intensity by tissue component			
	Fibrous cap	Lipid core	Calcification	Thrombus
T1	Intermediate	High	Low	Variable
T2	Intermediate	Low	Low	Variable
Proton density	Intermediate	High	Low	Variable
Time of flight	Intermediate	Low	Low	Variable

Algorithms have been drawn up to combine information from several scans. An example is shown as Table 1.

MULTISPECTRAL IMAGING

By improving tissue characterisation, multispectral MRI provides better lesion-type classification. A large and typical study by Cai and colleagues,[10] looking at the carotid arteries of 60 patients before endarterectomy, showed that multispectral CMR correlates well with the AHA classification with an accuracy of 80.2%.

Table 2 Conventional and modified American Heart Association classification of atherosclerotic plaque

Plaque type	Histological appearance	CMR plaque type	CMR appearance
Type I	Initial lesion with foam cells	Type I–II	Near-normal wall thickness, no calcification
Type II	Fatty streak with multiple foam cell layers		
Type III	Pre-atheroma with extracellular lipid pools	Type III	Diffuse intimal thickening or small eccentric plaque with no calcification
Type IV	Atheroma with a confluent extracellular lipid core	Type IV–V	Plaque with a lipid or necrotic core surrounded by fibrous tissue
Type V	Fibro-atheroma with possible calcification		
Type VI	Complex plaque with possible surface defect, haemorrhage, or thrombus	Type VI	Complex plaque with possible surface defects, haemorrhage, or thrombus
Type VII	Calcified plaque	Type VII	Calcified plaque
Type VIII	Fibrotic plaque without lipid core	Type VIII	Fibrotic plaque without lipid core and with possible small calcifications

Adapted from Cai et al.[10]

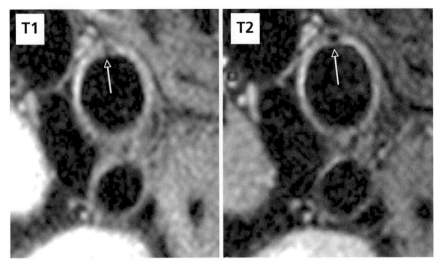

Fig. 6 Very early plaque on the posterior aspect of the right internal carotid artery. T1-weighted image (left) and T2-weighted image (right). The fibrous cap can be seen, overlying an area of calcification which is of low signal on both T1- and T2-weighted images.

Sensitivity ranged from 67–84%, with specificity between 90–100%.[10] The standard AHA plaque classification was adapted for CMR (Table 2; Figs 6 and 7).

FIBROUS CAP THICKNESS AND INTEGRITY

Fibrous cap rupture is the key event in the development of many of the clinical syndromes of atherosclerosis. It is usually presumed to have occurred and not

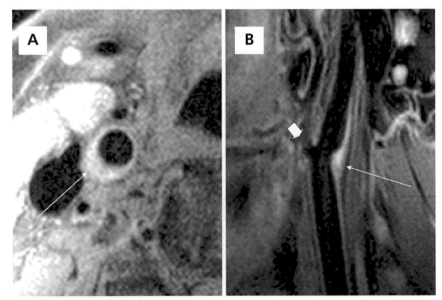

Fig. 7 T1-weighted, fast spin echo CMR image. A moderate plaque is seen in short axis (A) and in long axis (B) at the carotid bifurcation (long arrow). The origin of the external carotid artery can be seen (arrowhead). The plaque is of uniform intermediate signal indicating fibrous tissue. This is a very typical site for plaque development.

sought out specifically, as techniques like intravascular ultrasound (IVUS) are needed for its identification. The first CMR study to assess fibrous cap integrity was performed *ex vivo* in 1998. Using carotid endarterectomy specimens, and only one MRI weighting, Winn and co-workers[11] showed that CMR was 90% specific for identifying the presence of a fibrous cap, and 98% specific for detecting cap rupture, but the sensitivities were much lower (37% for presence of cap and 12% for identification of rupture). For a non-invasive method of plaque imaging, however, a high degree of sensitivity is essential, as the technique needs to identify patients with unstable plaque reliably. Fortunately, progress has been made over the last decade,[11] and improvements in resolution and multispectral imaging have enabled the thickness of the fibrous cap to be measured *in vivo*, giving an indication of plaque stability. In a study of 22 endarterectomy patients, CMR classification of fibrous cap as intact or ruptured correlated with histology with a sensitivity of 89% and a specificity of 96%. When plaques were subdivided into 'intact and thick' or 'intact and thin' or 'ruptured', CMR findings were 89% accurate.[12]

LIPID-RICH NECROTIC CORE

The presence of a lipid core is another marker of a vulnerable plaque. The size of the lipid core is also important, and may itself be an end-point in therapeutic trials. In 101 sections from 18 endarterectomy patients, the sensitivity and specificity of CMR for lipid-rich necrotic core were 98% and 100%, respectively. However, this analysis excluded lipid-rich necrotic cores that were subsequently found on histology to contain intraplaque haemorrhage. If these plaques were included, sensitivity and specificity dropped to 85% and 92%, respectively. Plaque haemorrhage is a challenge for CMR, but an important marker of instability.[13] Quantification of lipid core by CMR correlates well with histology.[14]

PLAQUE HAEMORRHAGE/THROMBUS IMAGING

As well as the thickness of the fibrous cap and the presence of a lipid-rich necrotic core, another indicator of plaque rupture or instability is the presence of haemorrhage or thrombus. If a haemorrhage has occurred into a plaque, then by definition the plaque is unstable. Adherent thrombus is also a sign of instability as it indicates that the plaque is in some way disrupted. Plaque haemorrhage is not a one-off event leading to vessel occlusion and a clinical syndrome. Although this does occur, small plaque haemorrhages can occur silently. Intraplaque haemorrhage is implicated in plaque growth and is a strong stimulus to repair (which leads to plaque expansion), inflammation and neovascularisation, weakening the plaque further. Thrombus has iron-containing breakdown products of haemoglobin, which have paramagnetic contrast properties. However, CMR of intraplaque haemorrhage presents a particular challenge because the signal intensity of the haemorrhage varies widely depending on its age. As shown in Table 3, a recent haemorrhage can be of high signal in all four of the common CMR weightings, while an old haemorrhage can be of low signal on all weightings, making it difficult to distinguish from calcification.

Table 3 MRI/histology criteria: intraplaque haemorrhage

Age of haem.	Erythrocytes	Histology	MRI		
			T1-w	T2-w/PDW	ToF
Fresh	Intact with intracellular methaemo-globin	Lymphocytes, neutrophils, scattered macrophages	Hyper-intense	Hypo-intense/ iso-intense	Hyper-intense
Recent	Lytic with extracellular methaemo-globin	Macrophage clusters, giant cells, cholesterol crystals, peripheral angiogenesis	Hyper-intense	Hyper-intense	Hyper-intense
Old	Amorphous	Amorphous debris with hemosiderin; no inflammatory reaction	Hypo-intense	Hypo-intense	Hypo-intense

haem. = haemorrhage; w = weighted; ToF = Time of flight

Adapted from Chu et al.[15]

In spite of these difficulties, Chu et al.[15] were able to identify intraplaque haemorrhage with a sensitivity of 90% and a specificity of 74% in 27 endarterectomy patients. Intraplaque haemorrhage was present in 77% of locations sampled. Haemorrhage into an atherosclerotic plaque can be subdivided into haemorrhage into the necrotic core without rupture of the fibrous cap, and haemorrhage or thrombus formation adjacent to the lumen (usually associated with a ruptured cap). This distinction has proved useful because haemorrhage without fibrous cap rupture has not been associated with clinical events whereas rupture with juxtaluminal thrombus or haemorrhage has, because it indicates on-going instability (erosion, rupture, ulceration) of the fibrous cap. CMR was able to differentiate between these two lesion types with an accuracy of 96%. In this study, the overall sensitivity and specificity of CMR for detection of thrombus had improved to 96% and 82%, respectively.[16]

USE OF CONTRAST AGENTS

In addition to multispectral imaging, the use of extrinsic intravenous contrast has improved plaque characterisation by CMR. The standard MRI contrast agent is gadolinium bound to a chelate. Gadolinium is a rare earth metal. It has a very short T1 time constant, giving water that comes into proximity with it high signal intensity on an appropriate MRI sequence.

Gadolinium is most commonly used for MR angiography (MRA), which is often performed in patients with carotid artery disease. It is also routinely used in CMR for imaging myocardial infarction and fibrosis. After injection, the contrast initially remains in the vascular space and so can demonstrate areas of vascularity in plaque, a marker of vulnerability. After the initial vascular phase, gadolinium chelate moves into the extracellular space, being more concentrated in areas where the extravascular space is expanded, such as in scar tissue, or the fibrous cap. In the Cai *et al.* study[14] of lipid rich necrotic core and fibrous cap, intravenous gadolinium contrast was used to improve tissue characterisation between the fibrous cap and the lipid core. After contrast, different types of fibrous cap could be differentiated. Of sections, 56% had collagen-rich fibrous caps. Of these, all those with moderate gadolinium enhancement were assessed histologically to be stable, whereas all those with strong enhancement after contrast had evidence of neovascularisation or inflammatory infiltrate. Of the 44% of patients with fibrous cap made of loose matrix, all had strong gadolinium enhancement (Fig. 8).[17]

CLINICAL CORRELATION

Developments in plaque imaging over the last 10 years have been rapid, but what effect have these advances had on patient care? Several studies have begun to show how a clinical role for this technology may develop, of which three are described for illustration. A 2002 study of fibrous cap rupture correlated carotid scan appearances with clinical history in 53 patients. Patients identified by CMR as having a ruptured fibrous cap were more likely to have had a transient ischaemic attack (TIA) or stroke than those with an intact, thick cap. Of patients with a ruptured plaque by CMR, 70% had symptoms, compared with 7% of patients with intact, thick caps. Compared

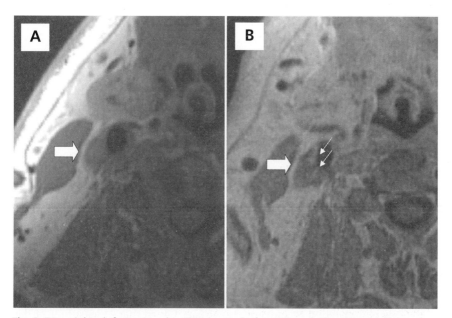

Fig. 8 T1-weighted, fast spin echo CMR image before (A) and after (B) gadolinium contrast. A large eccentric plaque in the right common carotid artery is shown (large arrows). Two small areas enhance after contrast administration (small arrows), suggesting regions of increased vascularity and possible plaque instability.

with patients with thick fibrous caps, patients with ruptured caps were 23 times more likely to have had a recent TIA or stroke.[18] As well as fibrous cap thickness, intraplaque haemorrhage has been correlated with clinical events, and also plaque growth. Of 29 patients with carotid plaque who were followed by serial CMR over 18 months, 14 had intraplaque haemorrhage by CMR at baseline. In these patients, vessel wall volume and lipid-rich necrotic core volume increased, but they stayed the same or reduced in patients without haemorrhage. In addition, plaques with haemorrhage were more likely to develop new plaque haemorrhages during follow-up (43% versus 0%), because of on-going plaque instability, indicating that plaque haemorrhage is a marker of vulnerable plaque.[19] Plaque haemorrhage has been correlated with clinical events in a larger study of 154 patients with asymptomatic 50–79% carotid stenosis by ultrasonography. There were 12 anterior circulation cerebrovascular events ipsilateral to the index carotid plaque over a mean of 38 months of follow-up after the CMR study. The hazard ratio (HR) for cerebrovascular accident (CVA) was 17.0 for plaque with thin or ruptured fibrous cap, and 5.2 for intraplaque haemorrhage, with an increase in hazard ratio of 2.6 for every 10-mm^2 increase in intraplaque haemorrhage area. There was also an increase in HR of 1.6 for every 10% increase in the plaque percentage of lipid-rich or necrotic core.[20]

Current guidelines for carotid endarterectomy are based on percentage stenosis as assessed by ultrasonography. The North American Symptomatic Carotid Endarterectomy Trial (NASCET) criteria state that carotid endarterectomy should be recommended to patients with symptomatic carotid stenosis of 70–99%.[21] CMR studies show that these criteria are a rather blunt tool for patient selection for an operation that carries considerable risks. Patients with unstable plaque but less than 70% stenosis are excluded, while patients with greater than 70% stenosis and stable plaque are recommended for surgery. In these patients, the unstable plaque may be further down the common carotid artery (as recent MR-PET work has shown). Improving patient selection for surgery improves outcomes as those most likely to benefit are operated, while those who are unlikely to benefit are excluded. CMR carotid plaque assessment has a key role to play in patients with TIA and stroke.

In the longer term, and with wider availability, this approach may prove of clinical use in other patients currently assessed by carotid ultrasonography, such as older patients being worked up for coronary artery bypass grafting. The ideal is to identify patients before symptoms develop. The numbers of 'at-risk' patients are so large that a CMR-based screening programme for unstable carotid plaque is not feasible. However, if reliable serum markers of plaque instability were available, the prospect would be more appealing. Recent practice in the US following the Asymptomatic Carotid Atherosclerosis Study (ACAS) was to offer carotid endarterectomy to patients with a carotid stenosis of 60–99%, who had had no symptoms.[22] In this trial, the event rate in the unoperated cohort was only 11% at 2.7 years, and it has been estimated that 40 operations were needed to prevent one stroke. Given that at least half of the 150,000 endarterectomies performed in the US each year are done for stenoses that have never been symptomatic, it is clear that CMR could have a clinical role.[23]

THERAPEUTIC STUDIES WITH CMR END-POINTS

As well as plaque characterisation, CMR plaque imaging parameters have been used as the primary end-points in clinical trials. Although a research application, these are some of the most exciting developments in the field of atherosclerosis research. Studies of this type have been among the first to show atherosclerosis regression. Similar studies with coronary intravascular ultrasonography (IVUS) require repeated cardiac catheterisation, with the associated risks, contrast dose and radiation exposure. External ultrasound studies are limited by poor reproducibility, usually requiring more patients. Quantitative studies require a method of reproducibly measuring the degree of atherosclerosis present. This is done for MR images by tracing the outer and inner arterial walls, and so measuring the lumen and vessel wall areas. This can be done for one 'slice' placed perpendicularly to an artery, ideally near a landmark (such as the carotid bifurcation) so that it can be easily repeated in subsequent studies. Each slice has a predetermined thickness (usually 2 mm in the carotid), so is a 3-D volume. If several contiguous slices are acquired, then the lumen and wall volume of an artery can be modelled along a set length of the artery. Increased sampling increases accuracy, and so reproducibility. The first example of a study of this type showed that simvastatin caused regression of atherosclerotic lesions in the aorta and carotid arteries of 18 patients followed for 1 year by CMR.[24] At 2 years, the results were expressed in terms of vessel wall thickness (similar to an ultrasound intima-media thickness [IMT]), and vessel wall area. There had been a 16% reduction in aortic vessel wall thickness (at the thickest point) and a 16% reduction in vessel wall area. There was no change in vessel wall thickness at the thinnest point. The same was found in the carotid artery, with a 19% reduction in vessel wall thickness, and an 18% reduction in the vessel wall area. Again, there was no difference in vessel wall thickness at the thinnest part. This illustrates a strength of the technique in that differential change around the arterial wall can be measured, which is not possible with the standardised ultrasonography technique. Simvastatin caused the vessel wall area to reduce by nearly one-fifth. The reduction in vessel wall area was not matched by a similar increase in lumen area. In fact, the increase in lumen area was comparatively modest at +6% in the aorta and +5% in the carotid. The arterial wall remodelled outwards in response to atherosclerosis, and in response to atherosclerosis regression, the vessel wall remodels inwards, with the lumen left comparatively unaffected.[25]

The power of this technique can be shown by a further study of plaque regression in patients randomised to simvastatin 80 mg or 20 mg. Although only 27 patients were randomised, the study demonstrated positive results in 6 months. Comparable ultrasonography studies often need to recruit several thousand patients and follow them for several years. Imaging the thoracic aorta, the authors showed a 12% reduction in plaque volume with high-dose statin, with no significant change in lumen volume. So, if this study had been performed with a purely luminographic technique, the results would have been negative.[26]

With improvements in imaging, studies of plaque regression are now starting to focus on individual plaque components rather than crude measures of overall vessel wall volume, area or thickness. An example of this approach is the Orion study. In this study comparing 40 mg with 5 mg rosuvastatin, the authors measured the carotid artery wall volume, but also the volume of the lipid core. The interim results show a reduction of the lipid core volume of 35.5%, although this did not quite achieve significance ($P = 0.06$).[27] Nevertheless, the approach seems likely to bear fruit, as reduction in the lipid core not only indicates plaque regression, but may also indicate stabilisation.

CORONARY VESSEL WALL IMAGING

The majority of the CMR work described so far has focused on the carotid artery partly because it is comparatively easy to image. The coronary artery is a more difficult target, but is of great interest to cardiologists. The coronary arteries are difficult to image by CMR because they are small, tortuous, not near the surface, and because they move with cardiac and respiratory motion. A coronary artery may have an external diameter of 5 mm, and yet move 5 cm with inspiration. CMR techniques are not yet sufficiently good to image the coronary artery wall with a single-shot imaging technique; therefore, the image needs to be built up over a number of cardiac cycles, for each of which the heart (and, therefore, the diaphragm) need to be in the same position. The first paper to demonstrate that CMR could characterise the coronary artery wall was published in 2000. The images were acquired during a breath-hold and imaging was performed over 12–18 cardiac cycles to get enough information to create an image. A special 'fat suppression' prepulse was used to reduce signal from the fat around the coronary artery so that the vessel wall could be clearly seen. Using coronary angiography as the gold standard, the authors demonstrated that CMR was able to identify a normal thin-walled vessel, and an eccentric plaque.[28] More recently, the first large study showing the clinical utility of this approach has been published.[29] In this study, CMR coronary artery vessel wall imaging was performed on 136 patients with type I diabetes, not previously known to have cardiovascular disease. Diagnostic quality coronary artery CMR images were obtained from 96% of patients. These authors did not correlate CMR findings with angiography as a gold standard because angiography was not indicated in this cohort. Instead, they measured the coronary artery wall thickness and the presence of stenoses by CMR and correlated these with diabetic nephropathy as indicated by proteinuria as an indicator of severity of diabetes. Coronary artery stenoses were identified in 10% of patients with nephropathy, and in no patients without. Also, the maximum right coronary artery wall thickness was 2.2 mm in patients with nephropathy and 1.6 mm in those without. Both differences were statistically significant. The authors describe this approach as measuring 'coronary plaque burden'. Previously, coronary artery calcification (CAC) scoring by computed tomography (CT) was also described in a similar way. A limitation of CAC by CT is that the test is normal unless these is calcification in the coronary arteries, so 'soft plaque' may be missed. Using CMR to assess the general degree of thickening of the coronary arteries is an appealing way of assessing the coronary plaque burden. Therapeutic studies assessing plaque regression in the coronary arteries may be possible.

NEWER APPROACHES

CMR provides good anatomical detail of atherosclerotic plaques, but it may be useful to combine CMR with other techniques which map functional and metabolical changes. Two methods used are multimodality imaging, and molecular imaging.

Positron emission tomography (PET) imaging uses a radioactive glucose isotope (^{18}F-fluorodeoxyglucose [^{18}FDG]), which is injected into the patient and taken up by metabolically active tissue, where it can be imaged by a PET scanner. The technique was originally developed for neuro-imaging and for identification of malignancy. In these scans, a common source of artefact was atherosclerotic plaques, particularly in the aorta, which were metabolically active and so took up ^{18}FDG. It was not possible to characterise the plaques in any detail from these images because of the low amount of anatomical detail and the comparatively poor spatial resolution of PET (about 5 mm).

Combining PET and CMR gives functional information from PET that can be transposed onto the anatomical map supplied by CMR. Combining the images requires co-registration, and it relies on the patient being in the same posture (a special cushion is used), and then various anatomical landmarks (such as the spinal cord) are identified on both scans. In a study of 12 patients with recent TIA and an ipsilateral high-grade carotid stenosis, CMR identified a lesion with high ^{18}FDG uptake at the site of the stenosis in 7 patients (58%). In the remaining 5 patients, ^{18}FDG uptake in the targeted lesion was low. In 3 of these 5 patients, MR-PET identified another different lesion with a high level of ^{18}FDG uptake, but without high-grade stenosis, in a vascular territory compatible with the patients' TIA.[30] This adds further credence to the paradigm that guidelines for carotid endarterectomy based purely on percentage stenosis fail to address a significant proportion of culprit lesions. This conclusion can be extrapolated to the coronary arteries.

Another approach is the use of molecular contrast agents. Ultra-small particles of iron oxide (USPIOs) have the combined properties of being taken up by macrophages, and of being visible by CMR, as iron particles cause low signal intensity on CMR images. Macrophages are present in inflamed (and, therefore, vulnerable) plaque. When USPIOs were injected into 30 patients before carotid endarterectomy, they were detectable in plaque in 24 of the 27 patients with analysable images. When this was compared with the presence of USPIOs in plaque at histology after surgery, CMR had a sensitivity and specificity of 93% and 64%, respectively, for the presence of USPIOs.[31] Using markers such as USPIOs to elucidate what is taking place at the cellular and molecular level is an approach that is rapidly spreading throughout the life sciences, with clinical developments to be expected.

CONCLUSIONS

CMR arterial wall imaging is a new addition to the array of tools available to image atherosclerosis. It is non-invasive and uses no ionising radiation. It is not limited to luminography, and has many advantages over ultrasonography. Detailed atherosclerotic plaque characterisation is currently possible in the carotid artery, and has been correlated with clinical events. In research, CMR arterial indices have been used as the primary end-points of therapeutic trials in atherosclerosis, and have been used to show plaque regression. Coronary artery wall imaging is also possible. Multimodality imaging, such as MR-PET, and molecular imaging are currently under active development and will further increase the importance of non-invasive imaging in the management of atherosclerosis.

Key points for clinical practice

- Cardiovascular magnetic resonance (CMR) is ideally suited to imaging atherosclerotic plaque because it is a non-invasive technique with excellent soft-tissue contrast.

- CMR can characterise atherosclerotic plaque morphology, composition and stability *in vivo*.

- CMR assessment of carotid plaque stability correlates with clinical events such as transient ischaemic attack and stroke.

- Arterial wall CMR has been used as the primary outcome measure of clinical trials where it has demonstrated plaque regression with statins.

- CMR of coronary artery plaque is possible and is in development.

- CMR can be combined with other imaging modalities such as positron emission tomography to assess atherosclerotic plaque at a functional level.

References

1. MacNamara JJ, Molot MA, Stremple JF, Cutting RT. Coronary artery disease in combat casualties in Vietnam. *JAMA* 1971; **216**: 1185–1187.
2. Glagov S, Weisenberg E, Zarins CK, Stanunavicius R, Kolettis GJ. Compensatory enlargement of human atherosclerotic coronary arteries. *N Engl J Med* 1987; **316**: 1371–1375.
3. Keenan NG, Pennell DJ, Mohiaddin RH. Glagov remodelling in the atherosclerotic carotid artery by cardiovascular magnetic resonance. *Heart* 2008; **94**: 228.
4. Ambrose JA, Tannenbaum MA, Alexopoulos D *et al*. Angiographic progression of coronary artery disease and the development of myocardial infarction. *J Am Coll Cardiol* 1988; **12**: 56–62.
5. Weishaupt D, Koechli VD, Marincek B. *How Does MRI Work?: An Introduction to the Physics and Function of Magnetic Resonance Imaging*, 2nd edn. Berlin: Springer, 2006.
6. Crooks L, Sheldon P, Kaufman L, Rowan W. Quantification of obstructions in vessels by nuclear magnetic resonance (NMR). *IEEE Trans Nucl Sci* 1982; **NS-29**: 1181–1185.
7. Herfkens RJ, Higgins CB, Hricak H *et al*. Nuclear magnetic resonance imaging of atherosclerotic disease. *Radiology* 1983; **148**: 161–166.
8. Serfaty JM, Chaabane L, Tabib A, Chevallier JM, Briguet A, Douek PC. Atherosclerotic plaques: classification and characterization with T2-weighted high-spatial-resolution MR imaging – an *in vitro* study. *Radiology* 2001; **219**: 403–410.
9. Toussaint J-F, LaMuraglia GM, Southern JF, Fuster V, Kantor HL. Magnetic resonance images lipid, fibrous, calcified, hemorrhagic, and thrombotic components of human atherosclerosis *in vivo*. *Circulation* 1996; **94**: 932–938.
10. Cai J-M, Hatsukami TS, Ferguson MS, Small R, Polissar NL, Yuan C. Multicontrast magnetic resonance imaging classification of human carotid atherosclerotic lesions with *in vivo*. *Circulation* 2002; **106**: 1368–1373.
11. Winn WB, Schmiedl UP, Reichenbach DD *et al*. Detection and characterization of atherosclerotic fibrous caps with T2-weighted MR. *Am J Neuroradiol* 1998; **19**: 129–134.
12. Hatsukami TS, Ross R, Polissar NL, Yuan C. Visualisation of fibrous cap thickness and rupture in human atherosclerotic plaque *in vivo* with high-resolution magnetic resonance imaging. *Circulation* 2000; **102**: 959–964.
13. Yuan C, Mitsumori LM, Ferguson MS *et al*. *In vivo* accuracy of multispectral magnetic resonance imaging for identifying lipid-rich necrotic cores and intraplaque haemorrhage

in advanced human carotid plaques. *Circulation* 2001; **104**: 2051–2056.

14. Cai J, Hatuskami TS, Ferguson MS *et al*. *In vivo* quantitative measurement of intact fibrous cap and lipid-rich necrotic core size in atherosclerotic carotid plaque. *Circulation* 2005; **112**: 3437–3444.

15. Chu B, Kampschulte A, Ferguson MS *et al*. Hemorrhage in the atherosclerotic carotid plaque: a high-resolution MRI study. *Stroke* 2004; **35**: 1079–1084.

16. Kampschulte A, Ferguson MS, Kerwin WS *et al*. Differentiation of intraplaque versus juxtaluminal hemorrhage/thrombus in advanced human carotid atherosclerotic lesions by *in vivo* magnetic resonance imaging. *Circulation* 2004; **110**: 3239–3244.

17. Cai J, Hatsukami TS, Ferguson MS *et al*. *In vivo* quantitative measurement of intact fibrous cap and lipid-rich necrotic core size in atherosclerotic carotid plaque: comparison of high-resolution, contrast-enhanced magnetic resonance imaging and histology. *Circulation* 2005; **112**: 3437–3444.

18. Yuan C, Zhang SX, Polissar NL *et al*. Identification of fibrous cap rupture with magnetic resonance imaging is highly associated with recent transient ischaemia attack or stroke. *Circulation* 2002; **105**: 181–185.

19. Takaya N, Yuan C, Saam T *et al*. Presence of intraplaque haemorrhage stimulates progression of carotid atherosclerotic plaques: a high-resolution magnetic resonance imaging study. *Circulation* 2005; **111**: 2768–2775.

20. Takaya N, Yuan C, Chu B *et al*. Association between carotid plaque characteristics and subsequent ischemic cerebrovascular events: a prospective assessment with MRI – initial results. *Stroke* 2006; **37**: 818–823.

21. North American Symptomatic Carotid Endarterectomy Trial Collaborators. Beneficial effect of carotid endarterectomy in symptomatic patients with high-grade carotid stenosis. *N Engl J Med* 1991; **325**: 445–453.

22. Executive Committee for the Asymptomatic Carotid Atherosclerosis Study. Endarterectomy for asymptomatic carotid artery stenosis. *JAMA* 1995; **273**: 1421–1428.

23. Rothwell PM, Goldstein LB. Carotid endarterectomy for asymptomatic carotid stenosis. *Stroke* 2004; **35**: 2425.

24. Corti R, Fayad ZA, Fuster V *et al*. Effects of lipid-lowering by simvastatin on human atherosclerotic lesions: a longitudinal study by high-resolution, non-invasive magnetic resonance imaging. *Circulation* 2001; **104**: 249–252.

25. Corti R, Fuster V, Fayad ZA *et al*. Lipid lowering by simvastatin induces regression of human atherosclerotic lesions: two years' follow-up by high-resolution non-invasive magnetic resonance imaging. *Circulation* 2002; **106**: 2884–2887.

26. Lima JAC, Desai MY, Steen H, Warren WP, Gautam S, Lai S. Statin-induced cholesterol lowering and plaque regression after 6 months of magnetic resonance imaging-monitored therapy. *Circulation* 2004; **110**: 2336–2341.

27. Saam T, Yuan C, Zhao XQ *et al*. Assessment of rosuvastatin treatment on carotid atherosclerosis in moderately hypercholesterolemic subjects using high-resolution MRI. Abstract, European Atherosclerosis Society Congress, Prague, April 2005.

28. Fayad ZA, Fuster V, Fallon JT *et al*. Noninvasive *in vivo* human coronary artery lumen and wall imaging using black-blood magnetic resonance imaging. *Circulation* 2000; **102**: 506–510.

29. Kim WY, Astrup AS, Stuber M *et al*. Subclinical coronary and aortic atherosclerosis detected by magnetic resonance imaging in type 1 diabetes with and without diabetic nephropathy. *Circulation* 2007; **115**: 228–235.

30. Davies JR, Rudd JHF, Fryer TD *et al*. Identification of culprit lesions after transient ischemic attack by combined ^{18}F fluorodeoxyglucose positron-emission tomography and high-resolution magnetic resonance imaging. *Stroke* 2005; **36**: 2642–2647.

31. Trivedi RA, Mallawarachi C, U-King-Im J-M *et al*. Identifying inflamed carotid plaques using *in vivo* USPIO-enhanced MR imaging to label plaque macrophages. *Arterioscler Thromb Vasc Biol* 2006; **26**: 1601–1606.

Jeremy P.R. Dick Jane E. Wainwright

11

The role of platelet antagonists in the management of cerebrovascular problems

Antiplatelet therapy is a cornerstone of preventive treatment in cardio- and cerebrovascular medicine. Aspirin (a cyclo-oxygenase inhibitor) is proven in both primary and secondary prevention of myocardial infarction, stroke and cardiovascular death, and is the mainstay of antiplatelet treatment.[1] Other antiplatelet agents such as dipyridamole (an antagonist of adenosine diphosphate [ADP]), clopidogrel (an irreversible thienopyridine ADP receptor antagonist), and glycoprotein IIb/IIIa antagonists also have a place in treatment and prevention of vascular events. However, the relative importance of these agents is significantly different in cerebrovascular and cardiovascular medicine. We will discuss possible reasons for these differences, in what is essentially the same disease process, in two different vascular beds.

The Antiplatelet and Antithrombotic Trialists' Groups evolved with the aim of maximising the information derived from the numerous small trials of antiplatelet agents. One of the many valuable outcomes from this collaboration has been an understanding of the magnitude of the antiplatelet treatment benefit. Among high-risk patients (those with acute or previous vascular disease or other predisposing condition), allocation to antiplatelet therapy reduces the chance of any serious vascular event by about one-quarter (non-fatal myocardial infarction by one-third and non-fatal stroke by one-quarter).

This chapter focuses on the role of the platelet in atherothrombotic disease, its physiology, activation pathways and the potential strategies for inhibition. We shall look at the role of the various agents currently available, focusing particularly on the reduction of recurrent cerebrovascular events.

Jeremy P.R. Dick MA MB BChir PhD FRCP (for correspondence)
Clinical Director of Greater Manchester Neuroscience Centre; Movement Disorder Neurologist and Lead Neurologist at South Manchester University Hospital Foundation Trust, UK.
E-mail: jeremy.dick@srft.nhs.uk

Jane E. Wainwright MD MRCP
Clinical Governance Lead for the Greater Manchester Neuroscience Centre Neurologists and Consultant Neurologist, Hope Hospital, Salford, UK E-mail: jane.wainwright@srft.nhs.uk

PLATELETS

PHYSIOLOGY

For survival, it is important for humans to have an efficient coagulation system to prevent unwanted bleeding. Coagulation depends on exposure of subendothelial elements (such as collagen) to activate the coagulation cascade.

In their resting state, within flowing blood, platelets are smooth discs (Fig. 1A). Healthy endothelium helps maintain this inactive state by the secretion of nitric oxide (NO) and prostacyclin (PGI$_2$). The endothelial surface also expresses CD39 which converts ADP, a powerful activator of platelets, into adenosine monophosphate (AMP).

Endothelial injury or damage exposes the platelet to numerous ligands such as von Willebrand factor and collagen, which bind their respective receptors

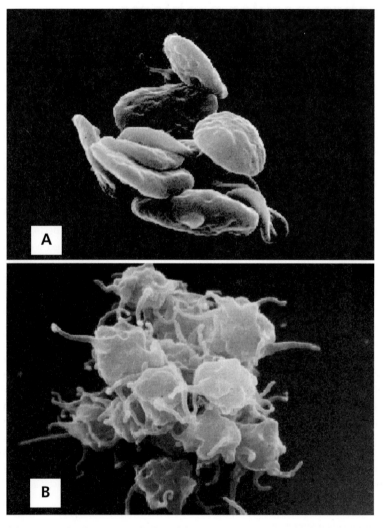

Fig. 1 (A) Resting platelets – smooth discs. (B) Activated platelets expressing pseudopodia. Figures downloaded from <www.perfusion.com> accessed 21 October 2007.

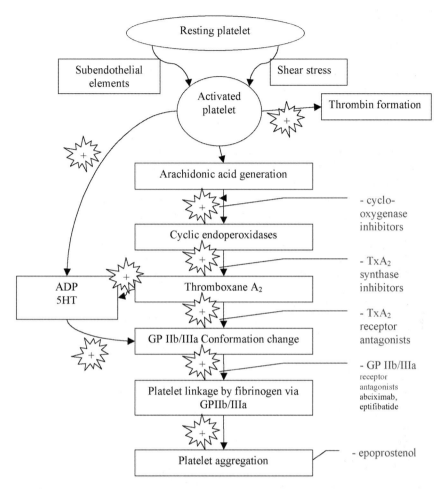

Fig. 2 Platelet activation cascade highlighting targets for platelet inhibition. ADP, adenosine diphosphate; 5HT, serotonin; GP, glycoprotein; Tx, thromboxane.

and trigger platelet activation. Activated platelets develop pseudopodia (Fig. 1B) which cross-link with other platelets. More importantly, they release adhesive proteins, coagulation and growth factors, and internal membrane proteins move to the surface (Fig. 1B). Release of these prothrombotic factors, such as thromboxane A_2 (TxA_2) and ADP, further activates platelets and amplifies the thrombotic process. Cross-linking, by means of fibrinogen binding to the glycoprotein (GP) IIb/IIIa receptor on platelets, leads to the formation of platelet aggregates. Several platelet surface proteins allow cross-talk with white blood and endothelial cells and are vital in the processes of wound healing and tissue remodelling. Both clinical and pathological studies show that increased levels of platelet activation are seen in the setting of acute or transient cerebral ischaemia and in cerebral infarction.[2]

Platelet activation has also been described in the setting of other vascular disorders – unstable angina, myocardial infarction, cardiopulmonary bypass and in relation to thrombolysis. Measurable platelet hyper-reactivity has been reported in association with vascular risk factors including hypertension,[3] cigarette smoking,[4] diabetes mellitus,[5] hyperlipidaemia,[6] and with emotional stress[7] or following strenuous exercise.[8]

The platelet activation cascade is illustrated in Figure 2. By understanding this activation cascade, we can focus on possible targets for its modification. For example, the thromboxane pathway may be inhibited by receptor antagonists (aspirin reduces formation of the natural agonist); the P2Y12 receptors (normally activated by ADP, some by ATP) can be inhibited by receptor antagonists (*e.g.* clopidogrel, prasugrel) and the protease activated receptors (PARs) which normally react to thrombin and bind fibrinogen provide a further target, currently under early investigation.

MEASURING PLATELET REACTIVITY

Assessing the effectiveness of platelet inhibition can be approached in a number of ways. The simplest measure of platelet function is the bleeding time. Other techniques for assessing platelet function include light aggregometry (the 'gold standard', though labour intensive and subject to variability), measurement of combined aggregation and adhesion, measurement of specific and non-specific platelet proteins and measurement of direct markers of platelet activity (flow cytometry).

Commercially available systems are being evaluated for clinical use; for example, the VerifyNow Rapid Platelet Function Assay (Accumetrics; San Diego, CA, USA) uses light aggregometry to assess the effectiveness of the specific antiplatelet agent used – a different assay for each agent. A second system, the PFA-100 (Dade-Behring Inc.; Deerfield, IL, USA), can be used at the bedside to assess platelet reactivity by measurement of the 'closure time' – this is the time taken for blood, drawn through a fine capillary, to block a membrane coated with collagen and epinephrine, or collagen and ADP.

However, there is no consensus regarding reference standards, and more work is needed in this area. Perhaps, in future, individual patients will undergo genetic analysis to define their personal prescription for platelet inhibitors with reactivity measured at baseline and after treatment, to assess efficacy.

ANTIPLATELET AGENTS

The numbers of agents in this group is ever-expanding; for simplicity, they have been divided into sub-groups defined by levels of evidence for their use and availability. Of course, as well as specific anti-platelet agents, a number of other drugs used in secondary prevention have been shown to have antiplatelet action, including statins,[9] angiotensin II receptor blockers[10] and fish oil.[11]

PROVEN AND IN ROUTINE CLINICAL USE

COX-1 inhibitors

Aspirin works by irreversibly acetylating the cyclo-oxygenase (COX)-1 enzyme, suppressing production of thromboxane A_2. Thromboxane A_2 is a potent agonist of platelet aggregation and aspirin reduces thrombus formation via this pathway. It does not have the same effect in all patients, and is subject to inter- and intra-individual variability. This has been shown to be clinically relevant – stroke patients with poor *in vitro* responses to aspirin have an increased risk of subsequent stroke compared with aspirin-sensitive patients (40% versus 4.4%; $P < 0.001$).[12]

Dipyridamole

Platelets possess three P2 receptors for adenine nucleotides: P2Y1 and P2Y12, which both interact with ADP, and P2X1, which interacts with ATP. Dipyridamole is a weak antiplatelet agent which acts as an ADP antagonist. In combination with aspirin, it has shown a small, but statistically significant, benefit over aspirin alone in secondary stroke prevention.

P2Y12 receptor antagonists

Thienopyridine ticlopidine, an antagonist of the platelet P2Y12 ADP receptor, reduces the incidence of vascular events in patients at risk, but it also has some important drawbacks, including: (i) a relatively high incidence of toxic effects; (ii) delayed onset of action; and (iii) high inter-individual variability in response. Another thienopyridine, clopidogrel, has superseded ticlopidine, because it is less toxic than ticlopidine (less neutropenia, less thrombocytopenia). It requires hepatic cytochrome P450 metabolism to release its active metabolite, which binds irreversibly through covalent modification to the P2Y12 receptor.

GPIIb/GPIIIa antagonists

Three GPIIb/GPIIIa receptor antagonists are approved for intravenous use in patients with unstable angina. Abciximab is a monoclonal antibody which causes long-lasting, non-competitive blockade of the GPIIb/GPIIIa receptor. Eptifibatide and tirofiban are rapidly acting GPIIb/GPIIIa receptor antagonists with a half-life of about 2 h. In cerebrovascular disorders, they may be used during endovascular treatment of aneurysms. Thus far, the oral preparations used in trial settings have been associated with increased rates of all-cause mortality and bleeding.

UNDERGOING PHASE III STUDIES

Thromboxane A$_2$ receptor antagonists

Thromboxane A$_2$ is an unstable metabolite of arachidonic acid formed by the cyclo-oxygenase pathway and released from activated platelets, monocytes and damaged vessel walls. It causes irreversible platelet aggregation, vasoconstriction and smooth muscle cell proliferation. In humans, oral administration of one such antagonist, terutroban, for 12 weeks (1–30 mg/day) has been reported to produce dose-proportional inhibition of *ex vivo* platelet aggregation.[13] Terutroban is currently in use in a phase III study in secondary prevention of atherothrombotic events.

Irreversible P2Y12 receptor antagonists

Prasugrel, a novel thienopyridine with a faster onset of action and 10 times the potency of clopidogrel, is under phase III investigation. Unlike clopidogrel, prasugrel is converted to its active metabolite in both hepatic and extrahepatic tissue, so its resistance pattern is likely to be different to clopidogrel. A phase II dose-finding study (JUMBO-TIMI 26) against clopidogrel, in patients undergoing elective or urgent percutaneous coronary intervention (PCI), showed no increase in adverse outcomes and a non-significant trend towards prasugrel benefit.[14] A phase III trial (TRITON-TIMI 38) in aspirin-treated patients with acute coronary syndromes and scheduled PCI, found a significant reduction in the composite end-point of vascular death, non-fatal myocardial infarction and non-fatal stroke (12.1% for clopidogrel versus 9.9% for prasugrel).[15] Stent thrombosis was reduced by 50% in the prasugrel group for both bare-metal and drug-eluting stents. These benefits were not without cost – a significant increase in both life-threatening and fatal bleeding events.

UNDER EARLY EVALUATION

Dual thromboxane A$_2$ inhibitors

Up to nine agents have been derived from torasemide, a loop diuretic. These act as both thromboxane A$_2$ (TxA$_2$) antagonists and TxA$_2$ synthase inhibitors, with no effect on COX-1 or COX-2 enzymatic activity. One such agent (BM-573) has undergone testing in an animal model and been shown to be a potent antithrombotic agent that does not affect bleeding time.[16]

Protease-activated receptor antagonists

In addition to stimulating fibrin production in the coagulation cascade, thrombin activates platelets via PAR receptors. PAR1 and PAR4 are expressed on the surface of human platelets, with the PAR1 receptor proposed as the principal thrombin receptor. At least two oral PAR1 receptor antagonists are currently in development: SCH 530348 and E5555. A recently completed phase II trial, Thrombin Receptor Antagonist in Percutaneous Coronary Intervention (TRA–PCI), has reported positive safety findings for SCH 530348. In the PCI cohort, treatment decreased (non-significantly) the incidence of death and major adverse cardiovascular events (5.9% versus 8.6% with placebo) without increasing major or minor bleeding.[17]

Reversible P2Y12 receptor antagonists

Two direct P2Y12 antagonists, cangrelor (intravenous) and AZD6140 (oral) are under study. They have a very rapid onset of action and are reversible. Phase II studies of safety and haemodynamic effects in patients undergoing PCI has shown cangrelor to be a promising agent, with a less prolonged bleeding time than abciximab.[18] Data from a phase II study of the safety, tolerability and initial efficacy of AZD6140 have shown no increase in major bleeding.[19] This agent is currently undergoing wider evaluation. These agents may be attractive alternatives to the classical thienopyridines, especially if very rapid inhibition of platelet aggregation (acute coronary or stroke situations) or its quick reversal are required. Inhibitors of the other platelet receptor for ADP (P2Y1) and of the receptor for ATP (P2X1) are also under development.

Phosphodiesterase-3 inhibitor

Another potential alternative, or adjunct, to current antiplatelet therapy is cilostazol, a phosphodiesterase-3 inhibitor, approved for the treatment of intermittent claudication. It is has an effect on the vascular endothelium in addition to its antiplatelet action and has been reported to reduce restenosis rates after coronary angioplasty and stenting. In patients who have had a cerebrovascular event, cilostazol monotherapy significantly reduces the risk of recurrent stroke.[20] In Japan, it is used routinely in secondary prevention of stroke, appearing to be more effective in patients with small vessel cerebrovascular disease.

ISCHAEMIC STROKE

THE SIZE AND NATURE OF THE PROBLEM

Stroke is common. Approximately 110,000 strokes occur every year in England and Wales, equating to one every 5 min. In 2002, four times as many women died from stroke as died from breast cancer, yet the relative public awareness of the two conditions is very different, and public awareness of stroke remains low despite a number of recent significant publications.

Historically, stroke has been seen as an inevitable consequence of growing old, with little to be done for those suffering an event, and it is true that one in four will suffer a stroke if we live to age 85 years. However, one-quarter of strokes affect those under the age of 65 years and there is now increasingly good evidence for active intervention. There are more than 900,000 stroke survivors living in England, half of whom are left dependent on others for activities of daily living. Stroke places, therefore, a heavy burden on society both financially and on the carers.

In reality, stroke is a medical emergency, as are transient ischaemic attacks (TIAs). The distinction between stroke and TIA is increasingly blurred, with TIA now appreciated as a much higher-risk condition than previously thought. Simply providing in-patient care on a dedicated stroke unit, rather than on a general medical ward, improves survival, reduces complications and increases the likelihood of a return to independent living. The main drug treatment leading to these improved outcomes is antiplatelet therapy.

CEREBROVASCULAR VERSUS CARDIOVASCULAR DISEASE

Cardiovascular and cerebrovascular disease have common risk factors – hypertension, smoking, dyslipidaemia, diabetes, increased body mass index, and physical inactivity. Indeed, ischaemic heart disease itself is a risk factor for stroke. For both vascular beds, antiplatelet agents are the mainstay of risk reduction. Trials of antiplatelet agents in the two patient groups have produced disparate results with regard to risk of event recurrence and bleeding complications. This has resulted in quite different antiplatelet regimens being recommended in routine clinical practice. Many theories are proposed for the differing results, including the varied pathologies seen in stroke compared with the more homogeneous pathology producing myocardial ischaemia.

The varied stroke subtypes are illustrated in Table 1. This shows the four distinct clinical stroke sub-groups as defined by the Oxfordshire Community Stroke Project group:[21] (i) those affecting the whole of the anterior (carotid)

Table 1 Stroke classification according to the Oxfordshire Community Stroke Project[21]

Subtype	Mechanism	Recur	Outcome
TACS (17%)	Embolic	–	Poor
PACS (34%)	Embolic	+	Good
LACS (25%)	Small vessel	+	Fair
POCS (24%)	Variable	±	Variable

circulation (total anterior circulation stroke, TACS); (ii) those affecting only part of the anterior circulation (partial anterior circulation stroke, PACS), (iii) those affecting the posterior circulation (posterior circulation stroke, POCS); and (iv) small vessel events, the so-called lacunar strokes (LACS). These subdivisions can be used to define stroke aetiology and prognosis and have become helpful in defining strategies to reduce recurrence risk. Unlike other subsequent schemata to define stroke sub-groups, no investigations are needed to define this classification.

PRIMARY PREVENTION

The effectiveness of aspirin in primary prevention is unclear. In one meta-analysis of 8 trials, aspirin was associated with a small increased risk of stroke (RR 1.07).[22] The Physicians' Health Study[23] found that, when employed in primary prevention in men, aspirin was associated with a small increased risk in haemorrhagic stroke, but no significant reduction in ischaemic stroke. The Women's Health Study[24] found that aspirin use was associated with a 17% reduction in the risk of stroke when compared with placebo. Both these latter studies used aspirin 75–100 mg every second day. Aspirin is clearly beneficial in stroke prevention in patients with symptomatic disease in other vascular beds.

TRANSIENT ISCHAEMIC ATTACK – AN EARLY OPPORTUNITY

Transient ischaemic attack (TIA) is defined as a clinical syndrome characterised by an acute loss of focal cerebral or ocular function with symptoms lasting less than 24 h. There are up to 70,000 per year UK-wide[25] and they are an accepted marker of stroke risk. TIAs precede up to 23% of completed strokes and, therefore, present a window of opportunity for targeting preventive treatment.[26] Computed tomography imaging is usually negative in patients with TIA, though the majority of patients will show evidence of tissue changes[27] on diffusion-weighted MR imaging. Hence, TIAs should be seen as mini-strokes and treated with the same urgency.

Although TIAs are an important warning of incipient stroke, the majority of patients with TIA do not go on to have a further event. Until recently, it was difficult to predict which patients were at highest risk of going on to completed stroke. However, the Oxford Vascular Study (OXVASC), using data from a previously identified population of patients with probable or definite TIA (Oxfordshire Community Stroke Project, OCSP[28]), derived a six-point score for

Table 2 The ABCD² scoring system – maximum score 7

ABCD² score variable [Choose appropriate single score from each section]	Score given
Age	
60 years or above	1
< 60 years	0
Blood pressure	
SBP > 140 mmHg or DBP > 90 mmHg	1
BP below these levels	0
Clinical features	
Any unilateral weakness (face/hand/arm/leg)	2
Speech disturbance (without motor weakness)	1
Duration of symptoms	
> 60 min	2
10–59 min	1
< 10 min	0
Diabetic	
Yes	1
No	0
Total	—

Low risk (0–3) – risk 1%, 1.2% and 3.1% at 2, 7 and 90 days.
Moderate risk (4–5) – risk 4.1%, 5.9% and 9.8% at 2, 7 and 90 days.
High risk (6–7) – 8.1%, 11.7% and 17.8% at 2, 7 and 90 days.

7-day risk. This 'ABCD' score was highly predictive of subsequent risk.[29] A similar scoring system was devised in the US (the California score[30]) and work to combine the two produced a refined 'ABCD²' score. This refined score was validated in a population of 4799 patients and shown to be highly predictive of 2-day stroke risk (Table 2).[31]

The ABCD² score allows identification of patients at highest risk of subsequent stroke. For instance, it is probably sensible to admit those with scores of 6 or 7 for immediate investigations, including carotid artery imaging perhaps leading to early endarterectomy in view of their high 48-h risk. This 'front-loading' of risk highlights the need for a major sea-change in provision of TIA/minor stroke services. Two recent studies (one UK-based, one based in France) assessed the impact of this urgent approach to management. Simple early treatments of TIA reduced risk of completed stroke by up to 80% from that predicted by ABCD². Treatments included antiplatelet agents, antihypertensives and statins, but also allowed early anticoagulation where appropriate for those in atrial fibrillation and early surgical intervention for those with carotid stenosis. The effect of the antiplatelet agents used cannot, of course, be teased out of the data, and the ABCD² scores in the two different studies were divergent (higher predicted risk for the Oxford population), but they do stress that the burden of stroke can be reduced by rapid and timely action.[32,33]

ACUTE STROKE TREATMENT

For patients presenting early (< 3 h), intravenous thrombolysis (using tissue plasminogen activator, tPA) is proven treatment.[34] However, outside the 3-h time window, the only proven treatment in acute stroke is aspirin. Pooled analysis of the two major trials in this area showed that aspirin produces a small, but real, reduction of about 10 deaths or recurrent strokes per 1000 during the first few weeks. This is, however, at the expense of two major extracranial bleeds per 1000 treated, even in the absence of concomitant heparin. Both trials suggest that aspirin should be started as soon as possible after the onset of acute ischaemic stroke.[35] The magnitude of risk reduction is comparable to that seen in long-term, low-dose aspirin treatment.[1]

It is accepted UK practice to use aspirin 300 mg once daily for the first 2 weeks following ischaemic stroke before stepping down to a 'maintenance' dose of antiplatelet therapy, currently a combination of aspirin and dipyiridamole. This should be continued for 2 years, with further 'step-down' to aspirin 75 mg once daily at that stage. Where there is true aspirin hyper-sensitivity, clopidogrel 75 mg once daily can be used in its place.

ANTIPLATELET STRATEGIES FOR LONG-TERM PREVENTION IN ISCHAEMIC STROKE

There is continuing enquiry into the most effective long-term regimen for prevention of recurrent stroke. Several studies have been published over the last few years and they can be confusing. We attempt to describe and to highlight the salient points made in these trials with respect to antiplatelet regimens.

MONOTHERAPY

Aspirin

A meta-analysis of aspirin versus control showed a relative risk reduction of 13% (95% CI, 6–19%) in prevention of serious vascular events, with no significant difference found between low- (< 100 mg) or high- (> 900 mg) dose aspirin. Lower doses were associated with fewer bleeding complications.[36] One Dutch group has reported 30 mg to be as effective as 283 mg in both prevention of stroke and serious vascular events.[37] Used in long-term prevention, doses of 75–150 mg appear as effective as higher doses, though it must be stressed that the absolute benefit of treatment is small and numbers needed to treat are 1000 to prevent 10 events. However, in patients undergoing coronary bypass surgery, low-dose aspirin (75 mg/day) has been suggested as less effective in preventing graft occlusion than medium-dose therapy (325 mg/day).[38] In UK stroke practice, 75 mg once daily is considered the minimum dose required.

Despite the proven benefits of aspirin, it does not prevent all further vascular events – indeed high-risk patients retain a significant risk of atherothrombotic events, with 10–20% suffering a recurrence within 5 years. In some patients, this high risk of recurrence has been attributed to the inability of aspirin to inhibit platelet aggregation.[1,39] However, many factors can

Table 3 Mechanisms of aspirin resistance

Clinical factors	Cellular factors	Genetic factors
Failure to prescribe	Insufficient COX-1 inhibition	Polymorphisms of COX-1 gene and GP IIb/IIIa receptor
Non-compliance	Over-expression of COX-2 mRNA	Polymorphisms of von Willebrand factor receptor and P2Y1 single nucleotide
Non-absorption	Erythrocyte-induced platelet activation	Polymorphisms of GP Ia/IIa collagen receptor gene
Interaction with NSAID	Increased norepinephrine	
Acute coronary syndrome	Generation of 8-iso-PGF$_{2\alpha}$	
Congestive heart failure	Resolvins	
Hyperglycaemia		
Catecholamine surge		

Derived from Wang et al.[40]

influence platelet aggregability, and recurrence could be attributed to many causes. Aspirin 'failure' may reflect clinical, cellular and genetic factors (Table 3).

Non-steroidal anti-inflammatory drugs (NSAIDs) compete for access to the active site of COX-1. Mature platelets express the COX-1 isoform only, but newly formed platelets, approximately 10% of circulating platelets, express the COX-2 isoform. During times of increased platelet turn-over, the quantity of newly formed platelets may be sufficient to produce significant quantities of COX-2-derived thromboxane. In such conditions, low- or medium-dose (81–325 mg) aspirin may inadequately inhibit platelets since it is more than 150-fold less potent in inhibiting COX-2 than COX-1. Currently, the role of COX-2 in the natural history of vascular events is controversial.

Dipyridamole

A recent Cochrane library review extracting data from 29 trials showed no change in numbers of vascular deaths in the dipyridamole-treated group but a relative risk reduction (RRR) of 12% (95% CI, 5–19%) in vascular events. The benefit is only seen in patients with prior cerebral ischaemia.[41]

Clopidogrel

The CAPRIE trial[42] compared clopidogrel (75 mg) and aspirin (325 mg). It took the recruitment of 19,185 patients to show a marginal benefit of clopidogrel over aspirin (RRR, 8.7%; 95% CI, 0.3–16.5%; $P = 0.043$) in preventing the composite end-point of vascular death, myocardial infarction or stroke. Subgroup analysis suggested that the margin of benefit was higher in the peripheral vascular disease group (relative benefit for clopidogrel – peripheral vascular disease +23.8%, recent stroke +7.3%, recent myocardial infarction –3.7%). The confidence intervals for the 'recent myocardial infarction' group (+7.3%) did not reach statistical significance though the study had not been powered to achieve this. In addition, the result for the 'recent myocardial' group was contrary to the result from the CURE study[43] though this could have been a chance observation. In UK stroke practice, clopidogrel is normally used as monotherapy only in those patients with true aspirin hypersensitivity.

As for aspirin, clopidogrel resistance is also an emerging entity and is likely, again, to be subject to clinical, cellular and genetic factors. Clopidogrel inhibits platelet aggregation by irreversible binding of its active metabolite to the P2Y12 ADP receptor on the platelet surface. Small studies in individuals undergoing coronary stenting with a 300-mg loading dose of clopidogrel have found highly variable responsiveness. Platelet aggregation and activation tests show interindividual variability in response to clopidogrel with 5–10% of patients not responding to its effects, and as many as 25% being only partially responsive to the drug.[44,45]

Possible causes of clopidogrel resistance include genetic polymorphisms of the platelet P2Y12 ADP receptor, defects in signalling pathways downstream from the receptor, heightened platelet reactivity before drug administration, and inadequate dosing. Drug–drug interactions that involve the cytochrome P450 system, and interindividual variability in baseline activity of the hepatic cytochrome P450 CYP3A4 system, may influence the conversion of clopidogrel to its active metabolite. For instance, rifampin, a CYP3A4 inducer, has been shown to enhance platelet inhibition when administered with clopidogrel.[46]

COMBINATION THERAPY

For patients who have an ischaemic cerebrovascular event despite aspirin, there is no evidence that increasing the dose provides additional benefit. In view of the differing mechanisms of action of the available antiplatelet agents, combining them would seem a logical approach and various combinations have been investigated.

Aspirin and dipyridamole

The European Stroke Prevention Study (ESPS-2)[47] randomised 6602 patients with stroke/TIA to one of four treatment arms (aspirin alone, dipyridamole alone, aspirin plus dipyridamole or matched placebo). After 2 years' treatment, the relative risk reduction versus placebo for stroke was 37% for dual therapy, 18.1% for aspirin and 16.3% for dipyridamole. Criticisms about data quality from some centres and the low dose of aspirin employed prevented widespread acceptance of these results, despite no extra gastrointestinal or intracranial haemorrhage risk with dual therapy. In addition, previous pooled studies had not found any advantage to adding dipyridamole.

Evidence from a subsequent study (European/Australasian Stroke Prevention In Reversible Ischaemia Trial, ESPRIT[48]) lent weight to this combination. The authors randomised 2739 patients with stroke/TIA to either aspirin or dipyridamole plus aspirin and demonstrated a similar marginal benefit to the combination. Intolerance to dipyridamole was common, with up to 34% of patients citing headache as their main reason for stopping treatment. Headache is due to a vasodilator effect and can be pronounced. Patients should be warned, though it often subsides after 1–2 weeks. Concern has been raised that this vasodilator effect could lead to 'steal' in critical coronary conditions, but no increase in cardiac events was observed.

If the annual risk for stroke in secondary prevention trials of patients with atherothrombotic disease is assumed to be ~5% per year, the addition of dipyridamole will save 10 further vascular events per 1000 patients treated per year.[49] More accurate natural history data (documenting risk in these populations) will be derived from the REACH registry. Currently, that registry suggests that, for patients with established atherothrombotic disease, 3.9% patients per year will experience a major event (myocardial infarction, stroke or cardiovascular death). This is 1.7% for those who only have 'risk factors'.

Aspirin and clopidogrel

In cardiological practice, this combination is proven in a number of situations. Here, dual interference in platelet pathways (often with thrombolytic drugs as well) yields improved outcomes, surprisingly with no overall increase in bleeding.

The Clopidogrel and Metoprolol in Myocardial Infarction Trial (COMMIT)[50] showed that adding 75 mg of clopidogrel to aspirin within 24 h of an acute myocardial infarction reduced the relative risk of in-hospital death by 7% and the composite risk (in-hospital death, repeated myocardial infarction, or stroke) by 9%, with no significant increase in bleeding.

The CURE (Clopidogrel in Unstable angina to prevent Recurrent Events) study[43] compared aspirin (75–325 mg) to combined treatment (aspirin plus clopidogrel, including a loading dose of clopidogrel) in patients with unstable angina. A composite endpoint (vascular death, myocardial infarction or stroke) was significantly less likely in the dual therapy group (relative benefit 20%, 95% CI, 10–28%). Subgroup analysis for those undergoing PCI showed a more striking benefit. In this subgroup, 59 patients on dual therapy and 86 patients on aspirin experienced vascular death, myocardial infarction or stroke (relative benefit 30%; $P = 0.03$). There was a significant increase in bleeding complications in the overall CURE study but not in the CURE-PCI study.

A parallel study (Clopidogrel for the reduction of events during observation, the CREDO study[51]) looked at this dual therapy in patients undergoing elective PCI (a lower-risk population). In 2116 patients, they found a 26.9% reduction in vascular death, myocardial infarction or stroke at 1 year.

These results contrast with those from the CHARISMA trial[52] in which the study group was 'relatively enriched with stroke patients'.[53] This trial randomized 15,603 patients with atherothrombotic disease, who were either symptomatic or merely had risk factors. In this study, there was no difference in primary outcome events (vascular death, myocardial infarction or stroke) between the two groups (534 events in the dual therapy group, and 573 in the aspirin group) with more bleeding in the dual therapy group. Subgroup analysis suggested a benefit for those who were classed as 'symptomatic' (had a recent vascular event, $n = 9478$) while the outcome in the 3284 asymptomatic patients was worse on dual therapy. Of course, such subgroup analyses are vulnerable to statistical criticism, but are of interest in 'hypothesis generation', such as: (i) is the benefit of antiplatelet therapy focused in the early post 'event' period, particularly for those with coronary artery atheroma?; and (ii) is the downside of aggressive antiplatelet therapy more substantial with time and with other patient subgroups?

Results from a primary cerebrovascular patient population offer a further contrast. The MATCH (Management of ATherothrombosis with Clopidogrel in High-risk patients) study[54] focused on a population of patients with cerebrovascular disease. Here 7599 stroke/TIA patients (with at least one additional risk factor) were randomised to either clopidogrel or clopidogrel with aspirin (75 mg each). A composite end-point (vascular death, myocardial infarction or stroke) may have been less likely in the clopidogrel group (RR 6.4%; 95% CI, –4.6 to 16.3%) but this did not achieve significance. The adverse effect profile in this trial was stronger in the combination arm who had more bleeding (96 life-threatening bleeds in the dual therapy group [2.6%] versus 49 in the aspirin alone group [1.3%]). Thus, on average, for every 1000 TIA/stroke patients there were 10 fewer recurrent ischaemic events per year (a similar effect to that of the aspirin plus dipyridamole combination) but 13 more life-threatening haemorrhages per year.

Many reasons for the 'failure' of MATCH have been proposed. These include the late randomisation of patients (patients were entered 15 days after their index event, after the period of highest risk had passed), the fact that clopidogrel was used as comparator (previous trials used an aspirin group), that there was no clopidogrel 'loading' and that almost half had small vessel disease. The over-representation of small vessel disease patients may also explain the relatively high risk of intracerebral haemorrhage in the combination group, as these patients have been shown on gradient echo MR to be at increased risk of asymptomatic intracerebral 'microbleeds'.[55]

OVERVIEW OF DUAL AND TRIPLE THERAPY

There are contrasting results from studies of dual antiplatelet therapy in the cardiovascular and the cerebrovascular arenas. Subjects tend to be recruited much earlier in cardiac studies (since there are established avenues for rapid referral) and the target pathology in these groups is a more homogeneously medium-sized vessel-atherothrombotic process.

There are trials of triple antiplatelet therapy in cardiac populations with no apparent excess of bleeding complications. The ISAR-REACT 2 study investigated patients with myocardial infarction requiring early PCI.[56] Triple therapy was associated with a 25% reduction in death or myocardial infarction in 2022 patients who were randomly assigned to either placebo or intravenous abciximab (a GPIIb/GPIIIa inhibitor) along with standard heparin, aspirin and clopidogrel. A smaller study, published in 2006, came to similar conclusions.[57] However, the recently reported TRITON-TIMI 38[15] was the first trial of dual-antiplatelet therapy (aspirin plus prasugrel) in patients with coronary artery disease to report an excess in fatal bleeding. Interestingly, subgroup analysis showed those with prior cerebrovascular disease to be at higher risk, highlighting that these patients are in some way 'different'.

In cerebrovascular patients, there is inevitably a more mixed vascular pathology, with high numbers of patients who have 'small vessel disease' (smaller than the medium-sized vessels affected in myocardial ischaemia) which is likely to skew study outcomes. Clinical delineation of stroke subtypes will be essential in future studies of novel antiplatelet strategies in subjects with prior cerebrovascular disease. It may be that we can only apply the lessons learned from cardiac populations to the subgroup of stroke patients with medium-to-large vessel arterial disease. Perhaps the commonest of these groups is those with carotid artery stenosis (CAS).

FUTURE DIRECTIONS

To have the power to detect treatment benefit in stroke, recent trials have needed to recruit large numbers of patients, often with only modest benefit. It has been suggested that transcranial Doppler detection of micro-embolic signals (MESs) could be used for pilot studies of newer agents or combinations. These MESs can be detected within the background waveform of flowing blood and have been shown to predict independently risk of subsequent stroke in patients with significant CAS, whether symptomatic or asymptomatic.[58] MESs have been shown to abate in response to intravenous aspirin and, more recently, with tirofiban.[59] They were used as a surrogate marker of embolic activity in the recent CARESS study,[60] examining the effect of addition of clopidogrel to aspirin in patients with CAS prior to endarterectomy. The positive results from this study have led to the recommendation that dual therapy (aspirin plus clopidogrel) be used in patients with significant CAS prior to endarterectomy. Use of this technique in future studies may allow more rapid evaluation of antiplatelet agents in smaller numbers of patients.

However, the main current goals for stroke prevention are logistical. Improved outcomes will follow increased awareness, more rapid referral and the establishment of acute stroke centres. Indeed, the frontiers of science and the real world are different places. Various national and international registries such as CRUSADE (Can Rapid Risk Stratification of Unstable Angina Patients Suppress ADverse Outcomes with Early Implementation of the ACC/AHA Guidelines), REACH (Reduction of Atherothrombosis for Continued Health) and GRACE (Global Registry of Acute Coronary Events) have all highlighted the variability of antiplatelet use across and within different health systems. Although aspirin uptake is consistently high, clopidogrel uptake is low (e.g. 39% in the US and 24% in Europe) and GPIIb/GPIIIa inhibitor use is even lower (e.g. 33% in the US and 9% in Europe). Nevertheless, trends seem to be improving; the European Heart Survey of the routine management of acute coronary syndromes has shown clopidogrel use increasing from 27.6% in 2000 to 67.4% in 2004. This was accompanied by a reduced 30-day mortality rate between the 2000 and the 2004 studies (42% down to 34%). It may be that longitudinal data from these registries will change our practice; however, in the interim, we shall continue to see aspirin as our antiplatelet cornerstone, despite its acknowledged limitations.

Key points for clinical practice

- Platelet reactivity is variable between and within subjects, and is triggered via a number of pathways.

- Numerous antiplatelet agents are available and vary in their mode of action.

- Antiplatelet agents are key in the prevention of recurrent cerebro-vascular events but must be used early (start within 24–48 h).

- Transient ischaemic attacks should be treated like stroke – as a medical emergency.

- Risk scores (ABCD^2) are important in predicting risk of further events.

- Stroke is a heterogeneous disease and strategies for prevention of further events need to be tailored.

- Antiplatelet agents should be used in combination with standard management of other vascular risk factors.

References

1. Antiplatelet Trialists' Collaboration. Collaborative overview of randomised trials of antiplatelet therapy. I. Prevention of death, myocardial infarction, and stroke by prolonged antiplatelet therapy in various categories of patients. *BMJ* 1994; **308**: 81–106.
2. Wu KK, Hoak JC. Increased platelet aggregates in patients with transient ischaemic attacks. *Stroke* 1975; **6**: 521–524.
3. Lip GY, Blann AD, Jones AF, Lip PL Beevers DG. Relation of endothelium, thrombogenesis and hemorheology in systemic hypertension to ethnicity and left ventricular hypertrophy. *Am J Cardiol* 1997; **80**: 1566–1571.
4. Hawkins RI. Smoking, platelets and thrombosis. *Nature* 1972; **236**: 450–452.
5. Sagel J, Colwell JA, Crook L, Laimins M. Increased platelet aggregation in early diabetes mellitus. *Ann Intern Med* 1975; **82**: 733–738.
6. Carvalho ACA, Colman RW, Lees RS. Platelet function in hyperlipoproteinaemia. *N Engl J Med* 1974; **290**: 434–438.
7. Levine SP, Towell BL, Suarez AM, Knieriem LK, Harris MM, George JN. Platelet activation and secretion associated with emotional stress. *Circulation* 1985; **71**: 1129–1134.
8. Wang J, Jen CJ, Kung H, Lin L, Hsiue T, Chen H. Different effects of strenuous exercise and moderate exercise on platelet function in men. *Circulation* 1994; **90**: 2877–2885.
9. Tirnaksiz E, Pamukcu B, Oflaz H, Nisanci Y. Effect of high dose statin therapy on platelet function; statins reduce aspirin resistant platelet aggregation in patients with coronary heart disease. *J Thromb Thrombolysis*. 2007; Oct 5 (e-pub ahead of print).
10. Yamada K, Hirayama T, Hasegawa Y. Antiplatelet effect of losartan and telmisartan in patients with ischaemic stroke. *J Stroke Cerebrovasc Dis* 2007; **16**: 225–231.
11. Din JN, Harding SA, Valerio CJ *et al*. Dietary intervention with oil rich fish reduces platelet-monocyte aggregation in man. *Atherosclerosis* 2007; Jun 16; (e-pub ahead of print).
12. Grotemeyer KH, Scharafinski HW, Husstedt IW. Two-year follow-up of aspirin responder and aspirin non responder. A pilot-study including 180 post-stroke patients. *Thromb Res* 1993; **71**: 397–403.
13. Gaussem P, Reny JL, Thalamas C *et al*. The specific thromboxane receptor antagonist S18886: pharmacokinetic and pharmocodynamic studies. *J Thromb Haemost* 2005; **3**: 1437–45.
14. Wiviott SD, Antman EM, Winters KJ *et al*. and JUMBO-TIMI 26 Investigators. Randomized comparison of prasugrel (CS-747, LY640315), a novel thienopyridine P2Y12

antagonist, with clopidogrel in percutaneous coronary intervention: results of the Joint Utilization of Medications to Block Platelets Optimally (JUMBO)-TIMI 26 trial. *Circulation* 2005; **111**: 3366–3373.

15. Wiviott SD, Braunwald E, McCabe CH *et al.* and TRITON-TIMI 38 Investigators. Prasugrel versus clopidogrel in patients with acute coronary syndromes. *N Engl J Med* 2007; **357**: 2001–2015.

16. Dogne JM, Hanson J, de Leval X *et al.* Pharmacological characterization of N-*tert*-butyl-N'-[2-(4'-methylphenylamino)-5-nitrobenzenesulfonyl]urea (BM-573), a novel thromboxane A_2 receptor antagonist and thromboxane synthase inhibitor in a rat model of arterial thrombosis and its effects on bleeding time. *J Pharmacol Exp Ther* 2004; **309**: 498–505.

17. Moliterno DJ, Becker RC, Jennings LK *et al.* for the TRA–PCI Study Investigators. Results from a multinational randomized, double-blind, placebo controlled study of a novel thrombin receptor antagonist SCH530348 in percutaneous coronary intervention. 56th Annual Session of the American College of Cardiology Annual Meeting, 24–27 March 2007, New Orleans, Louisiana. Abstract 2402–9.

18. Greenbaum AB, Grines CL, Bittl JA *et al.* Initial experience with an intravenous P2Y12 platelet receptor antagonist in patients undergoing percutaneous coronary intervention: results from a 2-part, phase II, multicenter, randomized, placebo- and active-controlled trial. *Am Heart J* 2006; **151**: 689–699.

19. Cannon CP, Husted S, Harrington RA *et al.* and DISPERSE-2 Investigators. Safety, tolerability, and initial efficacy of AZD6140, the first reversible oral adenosine diphosphate receptor antagonist, compared with clopidogrel, in patients with non-ST-segment elevation acute coronary syndrome: primary results of the DISPERSE-2 trial. *J Am Coll Cardiol* 2007; **50**: 1844–1851.

20. Matsumoto M. Cilostazol in secondary prevention of stroke: impact of the Cilostazol Stroke Prevention Study. *Atheroscler Suppl* 2005; **6**: 33–40.

21. Bamford J, Sandercock P, Dennis M, Burn J, Warlow C. Classification and natural history of clinically identifiable subtypes of cerebral infarction. *Lancet* 1991; **337**: 1521–1526.

22. Straus SE, Majumdar SR, McAlister FA. New evidence for stroke prevention: scientific review. *JAMA* 2002; **288**: 1388–1395.

23. Steering Committee of the Physicians' Health Study Research Group. Final report on the aspirin component of the ongoing Physicians' Health Study. *N Engl J Med* 1989; **321**: 129–135.

24. Ridker PM, Cook NR, Lee IM *et al.* A randomized trial of low-dose aspirin in the primary prevention of cardiovascular disease in women. *N Engl J Med* 2005; **352**: 1293–1304.

25. Giles M, Rothwell P. Substantial underestimation of the need for outpatient services for TIA and minor stroke. *Age Ageing* 2007 Jul 26 (e-pub ahead of print).

26. Rothwell PM, Warlow CP. Timing of TIAs preceding stroke: time window for prevention is very short. *Neurology* 2005; **36**: 817–820.

27. Kidwell CS, Alger JR, Di Salle F *et al.* Diffusion MRI in patients with transient ischemic attacks. *Stroke* 1999; **30**: 1174–1180.

28. Dennis MS, Bamford J, Sandercock PA, Warlow CP. Incidence of transient ischaemic attacks in Oxfordshire, England. *Stroke* 1989; **20**: 333–339.

29. Rothwell PM, Giles MF, Flossman E *et al.*. A simple score (ABCD) to identify individuals at high early risk of stroke after transient ischaemic attack. *Lancet* 2005; **366**: 29–36.

30. Johnston SC, Gress DR, Browner WS, Sidney S. Short-term prognosis after emergency-department diagnosis of transient ischemic attack. *JAMA* 2000; **284**: 2901–2906.

31. Claiborne Johnston S, Rothwell PM, Nguyen-Huynh MN *et al.* Validation and refinement of scores to predict very early stroke risk after transient ischaemic attack. *Lancet* 2007; **369**: 283–292.

32. Rothwell PM, Giles MF, Chandratheva A *et al.* on behalf of the Early use of Existing Preventive Strategies for Stroke (EXPRESS) study. Effect of urgent treatment of transient ischaemic attack and minor stroke on early recurrent stroke (EXPRESS study): a prospective population-based sequential comparison. *Lancet* 2007; Oct 8; (e-pub ahead of print).

33. Lavallee PC, Meseguer E, Abboud H *et al.* A transient ischaemic attack clinic with round-the-clock access (SOS-TIA): feasibility and effects. *Lancet Neurol* 2007; **6**: 953–960.

34. The National Institute of Neurological Disorders and Stroke rt-PA Stroke Study Group. Tissue plasminogen activator for acute ischemic stroke. *N Engl J Med* 1995; **333**: 1581–1587.

35. Chen ZM, Sandercock P, Pan HC *et al.* on behalf of the CAST and IST collaborative groups. Indications for early aspirin use in acute ischemic stroke: a combined analysis of 4000 randomized patients from the Chinese acute stroke trial and the international stroke trial. *Stroke* 2000; **31**: 1240–1249.

36. Algra A, van Gijn J. Cumulative meta-analysis of aspirin efficacy after cerebral ischaemia of arterial origin. *JNNP* 1999; **66**: 255.

37. The Dutch TIA Trial Study Group. A comparison of two doses of aspirin (30 mg versus 283 mg a day) in patients after transient ischaemic attack or minor ischaemic stroke. *N Engl J Med* 1991; **325**: 1261–1266.

38. Lim E, Ali Z, Ali A *et al.* Indirect comparison meta-analysis of aspirin therapy after coronary surgery. *BMJ* 2003; **327**: 1309.

39. Michos ED, Ardehali R, Blumenthal RS, Lange RA, Ardehali H. Aspirin and clopidogrel resistance. *Mayo Clin Proc* 2006; **81**: 518–526.

40. Wang TH, Bhatt DL, Topol EJ. Aspirin and clopidogrel resistance: an emerging clinical entity. *Eur Heart J* 2006; **27**: 647–654.

41. De Schryver EL, Algra A, van Gijn J. Dipyridamole for preventing stroke and other vascular events in patients with vascular disease. Cochrane Database Syst Rev. 2007;(3): CD001820.

42. CAPRIE Steering Committee. A randomised, blinded, trial of clopidogrel versus aspirin in patients at risk of ischaemic events (CAPRIE). *Lancet* 1996; **348**: 1329–1339.

43. The CURE Trial Investigators. Effects of clopidogrel in addition to aspirin in patients with acute coronary syndromes without ST segment elevation. *N Engl J Med* 2001; **345**: 494–502.

44. Muller I, Besta F, Schulz C, Massberg S, Schonig A, Gawaz M. Prevalence of clopidogrel non-responders among patients with stable angina pectoris scheduled for elective coronary stent placement. *Thromb Haemost* 2003; **89**: 783–787.

45. Serebruany VL, Steinhubl SR, Berger PB, Malinin AI, Bhatt DL, Topol EJ. Variability in platelet responsiveness to clopidogrel among 544 individuals. *J Am Coll Cardiol* 2005; **45**: 246–251.

46. Lau WC, Gurbel PA, Watkins PB *et al.* Contribution of hepatic cytochrome P450 3A4 metabolic activity to the phenomenon of clopidogrel resistance. *Circulation* 2004; **109**: 166–171.

47. Diener HC, Cunha L, Forbes C, Sivenius J, Smets P, Lowenthal A. European Stroke Prevention Study 2. (ESPS-2). Dipyridamole and acetylsalicylic acid in the secondary prevention of stroke. *J Neurol Sci* 1996; **143**: 1–13.

48. ESPRIT Study Group. Aspirin plus dipyridamole versus aspirin alone after cerebral ischaemia of arterial origin (ESPRIT): randomised controlled trial. *Lancet* 2006; **367**: 1665–1673.

49. Sudlow C. Give dipyridamole with aspirin instead of aspirin alone to prevent vascular events after ischaemic stroke or TIA. *BMJ* 2007; **334**: 901.

50. Chen ZM, Jiang LX, Chen YP *et al.*; COMMIT (ClOpidogrel and Metoprolol in Myocardial Infarction Trial) collaborative group. Addition of clopidogrel to aspirin in 45,852 patients with acute myocardial infarction: randomised placebo-controlled trial. *Lancet* 2005; **366**: 1607–1621.

51. Steinhubl SR, Berger PB, Mann 3rd JT *et al.*; CREDO Investigators. Clopidogrel for the Reduction of Events During Observation. Early and sustained dual oral antiplatelet therapy following percutaneous coronary intervention: a randomized controlled trial. *JAMA* 2002; **288**: 2411–2420.

52. Bhatt DL, Fox KA, Hacke W *et al.* Clopidogrel and aspirin versus aspirin alone for the prevention of atherothrombotic events (CHARISMA). *N Engl J Med* 2006; **354**: 1706–1717.

53. Howard G, McClure LA, Krakauer JW, Coffey CS. Stroke and the statistics of the aspirin/clopidogrel secondary prevention trials. *Curr Opin Neurol* 2007; **20**: 71–77.

54. Diener HC, Bogousslavsky J, Brass LM *et al.*; MATCH investigators. Aspirin and clopidogrel compared with clopidogrel alone after recent ischaemic stroke or transient ischaemic attack in high-risk patients (MATCH): randomised, double-blind, placebo-controlled trial. *Lancet* 2004; **364**: 331–337.

55. Cordonnier C, Al-Shahi Salman R, Wardlaw J. Spontaneous brain microbleeds: systematic review, subgroup analyses and standards for study design and reporting. *Brain* 2007; **130**: 1988–2003.

56. Kastrati A, Mehilli J, Neumann FJ *et al.*; Intracoronary Stenting and Antithrombotic Regimen Rapid Early Action for Coronary Treatment 2 (ISAR-REACT 2) Trial Investigators. Abciximab in patients with acute coronary syndromes undergoing percutaneous coronary intervention after clopidogrel pretreatment: the ISAR-REACT 2 randomized trial. *JAMA* 2006; **295**: 1531–1538.

57. Rasoul S, Ottervanger JP, de Boer MJ *et al.* A comparison of dual vs. triple antiplatelet therapy in patients with non-ST-segment elevation acute coronary syndrome: results of the ELISA-2 trial. *Eur Heart J* 2006; **27**: 1401–1407.

58. Molloy JE, Markus HS. Asymptomatic embolization predicts stroke and TIA risk in patients with carotid artery stenosis. *Stroke* 1999; **30**: 1440–1443.

59. Junghans U, Siebler M. Cerebral microembolism is blocked by tirofiban, a selective nonpeptide platelet glycoprotein IIb/IIIa receptor antagonist. *Circulation* 2003; **107**: 2717–2721.

60. Markus HS, Droste DW, Kaps M *et al.*. Dual antiplatelet therapy with clopidogrel and aspirin in symptomatic carotid stenosis evaluated using Doppler embolic signal detection: the Clopidogrel and Aspirin for Reduction of Emboli in Symptomatic Carotid Stenosis (CARESS) trial. *Circulation* 2005; **111**: 2233–2240.

Emma J. Birks

12

Ventricular assist devices: their current and evolving role

Heart failure is a major problem associated with high morbidity and mortality affecting over 900,000 people in the UK with 65,000 new cases every year. It is associated with a 40% 1-year mortality in newly diagnosed cases[1] with NYHA class IV having a 60% 1-year mortality. Heart failure costs the NHS £716 million per year and 1 million bed-days. The prognosis from heart failure is worse than that for myocardial infarction, carcinoma of the bowel, breast or prostate.[2]

Medical therapy with ACE inhibitors, β-blockers, angiotensin 2 inhibitors and aldosterone antagonists, together with resynchronisation therapy, has improved the survival of many with heart failure, but there remain a large group of patients who, despite optimal medical therapy, are in NYHA Class III/IV heart failure with a very poor prognosis. Unfortunately, the numbers of usable donor hearts available to perform heart transplantation for these patients in advanced heart failure has significantly decreased over recent years and now, across the UK, only a total of about 125 adult heart transplants are performed per year, a number totally inadequate for the population who require heart transplantation.

Left ventricular assist devices (LVADs) are rapidly evolving and increasingly used to treat patients with advanced heart failure. They are artificial hearts that assist the circulation and they are being inserted into an increasing number of patients with advanced heart failure. The LVAD technology itself is also evolving very quickly. They have been initially inserted as a bridge to transplantation in those patients with advanced heart failure with deteriorating clinical status who are unable to wait any longer for heart transplantation, being mostly inserted into patients who, despite

Emma J. Birks MRCP PhD
Consultant Cardiologist in Transplantation and Mechanical Circulatory Support, Royal Brompton and Harefield NHS Trust, Hill End Road, Harefield, Middlesex UB9 6JH, UK
E-mail: e.birks@imperial.ac.uk

inotropic ± intra-aortic balloon pump support, have deteriorating NYHA Class IV heart failure and usually also end-organ dysfunction. Not only are LVADs life saving in these deteriorating patients who might otherwise die before a donor heart becomes available, but they also improve secondary organ function prior to transplantation, reduce pulmonary hypertension and allow for improvement of nutritional status. The decrease in donors means that an increasing number of patients are requiring support with a left ventricular assist device for survival when their clinical status deteriorates.

There is also now compelling evidence that with LVAD unloading, recovery of the patient's myocardial function can occur, allowing device removal and avoiding the need for transplantation, (together with immunosuppression and its associated complications) and leaving the patient with an excellent quality of life. This means that the precious resource of a donor organ can be used for another needy individual. This indication, known as 'bridge to recovery' is a newer and expanding indication. The future use of these devices, particularly as survival continues to increase, is likely to extend to their much wider use as destination therapy, *i.e.* the insertion of the device life-long as an alternative to transplantation.

Early referral of the deteriorating patient and insertion of the LVAD before the onset of severe end-organ dysfunction is extremely important. Factors affecting early survival and reversal of organ dysfunction include chronicity of disease, intrinsic end-organ functional reserve, co-morbid conditions and age. Early intervention improves outcome – the stress of surgery superimposed on a fragile patient with advanced disease contributes to poor outcomes in the short- and long-term.

VENTRICULAR ASSIST DEVICES

The devices used have evolved over the years and are still rapidly evolving.[3] They can broadly be divided into first, second and third generation devices.

FIRST GENERATION DEVICES

The first generation ventricular assist devices are the pulsatile positive displacement pumps. The main ones are the HeartMate I, the Thoratec PVAD and the Novacor. The HeartMate I has been inserted in over 5000 patients; it is made of titanium with a polyurethane diaphragm and has a pusher-plate actuator. It can be powered pneumatically or electrically. A cannula is placed in the apex of the left ventricle and blood flows through a Dacron conduit, in which there is a porcine valve, to the pump and returns into a Dacron outflow graft through another porcine valve and returns to the ascending aorta (Fig. 1). The HeartMate I is unique because its blood pumping surface consists of titanium microspheres and a fibrillar textured inner surface that promotes the formation of a 'pseudo-intima' that seems to resist thrombogenesis. This means that with this pump the only anticoagulant needed is aspirin. Power is supplied by two external batteries (approximately the size of video camera batteries) and an external controller that weighs less than 300 g. The pumping can be performed in a 'fixed-rate' way or in an 'automatic' mode, in which stroke volume is maintained at 97% full and the rate is varied in response to

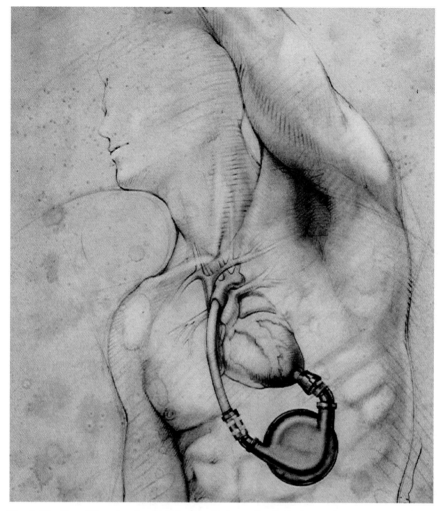

Fig. 1 The HeartMate I pulsatile left ventricular assist device.

preload. This device can pump 4–10 l/min. The HeartMate I has undergone several design improvements and evolved from the pneumatic to the vented electric, to the XVE. The percutaneous lead has been strengthened to reduce kinking and occlusion, improve fatigue resistance and improve patient comfort. The outflow graft has been adapted for 'bend relief' to prevent kinking and abrasion of the graft, and the diaphragm has been repositioned to prevent the diaphragm 'buckling', a major cause of diaphragm rupture. The valves have also been modified to prevent commissural dehiscence and incompetence, which previously limited the life-span of the pump. Also, the pump chamber pressure has been reduced, reducing stress on the valves, motor, bearings and diaphragm.

The Thoratec paracorporeal ventricular assist device (PVAD) has been inserted in over 3000 patients, it has a 65-ml stroke volume pumping chamber and two mechanical valves. It has the advantage that it can be used as an LVAD, RVAD or two together as a BIVAD. Alternating positive and negative

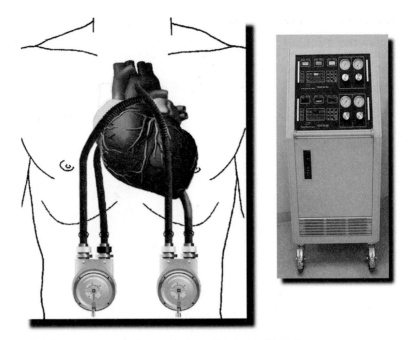

Fig. 2 The Thoratec pneumatic ventricular assist device (PVAD).

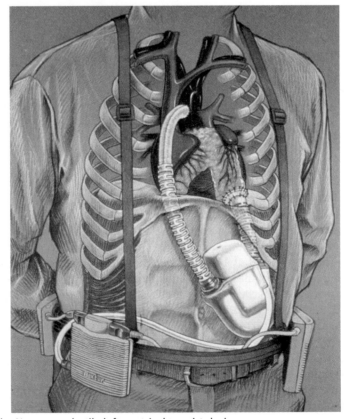

Fig. 3 The Novocor pulsatile left ventricular assist device.

air pressure by a console or portable pneumatic driver produces a beat rate of 40–110 bpm and a flow rate of 1.3–7.2 l/min. The PVAD is positioned outside the body (paracorporeal) on the anterior abdominal wall with cannulas crossing into the chest wall (Fig. 2). Warfarin (INR 2.5–3.5) and aspirin anticoagulation is required for this pump. There is also now an implantable version of this pump – the IVAD.

The Novacor LVAD (Fig. 3) has been implanted in over 1600 patients for durations of up to 6.1 years. It has a pump drive unit (PDU) which is implanted in the left upper quadrant of the abdomen and incorporates a dual pusher plate 70-ml stroke volume, sac-type blood pump with a smooth blood-contacting surface, coupled to a pulsed-solenoid energy converter drive. The PDU is implanted in a pocket in the left upper quadrant of the abdomen, the inflow cannula is inserted through the diaphragm into the left ventricular apex and the outflow graft is anastomosed to the ascending aorta. Pump flow, optimised through flow visualisation, is maintained through the pumping cycle, in contrast to the typical diaphragm pusher-plate pump. The normal operating module is fill-to-empty, although fixed-rate, single-stroke and synchronous counterpulsation are available. The early version of this pump had some thrombo-embolism problems but modification of the materials involved drastically improved this problem.[4]

The pulsatile volume-displacement devices provide excellent haemo-dynamic support and improve survival but have constraints, particularly the need for extensive surgical dissection, the presence of a large diameter lead (which is more prone to infection), an audible pump, the need for medium-large body habitus and limited long-term durability.

SECOND GENERATION DEVICES

The second generation axial flow pump devices are being increasingly used. These are continuous-flow, rotary pumps that have only one moving part, the rotor, unlike the first generation devices (and hence are expected to be more durable). They are also smaller (principally through elimination of the blood sac or reservoir necessary for a pulsatile system), quieter and tend to have a less traumatic surgical implantation. They have smaller drive-lines and, hence, tend to have lower rates of drive-line infection.

The HeartMate II device is a continuous-flow, axial blood pump (Fig. 4) with an internal rotor with helical blades that curve around a central shaft. As the blood flows around the pump rotor, the spinning action of the rotor, with its three curving blades, introduces a radial or tangential velocity to the blood flow and imparts kinetic energy to the blood, which then flows past the outlet stator vanes. The twisted shape of the outlet stator vanes converts the radial velocity of the blood flow to an axial direction. The pump weight is 350 g and it is approximately 7.0 cm in length and 4.0 cm at its largest diameter. It can generate up to 10 l/min of flow at a pressure of 100 mmHg. The axial flow design and absence of blood sac eliminates the need for venting (currently required for the first generation of implantable pump) thus reducing the size of the percutaneous drive lead and also eliminating the need for internal one-way valves. Again, blood drains through the inflow cannula in the apex of the left ventricle to the pump and returns back to the ascending aorta (Fig. 4).

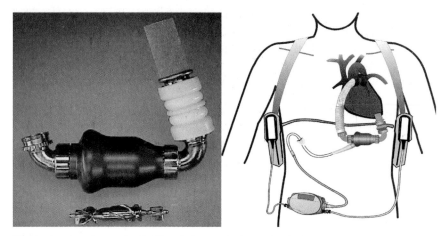

Fig. 4 The HeartMate II axial flow left ventricular assist device.

The Jarvik 2000 is a continuous-flow, axial-flow pump which has an intraventricular position with the whole pump sitting within the left ventricular cavity (Fig. 5). The pump weighs 85 g, measures 2.4 cm in diameter and is 5.5 cm long. The single moving component is the impeller located in the centre of the titanium housing. A brushless, direct-current motor, contained within the housing, creates the electromagnetic force necessary to rotate the impeller. Blood flow is directed through the outlet graft by stator blades located near the pump outlet and it returns to either the ascending or descending aorta. The pump can generate flows of up to 8 l/min maximum. Pump implantation with the outlet graft in the descending aorta can result in stasis and clot formation in the aortic root; therefore, an intermittent low-speed controller can be used which drops the pump speed for 9 s every minute to allow the aortic valve to open. Furthermore, many units, including our own,[5] anastomose the graft to the ascending and not the descending aorta; we have found no static complications in patients implanted in this way. Because this pump has no pocket, serious pump infections are rare.

The Berlin Heart Incor is also an axial flow pump. As blood passes into the Incor, it first passes the inducer which guides the laminar flow onto the actual

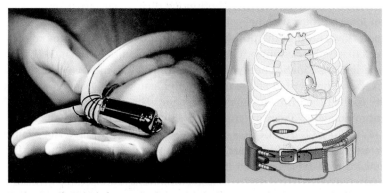

Fig. 5 The Jarvik 2000 left ventricular assist device. Note the intraventricular position of the device.

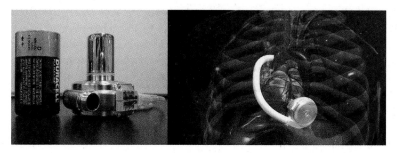

Fig. 6 The Heartware magnetic levitation (the rotor is magnetically levitated) ventricular assist device.

impeller which is suspended by a magnetic bearing and floats free of contact with other parts. The impeller operates between speeds of 5000–10,000 rpm. The stationary diffuser behind the rotor has specially aligned blades which reduce the rotational effect of the blood flow and add additional pressure to assist the transport of blood in the outflow cannula to the aorta.

The MicroMed-De-Bakey VAD is another axial flow rotary pump. It has an elbow-shaped inflow cannula that inserts into the left ventricular apex, a pump housing unit which houses the impeller (which is actuated by an electromagnet), a Dacron outflow conduit graft and an ultrasonic flow probe that encircles the outflow graft and provides direct, online measurements of pump flow.

THIRD GENERATION DEVICES

Heartware, Terumo and Ventrassist are magnetic levitation, third generation pumps that are now being tested in clinical use. Heartware has no bearings and hence is likely to have a very long durability, is much smaller than previous devices (Fig. 6) and easier surgically to implant. These third generation devices also tend to run at lower rpm which increases their durability. Although these third generation devices are only just starting to be used, they are anticipated to last for 5–10 years.

Patients on left ventricular assist devices are now discharged home into the community whilst on the devices. They and their 'companions' are trained about the device including what to do in the event of device failure.

CLINICAL ROLE OF VENTRICULAR ASSIST DEVICES

Left ventricular assist devices are being increasingly inserted into patients with advanced heart failure. Initially, this was mainly as a bridge to transplant, now it is also as a bridge to recovery and increasingly is likely to be as destination therapy.

BRIDGE TO TRANSPLANTATION

For patients with advanced medical urgency status 1A (United Network for Organ sharing classification), the death rate in 1999 was 58% compared to 20% for medical urgency status 1B and 13% for regular urgency status 2.[6] Hence,

LVAD and inotrope-supported patients stand to gain most from transplantation. LVAD insertion for bridge to transplantation is usually considered either because of cardiogenic shock and deteriorating clinical status (when it is felt the patient will not survive long enough to receive a donor organ) or if the patient develops secondary organ dysfunction such that transplantation becomes contra-indicated. Support from the device allows renal function, nutritional status and pulmonary vascular resistance to improve for subsequent transplantation, which usually takes several weeks or months. Transplantation should only be considered once these improvements have occurred.

In the multicentre evaluation of the HeartMate vented electric LVAD as a bridge to transplantation, 71% of 280 patients survived to transplantation or device removal.[7] In the Cleveland Clinic experience of 277 LVADs, 69% survived to transplantation.[8] From 60–75% survival to transplantation has been reported in other series.[9–11] However, these data are all from the first generation pumps which are associated with higher mortality. Data from the second generation pumps (which would be expected to have a better outcome due to their smaller size, easier surgical implantation, lower complication rates, *etc.*) are now becoming available. Recently, Miller *et al.*[12] published a prospective multicentre study of 133 NYHA Class IV patients on a transplant waiting list who underwent implantation of a HeartMate II device as a bridge to transplantation. All were on inotropic support (except 11% who were intolerant because of arrhythmias) and 41% were also intra-aortic balloon pump dependent. After 180 days, 100 (75%) patients had reached the principal outcome of transplantation, recovery or survival on on-going support with eligibility for transplantation. Patients on HeartMate II support had improvement in NYHA class, 6-min walk, functional status and quality of life. An additional 5 (4%) were alive but not yet eligible for transplantation and another 3 (2%) were alive but had had a device replacement, *i.e.* overall survival was 81% at 6 months. Interestingly, 4 patients removed themselves from the transplant waiting list as they preferred to continue mechanical support. The overall survival of patients who underwent transplantation, recovered their cardiac function or continued to receive mechanical circulatory support while remaining a candidate for transplantation was estimated to be 70% at 1 year.[12] These 133 patients, enrolled from March 2005 to May 2006, represented the primary cohort, enrolment continued and those enrolled between May 2006 and March 2007 represent the CAP (Continued Access Protocol Cohort), which consist of a further 164 patients; this group had an 88% survival at 180 days.[13]

A recent analysis[14] of 48,982 patients on the transplant waiting list in the US between 1990 and 2005 (era 1, 1990–1994; era 2, 1995–1999; era 3, 2000–2005) showed that the 1-year survival on the heart transplant waiting list has improved from 49.5% to 69% for status 1 patients (those who require continuous inotropic or mechanical circulatory support [IABP, LVAD, ECMO, total artificial heart] or ventilation, have a life expectancy < 7 days without transplantation or are considered a justifiable exceptional case) and from 81.8% to 89.4% for status 2 candidates (those who meet the general criteria for heart transplantation but do not meet status 1 criteria) between eras 1 and 3 (*i.e.* between 1990 and 2005). For status 2 candidates, demographics, aetiology and markers of severe heart failure did not substantially change throughout the period indicating that improved outcomes most likely represent improvements in heart failure therapy. In the current era of medical therapy, the 1-year survival of status 2 candidates without transplantation (81.4%) is approaching the outcome of heart transplantation.[15] However, caution must be extended as 40% of status 2 candidates listed in the early 2000s worsened and required upgrading to status 1.[16] In the most recent era (2000–2005), the majority of patients listed as UNOS status I candidates were hospitalised at the time of listing (82%), including 56% in the intensive care unit (ICU). The majority (71%) required continuous inotropic infusions or balloon pump support (12%) or were on mechanical circulatory support (23%). In comparison in era 1 (1990–1995), although 87% were hospitalised, only 20% were in the ICU, 14.6% required inotropes, 3.4% required balloon pump support and 8.4% were on mechanical circulatory support. Despite the improvements in survival of transplant candidates, the survival of status I patients continues to depend on urgent cardiac replacement therapy; 52.4% of those listed between 2000 and 2005 died within 6 months without heart transplantation. Although the use of mechanical circulatory support has increased and the presence of mechanical circulatory support on the day of listing as a bridge to heart transplantation had increased from 8.4% in era 1 to 22.8% in era 3, given the high 6-month mortality in this group without heart transplantation, it is likely that mechanical circulatory support is still being underused in this population.

BRIDGE TO RECOVERY

A small number of patients supported with a left ventricular assist device have shown significant improvement in their myocardial function[17] and there is now compelling evidence that prolonged, near-complete unloading of the left ventricle with the use of an LVAD is associated with structural reverse remodelling that can be accompanied by functional improvement.[18] This can be sufficient in some cases to allow explantation of the device;[17–21] however, the exact proportion of patients in which this is possible is unknown but has been reported to be only 5–24% in various series.[19–22] We have evolved a strategy which combines mechanical unloading using LVAD support with specific pharmacological interventions to: (i) maximise the incidence of recovery in patients with dilated cardiomyopathy; and (ii) improve durability of recovery following explantation.[18,23–25] Briefly, the pharmacological interventions of the first phase of the therapy are designed to act on component parts of the myocardium with the aim of reversing the pathological hypertrophy, remodelling and normalising cellular metabolic function. When maximal reverse remodelling, as judged by echocardiographic measurements of left ventricular dimensions with the pump switched off (under full heparinisation) has been achieved, clenbuterol is given as the second phase. This drug has been shown to induce physiological hypertrophy in several experimental models including those with pressure overload hypertrophy.[26,27] Using this strategy, it has been possible to promote recovery and allow removal of the pump in approximately two-thirds of patients.[18] Furthermore, these patients remain well 5 years later, suggesting this recovery is durable, and they have a good quality of life.[28] In these patients, we have also observed reversal of many molecular changes seen at the time of LVAD implantation.[29–33] Recovery of patients on an LVAD provides an ideal, and so far unique, opportunity to study the molecular mechanisms that occur during reverse remodelling as the patient recovers. Myocardial samples, obtained at the time of device insertion and removal, along with serum samples, provide an ideal opportunity to explore the myocardial and circulating factors involved in the recovery of human heart failure.

DESTINATION THERAPY

The future use of these devices, particularly as survival increases, is likely to lie in their wider use as destination therapy; this is already happening in the US. Successful experience in the bridge-to-transplant patients, particularly among those who had prolonged periods of support justified evaluating these devices as long-term or destination therapy for chronic heart failure.

A randomised trial (REMATCH, The Randomised Evaluation of Mechanical Assistance for the Treatment of Congestive Heart failure)[34] randomised 129 patients with end-stage failure at 20 experienced cardiac transplant centres to receive either optimal medical therapy (OMM) or a HeartMate I LVAD as permanent therapy. Patients were in NYHA Class IV for at least 60 of 90 days despite maximal medical therapy and they were ineligible for cardiac transplantation (age over 65 years, insulin-dependent diabetes with end-organ damage, chronic renal failure or significant irreversible co-morbidity). Median age was 69 years. The 1-year survival in the LVAD group was 52% compared to 25% in the OMM group and 2-year survival was 23% compared to 8% in the OMM group. Overall, all-cause mortality was reduced by 48%. Interestingly, 1-year survival for patients under 60 years of age was 74%. Both NYHA Class and quality of life were better at follow-up in the LVAD group. The survival benefit was particularly significant for those on inotropes (survival benefit $P = 0.0014$ for LVAD compared to OMM).[35] There was a significant improvement in survival for LVAD patients enrolled during the second half of the trial (1 January 2000 to July 2001) compared with the first half (May 1998 to 31 December 1999),[36] reflecting improvements in patient management and device modifications even throughout this period of the trial. The 1-year survival in the second half of the trial patients was 59% versus 44% in the first half ($P = 0.029$) and the 2-year survival was 38% versus 21%. The Minnesota Living with Heart Failure scores also improved significantly over the course of the trial.[36] Terminal heart failure caused the majority of deaths in the medical therapy group, whereas the most common cause of death in the device group was sepsis (41% of deaths) and failure of the device (17% of deaths).[34] The adverse event rate was also significantly lower as the trial progressed and the rates per patient-year of sepsis, renal failure and infection were significantly lower for those enrolled during the second half of the trial.[36] A further study of patients implanted with the first generation HeartMate I device at four high-volume centres following REMATCH from January 2003 to December 2004 showed improved 90% and 61% 30-day and 1-year survival, respectively.[37] The death rates due to sepsis and device failure were 8.3 times and 2.2 times lower than REMATCH, respectively. Overall, patients were 2.1 times less likely to experience an adverse event and there was a reduction of 66%, 63%, 89% and 92% in neurological dysfunction, sepsis, site infection and for combined and suspected device failure. respectively.

The INTrEPID trial is a prospective, non-randomised, clinical trial comparing outcome with the Novocor first generation pulsatile pump with medical therapy. Again, the LVAD-treated patients had superior survival rates at 6 months (46% versus 22%) and 12 months (27% versus 11%). Patients treated with medical therapy experienced no improvement in NYHA functional class whereas 85% of the LVAD patients had either no symptoms or minimal heart failure symptoms at the last assessment. Quality-of-life measures improved in the LVAD group.[4]

Introduction of axial flow and centrifugal designs have improved LVAD survival further and reduced complications; it has been proposed that there should now be a randomised trial of axial pumps versus OMM. A trial is currently underway randomising the pulsatile HeartMate I device against the HeartMate II continuous flow pump with a 1:2 randomisation.

The results of the REMATCH trial led to US FDA approval of the HeartMate VE for destination therapy in November 2002; in October 2003, the Center for Medicare and Medicaid services approved cover and re-imbursement of LVADs for this indication in the US.

BRIDGE TO DECISION

Despite the improvements in the field of mechanical circulatory support observed in the last few years, the group of patients who present with severe heart failure in an extremely critical condition or 'moribund' state are still a difficult group of patients to deal with, usually because of the presence of end-stage organ failure and/or uncertain neurological status in a ventilated patient. The outcome remains poor in these very critically ill patients. The Levitronix short-term VAD (Fig. 7) can be used as a 'bridge to decision' in these extremely sick patients who have contra-indications to the implantation of a long-term VAD or urgent transplantation at the time of presentation, if these

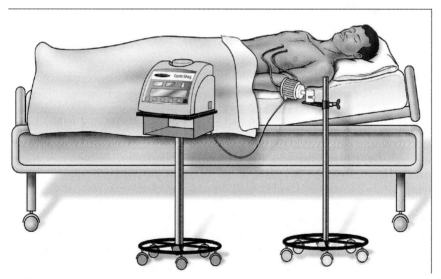

Fig. 7 The Levitronix Centrimag short-term device. Cannulation is from the left atrium to the aorta and the pump sits outside the body.

contra-indications are considered acute and potentially reversible prior to deciding if a more expensive device or transplant should be used. Using short-term, low-cost devices such as the Centrimag in this setting is very effective in stabilising the haemodynamic state, improving the end-organ function, extubating the patient to allow assessment of the neurological status and to provide an opportunity to assess further their clinical condition. Short-term, low-cost devices that can be inserted with minimal surgical invasiveness in such sick patients often with coagulopathy, provide immediate haemodynamic stability and recovery for future assessment of these patients either for bridge-to-transplantation, bridge-to-recovery or a long-term device. These patients can then be upgraded to a longer term device when their condition improves – usually extubated with normalised renal and liver function and with sepsis under control. Alternatively, some patients can be bridged straight to transplantation from the Levitronix device or straight to recovery, especially if they have a disease in which their myocardial function has the potential to recover in a short time (*e.g.* myocarditis or post myocardial infarction).

COMPLICATIONS OF VENTRICULAR ASSIST DEVICES

LVADs are not without complications. Early on, peri-operative haemorrhage, right heart failure and abdominal complications caused by the device can occur; later, infection, thrombo-embolism, haemolysis and device failure can be a problem. Earlier insertion of the LVAD before the development of multi-organ failure improves survival and lessens the risk of these complications. With evolving LVAD technology, some of these complications are now improving.

Early complications following device insertion include peri-operative haemorrhage (although this remains common, it is much less of a problem with the newer continuous flow pumps which involve a less traumatic surgical implantation than the bulkier pulsatile pumps), abdominal complications and right ventricular failure. Often, the underlying disease has a biventricular component; when the LVAD supports the left side of the heart and a normal cardiac output is returned to the right side, the right side can fail more and sometimes additional RVAD support is needed. Most commonly, this can be removed again after a short period. Abdominal complications caused by the device were common with the bulkier pulsatile devices, in particular the HeartMate I device which is inserted into the abdomen, and can lead to gastrointestinal obstruction, fistula and adhesions in some cases. However, these abdominal complications are rare with the axial flow pumps and with the devices that are not implanted into the abdomen.

Later complications include infection, thrombo-embolism, haemolysis and device failure. Infection can occur in the pump, in the pump pocket and around the drive-line. The smaller surface area of foreign material of the axial flow pumps, the minimal movement of the device inside the body and the smaller drive-line compared to the pulsatile pumps results in lower infection rates with the axial flow pump devices (0.37 versus 3.49 drive-line infections per patient year for the HeartMate II vs HeartMate 1 devices[12]). In terms of thrombo-embolism, pump thrombosis is a complication that can occur causing obstruction of the pump; it usually manifests as an increased power consumption of the pump which is seen as an increased wattage. Although it can be successfully treated with tyrofiban/tissue plasminogen activator, it is associated with a high mortality and can require a pump change. Although most thrombo-embolism is avoided by the anticoagulation these patients require, stroke can still be a problem – all devices except the HeartMate I require warfarin therapy. Although the regimen varies between units, the HeartMate II, Novocor and Heartware require an INR of 2–3 plus aspirin; the Jarvik 2000 and DeBakey require an INR of 2.5–3.5 plus aspirin; and the PVAD an INR of 2.5–3.5. As these patients are anticoagulated, bleeding complications (e.g. intracerebral haemorrhage) can occur and it is important to control the patient's blood pressure well to reduce the risk of an intracerebral bleed. Another recognised complication of continuous flow pumps is bleeding from arteriovenous malformations of the intestine that are found incidentally in normal adults;[38] this bleeding is worsened by the anticoagulation the patients require.

Device failure is another serious problem that can occur, particularly late after device insertion. There can be failure of the external components (which can usually be replaced) or of the internal components (which can be life-threatening). Device failure is more common with the first generation pulsatile pumps as they have more moving parts and also have valves which can degenerate leading to valvular regurgitation. However, they do have a hand-pump back-up system (manually operated by the patient or their carer, both of whom are trained in this procedure). Consequently, device failure can be associated with low morbidity and mortality,[39] if appropriately managed. In the REMATCH trial, device failure was the second most common cause of death in LVAD patients. Since then there have been many modifications to the HeartMate I device, which have significantly reduced the incidence of device failure. The second generation axial flow pumps have only one moving part, the rotor. They are expected to be more durable and appear to have a lower rate of device failure. The third generation magnetic levitation pumps have no bearings to wear out and are expected to be much more durable. The possibility of changing the device in device failure should be considered. Haemolysis is an unusual problem and is only usually significant enough to result in clinical compromise when it is due to thrombus in the pump.

The cost of LVAD implantation is high, but is already beginning to come down with costs in the postREMATCH era being much less than in REMATCH.[40,41] A large proportion of the cost of the devices is still spent on research and development of the devices. As the technology develops, survival increases and complications decrease, it is anticipated that their use will widen to involve increasing numbers of people with heart failure and probable cost reductions.

CONCLUSIONS AND EVOLVING ROLE

Insertion of left ventricular assist devices in patients with advanced heart failure with deteriorating clinical status is life-saving and they are now being inserted into an increasing number of patients. As the devices and patient management improve, the complications lessen and patient survival improves, justifying the earlier referral of patients for VAD implantation. Earlier referral of patients significantly reduces the risks of these complications, improves survival and long-term outcomes further; thus, the vicious circle of treating these patients with such a poor prognosis can be broken. Sustained reversal of severe heart failure (myocardial recovery) can be achieved with LVAD therapy, particularly when combined with pharmacological therapy. This can allow explantation of the device in a high proportion of patients with non-ischaemic cardiomyopathy avoiding the need for transplantation, immunosuppression and its associated complications, leaving the patient with a good quality of life and allowing the precious resource of a donor organ to be used for another needy individual.

These devices are rapidly evolving, which together with better patient management and selection is resulting in improved survival and a lower rate of complications and is also likely to lead to lower cost. The role of VADs as an alternative to transplantation (*i.e.* destination therapy) is likely to increase in the future for patients with advanced heart failure despite medical therapy. It appears that as device design, patient selection and management and the promptness of referral continue to improve, the outcome for many patients with advanced heart failure will improve further.

Key points for clinical practice

- Insertion of left ventricular assist devices in patients with advanced heart failure with deteriorating clinical status is life-saving and they are now being inserted into an increasing number of patients, particularly because of the decreasing availability of donor hearts.

- Patients are still being referred in a very advanced state and earlier referral of patients significantly improves survival and reduces the risks of complications.

- Ventricular assist devices were initially inserted as a bridge to transplantation in patients with advanced heart failure with deteriorating clinical status who were unable to wait any longer for heart transplantation. They are now also being inserted as 'destination therapy' (*i.e.* as an alternative to transplantation) and this use is likely to expand widely in the future.

- Sustained reversal of severe heart failure (myocardial recovery) can be achieved with ventricular assist device therapy, particularly when it is combined with pharmacological therapy which can allow explantation of the device in a proportion of patients with non-ischaemic cardiomyopathy avoiding the need for transplantation (including immunosuppression and its associated complications), leaving the patient with a good quality of life and allowing the precious resource of a donor organ to be used for another needy individual.

- The devices used have improved significantly over the years and are still rapidly evolving. They can broadly be divided into first, second and third generation devices.

- Second and third generation devices are designed to last longer and have less complications than the first generation devices.

- As the devices and patient management improve, the complications are decreasing and patient survival is improving, which justifies earlier referral of patients for ventricular assist device implantation.

References

1. Cowie MR, Wood DA, Coats AJ *et al.* Survival of patients with a new diagnosis of heart failure: a population based study. *Heart* 2000; **83**: 505–510.
2. Stewart S, MacIntyre K, Hole DJ, Capewell S, McMurray JJ. More 'malignant' than cancer? Five-year survival following a first admission for heart failure. *Eur J Heart Fail* 2001; **3**: 315–322.
3. Kirklin JK, Frazier OH. Developmental history of mechanical circulatory support. In: Frazier OH, Kirklin JK. (eds) *Mechanical Circulatory Support*. ISHLT Monograph Series. Amsterdam: Elsevier, 2006.
4. Rogers JG, Butler J, Lansman SL *et al.*; INTrEPID Investigators. Chronic mechanical circulatory support for inotrope-dependent heart failure patients who are not transplant candidates: results of the INTrEPID Trial. *J Am Coll Cardiol* 2007; **50**: 741–747.
5. Haj-Yahia S, Birks EJ, Rogers P *et al.* Midterm experience with the Jarvik 2000 axial flow left ventricular assist device. *J Thorac Cardiovasc Surg* 2007; **134**: 199–203.
6. Deng MC. Cardiac transplantation. *Heart* 2002; **87**: 177–184.
7. Frazier OH, Rose EA, Oz MC *et al.* Multicenter clinical evaluation of the HeartMate vented electric left ventricular assist system in patients awaiting heart transplantation. *J Thorac Cardiovasc Surg* 2001; **122**: 1186–1195.
8. Navia JL, McCarthy PM, Hoercher KJ *et al.* Do left ventricular assist device (LVAD) bridge-to-transplantation outcomes predict the results of permanent LVAD implantation? *Ann Thorac Surg* 2002; **74**: 2051–2062.
9. El-Banayosy A, Arusoglu L, Kizner L *et al.* Predictors of survival in patients bridged to transplantation with the Thoratec VAD device: a single-centre retrospective study on more than 100 patients. *J Heart Lung Transplant* 2000; **19**: 964–968.
10. Sun BC, Catanese KA, Spanier TB *et al.* 100 long-term implantable left ventricular assist devices: the Columbia Presbyterian interim experience. *Ann Thorac Surg* 1999; **68**: 688–694.
11. DeRose JJR, Michael A, Sun B *et al.* Implantable left ventricular assist devices: an evolving long-term cardiac replacement therapy. *Ann Surg* 1997; **226**: 461–470.
12. Miller LW, Pagani FD, Russell SD *et al.*; HeartMate II Clinical Investigators. Use of a continuous-flow device in patients awaiting heart transplantation. *N Engl J Med* 2007; **357**: 885–896.
13. Pagani F, Miller LW, Russell SD *et al.* Left ventricular assist device therapy with the HeartMate II continuous flow rotary pump as a bridge to heart transplantation. *Circulation* 2007; **116 (Suppl II)**: 540.
14. Lietz K, Miller LW. Improved survival of patients with end-stage heart failure listed for heart transplantation. *J Am Coll Cardiol* 2007; **50**: 1282–1290.
15. Taylor DO, Edwards LB, Boucek MM *et al.* Registry of the International Society for Heart and Lung Transplantation: twenty-fourth official adult heart transplant report 2007. *J Heart Lung Transplant* 2007; **26**: 769–781.
16. Mokadam NA, Ewald GA, Damiano RJ, Moazami N. Deterioration and mortality among patients with United Network for Organ Sharing status 2 heart disease: caution must be exercised in diverting organs. *J Thorac Cardiovasc Surg* 2006; **131**: 926–926.
17. Frazier OH, Benedict CR, Radovacevic B *et al.* Improved left ventricular function after chronic ventricular unloading. *Ann Thorac Surg* 1996; **62**: 675–682.
18. Birks EJ, Tansley PD, Hardy J *et al.* Left ventricular assist device and drug therapy for the reversal of heart failure. *N Engl J Med* 2006; **355**: 1873–1884.
19. Dandel M, Weng Y, Siniawski H, Potapov E, Lehmkuhl HB, Hetzer R. Long-term results in patients with idiopathic dilated cardiomyopathy after weaning from left ventricular assist devices. *Circulation* 2005; **112 (Suppl)**: I37–I45.
20. Simon MA, Kormos RL, Murali S *et al.* Myocardial recovery using ventricular assist devices: prevalence, clinical characteristics, and outcomes. *Circulation* 2005; **112 (Suppl)**: I32–I36.
21. Farrar DJ, Holman WR, McBride LR *et al.* Long-term follow-up of Thoratec ventricular assist device bridge-to-recovery patients successfully removed from support after recovery of ventricular function. *J Heart Lung Transplant* 2002; **21**: 516–521.
22. Mancini DM, Beniaminovitz A, Levin H *et al.* Low incidence of myocardial recovery

after left ventricular assist device implantation in patients with chronic heart failure. *Circulation* 1998; **98**: 2383–2389.

23. Yacoub MH. A novel strategy to maximise the efficacy of LVADs as a bridge to recovery. *Eur Heart J* 2001; **22**: 534–540.

24. Yacoub MH, Birks EJ, Tansley P, Henein MY, Bowles CT. Bridge to recovery: the Harefield approach. *J Congestive Heart Fail Circ Support* 2001; **2**: 27–30.

25. Yacoub MH, Tansley P, Birks EJ, Bowles CT, Banner NR, Khaghani A. A novel combination therapy to reverse end-stage heart failure. *Transplant Proc* 2001; **33**: 2762–2764.

26. Wong K, Boheler K, Bishop J *et al.* Pharmacological modulation pressure overload cardiac hypertrophy changes in ventricular function, extracellular matrix and gene expression. *Circulation* 1997; **96**: 2239–2246.

27. Wong K, Boheler KR, Bishop J *et al.* Clenbuterol induces cardiac hypertrophy with normal functional, morphological and molecular features. *Cardiovasc Res* 1998; **37**: 115–122.

28. George RS, Yacoub MH, Bowles CT *et al.* Quality of life following LVAD removal for myocardial recovery. *J Heart Lung Transplant.* 2007; 26: S161.

29. Birks EJ, Hall JL, Barton PJ *et al.* Gene profiling changes in cytoskeletal proteins during clinical recovery after left ventricular-assist device support. *Circulation* 2005; **112 (Suppl)**: I57–I64.

30. Hall JL, Birks EJ, Grindle S *et al.* Molecular signature of recovery following combination left ventricular assist device (LVAD) support and pharmacologic therapy. *Eur Heart J* 2007; **28**: 613–627.

31. Latif N, Yacoub MH, George R, Barton PJ, Birks EJ. Changes in sarcomeric and non-sarcomeric cytoskeletal proteins and focal adhesion molecules during clinical myocardial recovery after left ventricular assist device support. *J Heart Lung Transplant* 2007; **26**: 230–235.

32. Cullen ME, Yuen AH, Felkin LE *et al.* Myocardial expression of the arginine:glycine amidinotransferase gene is elevated in heart failure and normalized following recovery: potential implications for local creatine synthesis. *Circulation* 2006; **114**: 16–20.

33. Terracciano CMN, Harding SE, Tansley PT, Birks EJ, Barton PJR, Yacoub MH. Changes in sarcolemmal Ca entry and sarcoplasmic reticulum Ca content in ventricular myocytes from patients with end-stage heart failure following myocardial recovery after combined pharmacological and ventricular assist device therapy. *Eur Heart J* 2003; **24**: 1329–1339.

34. Rose EA, Gelijins AC, Moskowitz AJ *et al.* Long-term use of a left ventricular assist device for end-stage heart failure. *N Engl J Med* 2001; **345**: 1435–1443.

35. Stevenson LW, Miller LW, Desvigne-Nickens P *et al.* Left ventricular assist device as destination for patients undergoing intravenous inotropic therapy. A subset analysis from REMATCH (Randomized Evaluation of Mechanical Assistance for the Treatment of Congestive Heart Failure). *Circulation* 2004; **110**: 975–981.

36. Park SJ, Tector A, Piccioni W *et al.* Left ventricular assist devices as destination therapy: a new look at survival. *J Thorac Cardiovasc Surg* 2005; **129**: 9–17.

37. Long JW, Kfoury AG, Slaughter MS *et al.* Long term destination therapy with the HeartMate XVE left ventricular assist device: improved outcomes since the REMATCH study. *Congest Heart Fail* 2005; **11**: 155–156.

38. Letsou GV, Shah N, Gregoric ID, Myers TJ, Delgado R, Frazier OH. Gastrointestinal bleeding from arteriovenous malformations in patients supported by the Jarvik 2000 axial-flow left ventricular assist device. *J Heart Lung Transplant* 2005; **24**: 105–109.

39. Birks EJ, Tansley PD, Yacoub MH *et al.* Incidence and clinical management of life-threatening left ventricular assist device (LVAD) failure. *J Heart Lung Transplant* 2004; **23**: 964–969.

40. Oz MC, Gelijins AC, Miller L *et al.* Left ventricular assist devices as permanent heart failure therapy. The price of progress. *Ann Surg* 2003; **238**: 577–585.

41. Miller LW, Nelson KE, Bostic RR, Tong K, Slaughter MS, Long JW. Hospital costs for left ventricular assist devices for destination therapy: lower costs for implantation in the post-REMATCH era. *J Heart Lung Transplant* 2006; **25**: 778–784.

Martin K. Rutter James B. Meigs
Peter W.F. Wilson

13

Cardiovascular risk and the metabolic syndrome

In 1923, Kylin, a Swedish physician, provided the first description of the within-subject clustering of risk factors that increase the risk for type 2 diabetes and cardiovascular disease (CVD).[1] This phenomenon, now known as the metabolic syndrome,[2] has generated much interest and debate by physicians and scientists. The fact that clustering occurs is widely accepted,[3] though the underlying cause(s) remain uncertain. What we do understand about causation is that obesity, insulin resistance and inflammation are important factors that link the healthy individual with the metabolic syndrome and the subsequent development of type 2 diabetes mellitus and CVD.

In this review, we describe how the presence of metabolic syndrome influences CVD risk. Our review has focused on published studies up to October 2007 referring to incident CVD in relation to the National Cholesterol Education Program Adult Treatment Panel III (NCEP) definition of the metabolic syndrome.[2,4]

CVD RISK ASSOCIATED WITH METABOLIC SYNDROME

The first reports of CVD risk associated with metabolic syndrome were based on relatively small numbers of cardiovascular events[5] and suggested that

Martin K. Rutter MD (for correspondence)
Consultant Physician and Honorary Senior Lecturer,Cardiovascular Research Group, Division of Cardiovascular and Endocrine Sciences, University of Manchester and Manchester Diabetes Centre, Manchester Royal Infirmary, Oxford Road, Manchester M13 9WL, UK
E-mail: martin.rutter@cmmc.nhs.uk

James B. Meigs MD MPH
Associate Professor of Medicine, Harvard Medical School; Associate Physician, General Medicine Division, Department of Medicine, Massachusetts General Hospital Boston, Massachusetts, USA

Peter W.F. Wilson MD
Professor of Medicine and Public Health Emory University; Director of Epidemiology and Genomic Medicine, Altanta VA Medical Centre, GA, USA

metabolic syndrome was associated with a substantially high CVD risk. These impressive results have generally not been replicated in more recent larger studies. Most,[5-42] but not all,[43] studies had shown greater CVD risk in subjects with metabolic syndrome. Only now is the degree to which risk is increased becoming clearer and are the precise reasons for the associated risk being understood.

The degree to which metabolic syndrome increases CVD risk has been estimated by Ford[44] in a meta-analysis of 12 prospective studies. In this analysis, the presence of metabolic syndrome was associated with an increased CVD risk of 1.7-fold after adjustment for a variable number of cardiovascular risk factors. Ford estimated the proportion of vascular events attributed to baseline metabolic syndrome (population-attributable fraction) and found that the population-attributable fraction for all-cause mortality associated with metabolic syndrome was approximately 6%, and for CVD the corresponding figure was only 12%. He concluded that the 'metabolic syndrome does an unremarkable job of predicting all-cause mortality (estimated summary relative risk, ~1.2–1.4) and only a modest job of predicting CVD (estimated summary relative risk, ~1.7–1.9)'. Another meta-analysis including data from 21 studies provided a very similar risk for CVD.[45]

At first glance, it is rather surprising that metabolic syndrome does not perform better as a CVD risk factor, especially since the definitions of the metabolic syndrome include several established CVD risk factors. However, it should be remembered that the metabolic syndrome definitions have not been developed from statistical modelling of population-based data designed to maximise CVD risk prediction. There are several potential explanations for the limited performance of metabolic syndrome in CVD risk prediction. First, metabolic syndrome definitions do not include some established and powerful CVD risk factors (age, gender, smoking and LDL-cholesterol). Second, considering metabolic syndrome risk factors as equally-weighted categorical variables that are defined at relatively low thresholds, and limiting the diagnosis to three or more of these factors are likely to be important. Subjects with one or two components may be at significantly elevated risk but remain in the reference group, thus reducing the relative risk associated with metabolic syndrome.[44] The relatively low CVD risk associated with metabolic syndrome might suggest that the underlying pathophysiological cause of the risk factor clustering is, in itself, a weak CVD risk factor.

The CVD risk associated with the metabolic syndrome may well be underestimated by recently-performed shorter-term studies. The Framingham study has shown a 50% increase in the prevalence of the metabolic syndrome over an 8-year period starting in the early 1990s.[23] The world-wide increasing prevalence of obesity will lead to an increased prevalence of metabolic syndrome and a rise in the associated CVD. There have been few studies performed to assess the long-term CVD risk associated with metabolic syndrome but there are emerging data to suggest that the CVD risk associated with metabolic syndrome may persist and be independent of at least some traditional CVD risk factors.[25,32]

INFLUENCE OF GENDER

The influence of gender on CVD risk associated with metabolic syndrome has been examined in several studies that have shown different results.

We examined 3323 middle-aged Framingham Heart Study subjects free of diabetes or CVD at baseline for 8-year incident CVD in relation to the presence of baseline metabolic syndrome.[23] The study showed that, in men, the age-adjusted relative risk for incident CVD associated with baseline metabolic syndrome was 2.9, and for coronary heart disease (CHD) events was 2.5. However, in women, the corresponding event rates and relative risks were lower at 2.3 and 1.5, respectively. In men, the age-adjusted population-attributable fraction was approximately 30% for both CVD and CHD; in women, the corresponding values were much lower at 16% for CVD and 8% for total CHD. The low risk of CVD in women in this study was attributed to the fact that many of the women were pre-menopausal or peri-menopausal during the study. Another study from Singapore showed that the adverse impact of metabolic syndrome or type 2 diabetes mellitus was greater among men than women.[46]

An analysis of the National Health and Nutrition Examination Survey (NHANES) II data has shown no significant gender interaction in the CVD risk associated with metabolic syndrome.[14] Within the Hoorn study population, Dekker and co-workers[18] showed that the presence of metabolic syndrome was associated with a similar increased risk of CVD in both genders; however, in men, CVD events were more often fatal and in women the CVD outcome was more often non-fatal.

In contrast, several other studies[15,19,20,24,35,40] and a recent meta-analysis[45] have suggested that metabolic syndrome could be more predictive of CVD events in women than in men. Another paper from Framingham investigators showed that metabolic syndrome has a larger population-attributable risk for stroke in women than in men.[29]

If the presence of metabolic syndrome does increase the relative CVD risk in women more than in men, then one possible mechanism might be through inflammation. In separate analysis of Framingham data, we showed that C-reactive protein was more strongly related to the features of metabolic syndrome in women than in men.[13] This study was underpowered to assess the effect of gender on CVD risk associated with metabolic syndrome, no major effect was evident, and a gender interaction term was not significant in this analysis.

Clearly, more research is needed to clarify the factors that influence the gender interaction in the CVD risk associated with metabolic syndrome. Prevalent diabetes, and the development of diabetes in some of the cohorts, could explain some of the discrepant results since diabetes carries a higher relative risk for CVD in women than it does in men.

INFLUENCE OF DIABETES AND CVD

Current definitions of the metabolic syndrome include subjects with diabetes and CVD and this has obvious implications for disease prediction.

Prevalent diabetes
Metabolic syndrome is significantly related to the presence of diabetes; about one-third of those with metabolic syndrome also have diabetes and about 60–95% with type 2 diabetes also meet criteria for metabolic syndrome.[14,47]

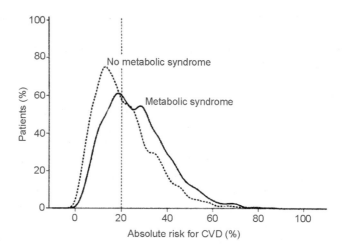

Fig. 1 Kernel density plots of the distribution of estimated 10-year absolute CVD risk for UKPDS patients with newly diagnosed type 2 diabetes mellitus classified by the presence or absence of metabolic syndrome defined according to ATP-III criteria. Vertical dotted line denoted 20% 10-year risk.[47] [Reprinted with permission: from Cull CA et al.[47] © 2007 Lippincott Williams & Wilkins]

Studies that have quantified the CVD risk associated with the metabolic syndrome have often included subjects with diabetes; therefore, risk estimates have been higher than they would have been if subjects with diabetes had been excluded.

Ford's meta-analysis and another more recently[45] have provided an estimate of how the presence of diabetes at baseline influences the CVD risk associated with the metabolic syndrome. In five prospective studies[7,9,12,15,16] that included subjects with diabetes, Ford showed that the relative risk for incident CVD associated with metabolic syndrome was 2.0 (range, 1.4–3.0). However, in seven studies[5,10,11,13,15,20,43] that excluded subjects with diabetes, the relative risk was lower at 1.6 (range, 1.3–1.9) indicating that a substantial proportion of the CVD risk associated with metabolic syndrome is attributable to the presence of diabetes at baseline.

Similarly, in an analysis of data from the NHANES II, Malik and co-workers[14] showed that those with metabolic syndrome but without diabetes had an a hazard ratio of CHD mortality of 1.7 but those with metabolic syndrome and diabetes had a hazard ratio of 2.9.

Since there are clear guidelines for the clinical management of type 2 diabetes mellitus, the additional diagnosis of metabolic syndrome has little utility for the practising clinician, especially since some data,[17,48] but not all,[47] suggest that metabolic syndrome may not have prognostic significance for CVD events in subjects with diagnosed diabetes. A recent analysis from the United Kingdom Prospective Study (UKPDS) has indicated that, in patients with type 2 diabetes mellitus, the presence of metabolic syndrome increased the CVD risk by approximately one-third.[47] However, there was a significant overlap in estimated 10-year CVD risks between patients with and without metabolic syndrome (Fig. 1). The authors argued that in type 2 diabetes mellitus the diagnosis of metabolic syndrome holds limited clinical value for CVD risk stratification.

These arguments create a case for the exclusion of subjects with diabetes from the definition of metabolic syndrome.

Incident diabetes

Metabolic syndrome is a stronger risk factor for incident diabetes than for incident CVD, and it is quite possible that the CVD risk associated with metabolic syndrome is partly explained by the development of type 2 diabetes mellitus. In other words, the subjects who develop CVD are largely those who develop type 2 diabetes mellitus on the way. There are limited numbers of studies that have tested this hypothesis. However, such an analysis was performed by Framingham investigators who showed that excluding subjects who developed type 2 diabetes mellitus during follow-up had no significant effect on the relative risk of incident CVD associated with baseline metabolic syndrome.[21]

Prevalent CVD

Some studies have included subjects with prevalent CVD.[11] which may also influence the CVD risk associated with metabolic syndrome. As in the case of established diabetes, we have clear guidelines for the management of subjects with CVD; therefore, the utility of including subjects with CVD in the definition of metabolic syndrome is questionable.

INFLUENCE OF METABOLIC SYNDROME COMPONENTS ON CVD RISK

Data from the Framingham study have demonstrated that one of the consequences of risk factor clustering is that the CVD risk associated with two or more components of metabolic syndrome being present is similar to the CVD risk associated with three or more components.[23] This suggests that even a modest degree of risk factor clustering can adequately capture the CVD risk associated with this phenotype. In another population-based study, Malik and co-workers[14] have shown that even those with one or two metabolic syndrome components have increased risks for CHD and CVD mortality when compared to subjects without metabolic syndrome components.

Does metabolic syndrome predict CVD risk beyond the sum of its parts?

This controversial question has been keenly debated over the past couple of years.[49,50] Khan and co-workers[50] have identified three cross-sectional studies[51–53] and two prospective studies[10,20] all indicating that the CVD risk associated with metabolic syndrome was no greater than the CVD risk associated with sum of its component parts. Similar findings have been shown in an analysis of prospective data from more recent studies.[18,31] In defence of these robust arguments, Grundy[49] has stressed the importance of multiplicative risk, and the hidden risk associated with the prothrombotic state, inflammation, hypertriglyceridaemia and other 'unmeasured risk factors' that are observed in subjects with metabolic syndrome. He has also argued that the long-term CVD risk associated with metabolic syndrome may have been underestimated by published studies. A recent study from a large, community-based sample of middle-aged men has suggested that the presence of metabolic syndrome at baseline is indeed predictive of 30-year CVD risk independently of traditional CVD risk factors.[32] An 18-year follow-up of men in the Multiple Risk Factor Intervention Trial has shown similar results though relative risks for CVD associated with baseline metabolic syndrome were very modest and lost statistical significance after serial adjustment for other CVD risk factors.[25] Neither study adjusted for the development of diabetes during follow-up. Clearly, further studies of the long-term impact of metabolic syndrome are required.

One strategy to answer the question as to whether risk factor clustering in the metabolic syndrome increases CVD risk information beyond the sum of the component parts would be to show that one or more traits modified CVD risk in combination with others. Few studies have had the power to look at interactions among traits predicting CVD. In the one such study, Golden and co-workers[51] used data from about 12,000 Atherosclerosis Risk in Communities Study participants to assess whether combinations of hypertension, hyperinsulinaemia, obesity, hypertriglyceridaemia, low HDL-cholesterol, and hyperglycaemia were associated with increased thickness of carotid intima media thickness. Most combinations of traits had additive effects on carotid intima media thickness, but trait combinations including hypertension and hypertriglyceridaemia showed evidence of an interactive, synergistic effect.

In aggregate, current data do not strongly support more than an additive effect of metabolic syndrome traits on CVD risk, consistent with the same relationship embodied in the Framingham risk score.

VALUE OF FRAMINGHAM RISK SCORE AND/OR METABOLIC SYNDROME FOR CVD RISK PREDICTION

How should the practicing physician assess CVD risk in the general population? To help answer this question, we need to consider measures of test performance other than relative risk which provides little information about the ability of a diagnosis, such as metabolic syndrome, to identify correctly individuals who will develop disease. The area under the receiver–operator characteristic curve provides such information, and is a function of a test's sensitivity (the probability that a test correctly identifies an individual with subsequent disease, or the true-positive rate) and false-positive rate. The area under the receiver–operator curve is the probability that a test correctly discriminates subjects developing an outcome from those without an outcome, where 0.5 is chance discrimination and 1.0 is perfect discrimination.

Is metabolic syndrome better or worse than the Framingham risk score?
Several studies have compared the performance of the Framingham risk score and metabolic syndrome in CVD prediction[11,17,20,22] and only one[11] has shown that the metabolic syndrome offers any advantage over the Framingham risk score. The population-based study by Stern and co-workers[17] is most informative on this issue. In this study, 2941 San Antonio Heart Study subjects who were free from CVD were examined for incident CVD in relation to baseline metabolic syndrome and Framingham risk score. The authors found that baseline metabolic syndrome had true-positive and false-positive rates for

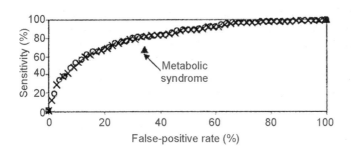

Fig. 2 Receiver–operator curve curves for the prediction of CVD in the San Antonio Heart Study. The Framingham risk score (X) and the models combining metabolic syndrome with Framingham risk score (open circles) are compared with the sensitivity and false-positive rate of metabolic syndrome (filled triangles). Adapted from Stern *et al.*[17]: © 2004 American Diabetes Association reprinted with permission from *The American Diabetes Association.*

CVD of 67% and 34%, respectively. When the true-positive rate for CVD was fixed at 67%, the authors found that the false-positive rate of the baseline Framingham risk score was better than metabolic syndrome at 20%; when the false-positive rate was fixed at 34%, the true-positive rate for CVD was also better than metabolic syndrome at 81% (Fig. 2). The area under the receiver–operator curve of the Framingham risk score was 0.816; considering both the Framingham risk score and the metabolic syndrome together gave a similar area under the receiver–operator curve (0.811). These data mean that the Framingham risk score identifies subjects at future risk of CVD more accurately than the diagnosis of metabolic syndrome. Further assigning a diagnosis of the metabolic syndrome tells us no more about future disease risk than we would already have known on the basis of information from the prediction rules. Stern and colleagues[17] concluded that the metabolic syndrome is inferior to established rules for CVD prediction.

The only study to show that metabolic syndrome has potential advantage over Framingham risk score for CVD prediction is a study of placebo-treated subjects from the Scandinavian Simvastatin Survival Study (4S) and the Air Force/Texas Coronary Atherosclerosis Prevention Study (AFCAPS/TexCAPS). In this *post hoc* analysis, metabolic syndrome was a significant predictor of incident CVD after adjustment for the Framingham risk score.[11] Subjects in these studies were selected based on the presence of dyslipidaemia and in the case of 4S, prior CHD; therefore, patient selection might explain why the results of this study were not replicated in the other population-based studies of lower-risk subjects.[17,20,22]

Therefore, for CVD risk prediction in the general population, the evidence strongly indicates that practicing physicians should continue to use the Framingham risk score and not the metabolic syndrome for the most precise estimation of individual CVD risk.

Do unique metabolic syndrome risk factors (obesity, triglycerides, and glucose) add to CVD risk estimated by the Framingham risk score?

This important question has been addressed by prospective analyses of population-based data from the Framingham Heart Study.[48] This analysis showed that when the Framingham risk score[54] and unique metabolic syndrome risk factors were combined, either as continuous or categorical variables, the ability of CVD prediction models did not improve. This important analysis suggests that the CVD risk information associated with the unique metabolic syndrome risk factors is adequately 'captured' by the variables present in the Framingham risk score. Since the Framingham risk score was developed from the Framingham population, one would expect that it would perform well in this setting and it might be argued that this analysis was biased against the metabolic syndrome definition. However, similar analyses have been performed in other studies[17,20] and provided identical results (Fig. 2).

INFLUENCE OF DIFFERENT METABOLIC SYNDROME DEFINITIONS ON CVD RISK

Several prospective studies have compared the risk of incident CVD according to different definitions of the metabolic syndrome. In the Kuopio Ischaemic Heart Disease Risk Factor Study of 1209 Finnish men, the World Health Organization (WHO) definition performed better than NCEP.[5] This was a study of middle-aged men in whom the prevalence of metabolic syndrome was rather low and the event numbers rather small. In the San Antonio Heart Study of Mexican-Americans and non-Hispanic whites, NCEP-defined metabolic syndrome was predictive of all-cause mortality and cardiovascular mortality. On the other hand, WHO-defined metabolic syndrome was predictive of cardiovascular mortality but not of all-cause mortality.[15] Dekker and co-workers showed that the NCEP definition was associated with an approximately 2-fold risk of all CVD end-points in men and of non-fatal CVD in women, after adjustment for age only. The hazard ratios associated with the WHO, European Group for the Study of Insulin Resistance (EGIR), and American Association of Clinical Endocrinologists definitions for all end-points were just slightly lower.[18] We recently examined Framingham offspring cohort subjects without diabetes or CVD at baseline for 11-year CVD associated with several metabolic syndrome definitions. When compared to subjects without metabolic syndrome, the relative risks for CVD were similar for all definitions (NCEP, 1.8 [95% CI, 1.4–2.3]; International Diabetes Federation, 1.7 [95% CI, 1.3–2.3]; and EGIR, 2.1 [95% CI, 1.6 –2.7]).[55]

In summary, there are no striking differences between the different metabolic syndrome definitions in CVD risk prediction.

SHOULD C-REACTIVE PROTEIN BE ADDED TO THE METABOLIC SYNDROME DEFINITION?

There has been interest in the value of adding C-reactive protein to the metabolic syndrome definition in order to improve population CVD prediction.[56] Although several studies suggest that metabolic syndrome and C-reactive protein are independent CVD risk factors, there are no data showing that adding C-reactive protein to metabolic syndrome variables improves CVD risk prediction at the population level. The standard statistical tests used to assess improvements in population risk are an increase in the area under the receiver–operator curve (see above) or 'c-statistic' (analogous to the area under the receiver–operator curve). Framingham investigators have performed a prospective analysis of Framingham Offspring Study subjects to address this issue.[13] This analysis showed that, although C-reactive protein and metabolic syndrome were independent CVD risk factors, the inclusion of both variables in the multivariable model produced no significant increase in the c-statistic when compared with that obtained using metabolic syndrome on its own. The explanation for this apparent paradox has been provided in a recent study showing that for a risk factor to be effective for population risk stratification, the associated hazards ratio has to be 'of a magnitude rarely seen in epidemiological studies'.[57] Therefore, for population CVD risk prediction, there is no practical value of adding C-reactive protein to the metabolic syndrome definition. Further research should aim to establish whether combining C-reactive protein and metabolic syndrome data could have utility in the risk assessment of individual patients.

ASSESSMENT OF CVD RISK IN SUBJECTS WITH METABOLIC SYNDROME

Subjects with metabolic syndrome but without diabetes

Wong and co-workers[58] showed that subjects with metabolic syndrome but without diabetes or CVD are at increased CHD risk as assessed by Framingham risk function, and are likely to benefit from risk factor modification. It would seem very reasonable that Framingham risk score be used in such subjects.

Subjects with diabetes and metabolic syndrome

The diagnosis of diabetes in an individual should prompt the physician to manage CVD risk actively according to established guidelines. Should a more accurate estimation of CVD risk in subjects with type 2 diabetes mellitus be required, then the Framingham risk score or the UKPDS risk engine would be appropriate tools.[59,60] However, this assessment would be unlikely to lead to a change in therapy because aggressive risk factor modification can be justified in the large majority of subjects with type 2 diabetes mellitus regardless of the risk estimated by either method. The only clinical test that might influence therapy might be an assessment of renal function by urine dipstick, estimated creatinine clearance and/or micro-albuminuria testing. The finding of micro-albuminuria or diabetic nephropathy should prompt angiotensin receptor blocker or angiotensin concerting enzyme inhibitor therapy and lower target levels for blood pressure.

There is scant evidence to justify screening for asymptomatic cerebral or coronary artery disease in subjects with type 2 diabetes mellitus. This applies whether or not these subjects also have the metabolic syndrome. The American Heart Association[61] and the US Preventive Task Force[62] have strongly discouraged CHD screening in asymptomatic subjects with type 2 diabetes mellitus. Only one small randomised study has shown benefit from revascularisation in asymptomatic subjects with type 2 diabetes mellitus screened for CHD.[63] This study needs to be replicated in larger groups with rigorous analysis of the psychological and physical benefits and cost-effectiveness. Although some authorities in the field have advocated non-invasive screening for CHD in subjects with diabetes, it is the firm opinion of the authors that screening guidelines should remain conservative until carefully performed studies show clear evidence of clinical benefit.

CONCLUSIONS

Clustering of metabolic syndrome components within individuals helps in the identification of subjects who are at increased risk for both CVD and diabetes. However, CVD risk in subjects with and without metabolic syndrome should continue to be estimated using the Framingham risk score. Current metabolic syndrome definitions perform a modest job of predicting CVD and further refinements to the definition are expected. The CVD risk associated with metabolic syndrome is influenced by inclusion of subjects with diabetes and CVD at baseline, and by the development of diabetes during follow-up; this might partly explain why metabolic syndrome appears to be a stronger risk factor for CVD in women than in men. CVD risk associated with metabolic syndrome does not appear to be greater than the sum of its parts but the long-term CVD risk associated with metabolic syndrome is an area for future research. Adding C-reactive protein to metabolic syndrome variables does not improve population CVD risk prediction.

Life-style intervention and treatment of specific abnormal metabolic syndrome components is appropriate until a better understanding of the pathogenesis of metabolic syndrome is available. At such time, we may be able to target the underlying causes of the syndrome and ultimately prevent the development of both CVD and diabetes.

ACKNOWLEDGEMENT

JBM was supported by NIDDK K24 DK080140.

Key points for clinical practice

- Clustering of metabolic syndrome components within individuals has been recognised for many years.
- Subjects with metabolic syndrome are at increased risk for both cardiovascular disease (CVD) and diabetes.
- CVD risk associated with metabolic syndrome is influenced by the inclusion of subjects with diabetes and CVD at baseline, and by the development of diabetes during follow-up.
- Metabolic syndrome is probably a stronger risk factor for CVD in women than in men.
- CVD risk associated with metabolic syndrome does not appear to be greater than the sum of its parts.
- Adding C-reactive protein to metabolic syndrome variables does not improve population CVD risk prediction.

Key points for clinical practice (continued)

- The Framingham risk function is the most appropriate method for assessing CVD risk in subjects with or without metabolic syndrome.

- Life-style intervention and treatment of specific abnormal metabolic syndrome components is appropriate until a better understanding of the pathogenesis of metabolic syndrome is available.

- Targeting the underlying causes of the syndrome may ultimately prevent the development of both CVD and diabetes.

References

1. Kylin E. Studien ueber das Hypertonie-Hyperglykamie-Hyperurikamiesyndrom. *Zentralbl Innere Med* 1923; **44**.

2. Executive Summary of The Third Report of The National Cholesterol Education Program (NCEP) Expert Panel on Detection, Evaluation, And Treatment of High Blood Cholesterol In Adults (Adult Treatment Panel III). *JAMA* 2001; **285**: 2486–2497.

3. Wilson PW, Kannel WB, Silbershatz H *et al*. Clustering of metabolic factors and coronary heart disease. *Arch Intern Med* 1999; **159**: 1104–1109.

4. Grundy SM, Cleeman JI, Daniels SR *et al*. Diagnosis and management of the metabolic syndrome: an American Heart Association/National Heart, Lung, and Blood Institute scientific statement: executive summary. *Circulation* 2005; **112**: e285–e290.

5. Lakka HM, Laaksonen DE, Lakka TA *et al*. The metabolic syndrome and total and cardiovascular disease mortality in middle-aged men. *JAMA* 2002; **288**: 2709–2716.

6. Isomaa B, Almgren P, Tuomi T *et al*. Cardiovascular morbidity and mortality associated with the metabolic syndrome. *Diabetes Care* 2001; **24**: 683–689.

7. Onat A, Ceyhan K, Basar O *et al*. Metabolic syndrome: major impact on coronary risk in a population with low cholesterol levels – a prospective and cross-sectional evaluation. *Atherosclerosis* 2002; **165**: 285–292.

8. Bonora E, Kiechl S, Willeit J *et al*. Carotid atherosclerosis and coronary heart disease in the metabolic syndrome: prospective data from the Bruneck study. *Diabetes Care* 2003; **26**: 1251–1257.

9. Ridker PM, Buring JE, Cook NR *et al*. C-reactive protein, the metabolic syndrome, and risk of incident cardiovascular events: an 8-year follow-up of 14 719 initially healthy American women. *Circulation* 2003; **107**: 391–397.

10. Sattar N, Gaw A, Scherbakova O *et al*. Metabolic syndrome with and without C-reactive protein as a predictor of coronary heart disease and diabetes in the West of Scotland Coronary Prevention Study. *Circulation* 2003; **108**: 414–419.

11. Girman CJ, Rhodes T, Mercuri M *et al*. The metabolic syndrome and risk of major coronary events in the Scandinavian Simvastatin Survival Study (4S) and the Air Force/Texas Coronary Atherosclerosis Prevention Study (AFCAPS/TexCAPS). *Am J Cardiol* 2004; **93**: 136–141.

12. Katzmarzyk PT, Church TS, Blair SN. Cardiorespiratory fitness attenuates the effects of the metabolic syndrome on all-cause and cardiovascular disease mortality in men. *Arch Intern Med* 2004; **164**: 1092–1097.

13. Rutter MK, Meigs JB, Sullivan LM *et al*. C-reactive protein, the metabolic syndrome, and prediction of cardiovascular events in the Framingham Offspring Study. *Circulation* 2004; **110**: 380–385.

14. Malik S, Wong ND, Franklin SS *et al*. Impact of the metabolic syndrome on mortality from coronary heart disease, cardiovascular disease, and all causes in United States adults. *Circulation* 2004; **110**: 1245–1250.

15. Hunt KJ, Resendez RG, Williams K *et al*. National Cholesterol Education Program versus

World Health Organization metabolic syndrome in relation to all-cause and cardiovascular mortality in the San Antonio Heart Study. *Circulation* 2004; **110**: 1251–1257.

16. Ford ES. The metabolic syndrome and mortality from cardiovascular disease and all-causes: findings from the National Health and Nutrition Examination Survey II Mortality Study. *Atherosclerosis* 2004; **173**: 309–314.

17. Stern MP, Williams K, Gonzalez-Villalpando C *et al*. Does the metabolic syndrome improve identification of individuals at risk of type 2 diabetes and/or cardiovascular disease? *Diabetes Care* 2004; **27**: 2676–2681.

18. Dekker JM, Girman C, Rhodes T *et al*. Metabolic syndrome and 10-year cardiovascular disease risk in the Hoorn Study. *Circulation* 2005; **112**: 666–673.

19. Girman CJ, Dekker JM, Rhodes T *et al*. An exploratory analysis of criteria for the metabolic syndrome and its prediction of long-term cardiovascular outcomes: the Hoorn study. *Am J Epidemiol* 2005; **162**: 438–447.

20. McNeill AM, Rosamond WD, Girman CJ *et al*. The metabolic syndrome and 11-year risk of incident cardiovascular disease in the atherosclerosis risk in communities study. *Diabetes Care* 2005; **28**: 385–390.

21. Rutter MK, Meigs JB, Sullivan LM *et al*. Insulin resistance, the metabolic syndrome, and incident cardiovascular events in the Framingham Offspring Study. *Diabetes* 2005; **54**: 3252–3257.

22. Wannamethee SG, Shaper AG, Lennon L *et al*. Metabolic syndrome vs Framingham Risk Score for prediction of coronary heart disease, stroke, and type 2 diabetes mellitus. *Arch Intern Med* 2005; **165**: 2644–2650.

23. Wilson PW, D'Agostino RB, Parise H *et al*. Metabolic syndrome as a precursor of cardiovascular disease and type 2 diabetes mellitus. *Circulation* 2005; **112**: 3066–3072.

24. Butler J, Rodondi N, Zhu Y *et al*. Metabolic syndrome and the risk of cardiovascular disease in older adults. *J Am Coll Cardiol* 2006; **47**: 1595–1602.

25. Eberly LE, Prineas R, Cohen JD *et al*. Metabolic syndrome: risk factor distribution and 18-year mortality in the multiple risk factor intervention trial. *Diabetes Care* 2006; **29**: 123–130.

26. Jeppesen J, Hansen TW, Rasmussen S, Ibsen H, Torp-Pedersen C. Metabolic syndrome, low-density lipoprotein cholesterol, and risk of cardiovascular disease: a population-based study. *Atherosclerosis* 2006; 189: 369–374.

27. Juutilainen A, Lehto S, Ronnemaa T *et al*. Proteinuria and metabolic syndrome as predictors of cardiovascular death in non-diabetic and type 2 diabetic men and women. *Diabetologia* 2006; **49**: 56–65.

28. Lorenzo C, Williams K, Hunt KJ *et al*. Trend in the prevalence of the metabolic syndrome and its impact on cardiovascular disease incidence: the San Antonio Heart Study. *Diabetes Care* 2006; **29**: 625–630.

29. Najarian RM, Sullivan LM, Kannel WB *et al*. Metabolic syndrome compared with type 2 diabetes mellitus as a risk factor for stroke: the Framingham Offspring Study. *Arch Intern Med* 2006; **166**: 106–111.

30. Reinhard W, Holmer SR, Fischer M *et al*. Association of the metabolic syndrome with early coronary disease in families with frequent myocardial infarction. *Am J Cardiol* 2006; **97**: 964–967.

31. Saely CH, Koch L, Schmid F *et al*. Adult Treatment Panel III 2001 but not International Diabetes Federation 2005 criteria of the metabolic syndrome predict clinical cardiovascular events in subjects who underwent coronary angiography. *Diabetes Care* 2006; **29**: 901–907.

32. Sundstrom J, Riserus U, Byberg L *et al*. Clinical value of the metabolic syndrome for long term prediction of total and cardiovascular mortality: prospective, population based cohort study. *BMJ* 2006; **332**: 878–882.

33. Chien KL, Hsu HC, Lee YT, Chen MF. Renal function and metabolic syndrome components on cardiovascular and all-cause mortality. *Atherosclerosis* 2007; [E-pub ahead of print].

34. de Simone G, Devereux RB, Chinali M *et al*. Prognostic impact of metabolic syndrome by different definitions in a population with high prevalence of obesity and diabetes: the Strong Heart Study. *Diabetes Care* 2007; **30**: 1851–1856.

35. Hunt KJ, Williams K, Hazuda HP *et al*. The metabolic syndrome and the impact of diabetes on coronary heart disease mortality in women and men: the San Antonio Heart Study. *Ann Epidemiol* 2007; **17**: 870–877.
36. Iso H, Sato S, Kitamura A *et al*. Metabolic syndrome and the risk of ischemic heart disease and stroke among Japanese men and women. *Stroke* 2007; **38**: 1744–1751.
37. Liu J, Grundy SM, Wang W *et al*. Ten-year risk of cardiovascular incidence related to diabetes, prediabetes, and the metabolic syndrome. *Am Heart J* 2007; **153**: 552–558.
38. Lorenzo C, Williams K, Hunt KJ *et al*. The National Cholesterol Education Program – Adult Treatment Panel III, International Diabetes Federation, and World Health Organization definitions of the metabolic syndrome as predictors of incident cardiovascular disease and diabetes. *Diabetes Care* 2007; **30**: 8–13.
39. Klausen KP, Parving HH, Scharling H *et al*. The association between metabolic syndrome, microalbuminuria and impaired renal function in the general population: impact on cardiovascular disease and mortality. *J Intern Med* 2007; **262**: 470–478.
40. Pischon T, Hu FB, Rexrode KM, Girman CJ, Manson JE, Rimm EB. Inflammation, the metabolic syndrome, and risk of coronary heart disease in women and men. *Atherosclerosis* 2007; [E-pub ahead of print].
41. Wang J, Ruotsalainen S, Moilanen L *et al*. The metabolic syndrome predicts cardiovascular mortality: a 13-year follow-up study in elderly non-diabetic Finns. *Eur Heart J* 2007; **28**: 857–864.
42. Zhao D, Grundy SM, Wang W *et al*. Ten-year cardiovascular disease risk of metabolic syndrome without central obesity in middle-aged Chinese. *Am J Cardiol* 2007; **100**: 835–839.
43. Resnick HE, Jones K, Ruotolo G *et al*. Insulin resistance, the metabolic syndrome, and risk of incident cardiovascular disease in nondiabetic American Indians: the strong heart study. *Diabetes Care* 2003; **26**: 861–867.
44. Ford ES. Risks for all-cause mortality, cardiovascular disease, and diabetes associated with the metabolic syndrome: a summary of the evidence. *Diabetes Care* 2005; **28**: 1769–1778.
45. Galassi A, Reynolds K, He J. Metabolic syndrome and risk of cardiovascular disease: a meta-analysis. *Am J Med* 2006; **119**: 812–819.
46. Mak KH, Ma S, Heng D *et al*. Impact of sex, metabolic syndrome, and diabetes mellitus on cardiovascular events. *Am J Cardiol* 2007; **100**: 227–233.
47. Cull CA, Jensen CC, Retnakaran R *et al*. Impact of the metabolic syndrome on macrovascular and microvascular outcomes in type 2 diabetes mellitus: United Kingdom Prospective Diabetes Study 78. *Circulation* 2007; **116**: 2119–2126.
48. Grundy SM, Brewer Jr HB, Cleeman JI *et al*. Definition of metabolic syndrome: Report of the National Heart, Lung, and Blood Institute/American Heart Association conference on scientific issues related to definition. *Circulation* 2004; **109**: 433–438.
49. Grundy SM. Metabolic syndrome: connecting and reconciling cardiovascular and diabetes worlds. *J Am Coll Cardiol* 2006; **47**: 1093–1100.
50. Kahn R, Buse J, Ferrannini E *et al*. The metabolic syndrome: time for a critical appraisal. Joint statement from the American Diabetes Association and the European Association for the Study of Diabetes. *Diabetologia* 2005; **48**: 1684–1699.
51. Golden SH, Folsom AR, Coresh J *et al*. Risk factor groupings related to insulin resistance and their synergistic effects on subclinical atherosclerosis: the atherosclerosis risk in communities study. *Diabetes* 2002; **51**: 3069–3076.
52. Alexander CM, Landsman PB, Teutsch SM *et al*. NCEP-defined metabolic syndrome, diabetes, and prevalence of coronary heart disease among NHANES III participants age 50 years and older. *Diabetes* 2003; **52**: 1210–1214.
53. Yarnell JW, Patterson CC, Bainton D *et al*. Is metabolic syndrome a discrete entity in the general population? Evidence from the Caerphilly and Speedwell population studies. *Heart* 1998; **79**: 248–252.
54. Wilson PW, D'Agostino RB, Levy D *et al*. Prediction of coronary heart disease using risk factor categories. *Circulation* 1998; **97**: 1837–1847.
55. Meigs JB, Rutter MK, Sullivan LM, Fox CS, D'Agostino Sr RB, Wilson PW. Impact of insulin resistance on risk of type 2 diabetes and cardiovascular disease in people with metabolic syndrome. *Diabetes Care* 2007; **30**: 1219–1225.

56. Ridker PM, Wilson PW, Grundy SM. Should C-reactive protein be added to metabolic syndrome and to assessment of global cardiovascular risk? *Circulation* 2004; **109**: 2818–2825.
57. Pepe MS, Janes H, Longton G *et al*. Limitations of the odds ratio in gauging the performance of a diagnostic, prognostic, or screening marker. *Am J Epidemiol* 2004; **159**: 882–890.
58. Wong ND, Pio JR, Franklin SS *et al*. Preventing coronary events by optimal control of blood pressure and lipids in patients with the metabolic syndrome. *Am J Cardiol* 2003; **91**: 1421–1426.
59. Kothari V, Stevens RJ, Adler AI *et al*. UKPDS 60: risk of stroke in type 2 diabetes estimated by the UK Prospective Diabetes Study risk engine. *Stroke* 2002; **33**: 1776–1781.
60. Stevens RJ, Kothari V, Adler AI *et al*. The UKPDS risk engine: a model for the risk of coronary heart disease in type II diabetes (UKPDS 56). *Clin Sci (Lond)* 2001; **101**: 671–679.
61. Redberg RF, Greenland P, Fuster V *et al*. Prevention Conference VI: Diabetes and Cardiovascular Disease: Writing Group III: risk assessment in persons with diabetes. *Circulation* 2002; **105**: e144–e152.
62. US Preventive Services Task Force. Screening for coronary heart disease: recommendation statement. *Ann Intern Med* 2004; **140**: 569–572.
63. Faglia E, Manuela M, Antonella Q et al. Risk reduction of cardiac events by screening of unknown asymptomatic coronary artery disease in subjects with type 2 diabetes mellitus at high cardiovascular risk: an open-label randomized pilot study. *Am Heart J* 2005; **149**: e1–e6.

K. Edward McLaughlin Finn G. Farquharson

14

Recent advances in surgery of the thoracic aorta

Management of thoracic aortic disease represents a formidable challenge. Accurate diagnosis, careful monitoring and medical and surgical therapy are important components of the treatment of these conditions. Surgical procedures are undertaken in order to prevent the complications of aortic rupture, dissection or death. In recent years, there have been significant developments in the understanding and management of these important conditions.

PATHOGENESIS OF AORTIC ANEURYSMS

Much work has been undertaken to investigate the pathogenesis of thoracic aortic disease. One area of interest concerns the study of matrix metalloproteinases (MMPs). MMPs are a group of over 20 zinc-dependent proteolytic enzymes which have been demonstrated to have a major role in the synthetic–lytic equilibrium of connective tissue. These enzymes are produced in the aortic wall and in the inflammatory cells. They are involved in the turn over of extracellular matrix (ECM) by breakdown of proteins such as elastin and collagen. MMPs are regulated by a tissue inhibitor of metalloproteinases (TIMPs). Thoracic aortic aneurysms are associated with destruction of the extracellular matrix and fragmentation of the elastic lammellae of the media, reduced elastin production and disordered collagen formation. Recent studies have examined the potential for altered metabolism of extracellular matrix as a precursor to major aortic disease. MMP expression is increased in thoracic aortic aneurysm and in thoracic aortic dissection compared to controls. There

K. Edward McLaughlin MD FRCS (for correspondence)
Consultant Cardiothoracic Surgeon, Manchester Heart Centre, Manchester Royal Infirmary, Oxford Road, Manchester M13 9WL, UK
E-mail: kenneth.mclaughlin@cmmc.nhs.uk

Finn G. Farquharson MBBS MSc FRCR
Consultant Vascular Radiologist, Manchester Royal Infirmary, Oxford Road, Manchester M13 9WL, UK

are also alterations in TIMP expression, suggesting a shift towards proteolysis. These changes are more marked in thoracic aortic dissection.[1] A genetic component for the pathogenesis of the aortic aneurysm has also been explored by comparing the level of MMP activity and level of TIMP in thoracic aortic aneurysm in patients with bicuspid and tricuspid aortic valves. An increased level of activity of MMPs was identified in the walls of aneurysms from patients with a bicuspid aortic valve. This may suggest a mechanism by which patients with a bicuspid aortic valve are predisposed to the histological abnormalities of elastic lammellae within the aorta and loss of normal elastic properties of the proximal aorta, leading to aneurysm formation.[2] Bicuspid aortic valves are associated with a reduction in expression of endothelial nitric oxide synthase in the ascending aorta and there is evidence of a relationship between endothelial nitric oxide synthase and the development of aneurysmal dilatation of the aorta.[4]

GENETIC ASPECTS OF THORACIC AORTIC DISEASE

The genetic aspects of thoracic aortic disease other than connective tissue disorders such as Marfan and Ehlers–Danlos syndromes are gradually being explored. The growing body of evidence implicating MMPs in the role of aortic aneurysm formation has led to investigation of the genetic aspect of these proteins. A single nucleotide polymorphism in the MMP-9 gene has been shown to be more frequent in patients with thoracic aortic aneurysm and thoracic aortic dissection than in control subjects. This raises the possibility of a genetic tool to assess an individual's risk of thoracic aortic dissection or thoracic aortic aneurysm by analysis of their DNA for specific single nucleotide polymorphism patterns.[3]

A recently characterised connective tissue disorder, known as Loeys–Dietz syndrome has features of premature, very aggressive, aortic aneurysm formation and aortic dissection. The syndrome shows autosomal dominant inheritance with variable clinical expression. Phenotypic features include aortic aneurysm, aortic dissection, widely spaced eyes (hypertelorism), bifid uvula or cleft palate or both, generalised arterial tortuosity and aneurysms throughout the arterial tree.[5]

Mutations in the gene encoding transforming growth factor beta (TGF-β) receptors 1 and 2 (TGFBR1 and TGFBR2) have been identified and are believed to cause the Loeys–Dietz syndrome phenotype. The alteration in TGFBR1 and TGFBR2 leads to increased production of the cytokine TGF-β in blood vessels. This, in turn, leads to excessive production of collagen, reduction of elastin and disorganisation of elastic fibres. Although there are some similarities with other connective tissue disorders (such as Marfan syndrome), patients with Loeys–Dietz syndrome demonstrate marked genotypic and phenotypic features. Early clinical experience demonstrates that Loeys–Dietz syndrome is a highly lethal condition with aggressive formation of aneurysms throughout the arterial tree and a marked tendency to rupture and dissection at a younger age and at smaller aortic dimensions than other connective tissue disorders. Early recognition and meticulous surveillance with prophylactic interventions at an early stage are warranted. Careful, life-long follow-up is also mandatory.[5,6]

NATURAL HISTORY OF THORACIC AORTIC ANEURYSMS

Although considerable literature exists with regard to the surgical treatment options in the management of thoracic aortic disease, high-quality scientific evidence to support clinical decision making in aortic surgery is relatively new. Evidence has now accumulated to demonstrate clearly the lethal nature of thoracic aortic aneurysmal disease and to inform decisions on surgical management.

Growth rates of thoracic aortic aneurysms average 0.1 cm per year (0.07 cm for ascending aorta and 0.19 cm for descending aorta). The yearly event rates for a patient with an aortic aneurysm of 6 cm or over include a risk of rupture of 3.7% and risk of rupture or dissection of 6.9% per year. The risk of death, rupture or dissection is 15.6% per year. Elective surgical repair prior to aortic catastrophe restores life expectancy.[7] More recently, a new measurement, aortic size index (ASI), has been developed which takes into account patient size in addition to aortic size, in estimating risk of aortic complications. Aortic size index equals aortic diameter (cm) divided by body surface area (m^2). Using ASI, three categories of risk have been identified. Patients with ASI less than 2.75 cm/m^2 have a low risk of rupture, dissection or death (yearly incidence of 4%). Those with an ASI of 2.75–4.25 cm/m^2 are at moderate risk of approximately 8% a year. Those with an ASI greater than 4.25 cm/m^2 have a yearly rate of rupture, dissection or death as high as 20–25%. This work supports the view that most patients benefit from aortic repair before the aorta reaches a diameter of 6 cm; however, surgical intervention may be justified in smaller patients with aortic diameters which are significantly smaller.[8]

AORTIC ROOT SURGERY

For patients with disease of the aortic valve and the aortic root, replacement of the aortic root and valve with a composite valved graft has become the standard procedure. In this operation, a valve prosthesis (most frequently a mechanical valve) attached to a tube of woven Dacron is implanted and the coronary arteries are re-implanted into the side of the graft with buttons of aortic wall. Successful surgery treats the valve disease and eliminates the risk of rupture, dissection or death as a result of proximal aortic aneurysm. Experienced centres expect to perform the procedure with a 30-day mortality of less than 5% and excellent long-term survival has been demonstrated.[9–11] There are, however, situations in which a mechanical valve with life-long requirement of warfarin is less attractive. Other options which are available include replacement of aortic root with homograft incorporating donor aortic valve and proximal aorta and a Ross procedure (pulmonary autograft). Issues such as limited availability of homografts and procedure complexity associated with the Ross procedure restrict the wide-spread application of these techniques. For a significant number of patients who require aortic root replacement, a tissue valve is preferable to a mechanical prosthesis, particularly with respect to anticoagulation with warfarin. Composite aortic root replacement has been performed with a bovine pericardial stented tissue valve and a Dacron tube graft. The conduit is constructed intra-operatively after excision of the native aortic valve. This allows patients, particularly the elderly and those intolerant of anticoagulants, to have aortic root replacement with the known advantages of a tissue valve.[12,13] Excellent intra-operative and long-term results have been demonstrated with this technique. In a consecutive series of 275 cases, re-operation for valve failure occurred in only 1 patient, at 12 years' postoperatively.[13] A biological valved conduit is now available which is constructed in a range of sizes and incorporates a stentless porcine tissue valve and a new trilaminate material conduit. The tube graft component is constructed in such a way as to replicate the sinuses of Valsalva to closely match aortic root anatomy (Biovalsalva Porcine Aortic Valved Conduit; Vascutek, Inchinnan, Renfrewshire, UK).

VALVE-SPARING AORTIC ROOT REPLACEMENT

While aortic root replacement with a composite valved graft (usually incorporating a mechanical valve) remains the gold standard for management of aortic root pathology, newer alternative strategies have been proposed. In order to avoid the well-recognised problems of life-long anticoagulant therapy, thrombo-embolism and prosthetic valve endocarditis, 'valve-sparing', aortic root replacement procedures have been described. Two techniques aim to achieve this – 'remodelling', developed by Sir Magdi Yacoub and 're-implantation' by Tirone David.[14] The remodelling method uses a tube graft tailored to replace each of the aortic sinuses. The re-implantation method replaces the entire aortic root within a Dacron tube graft. Excellent short- and mid-term results have been demonstrated in experienced centres.[15,16] There has been concern as to whether these techniques will be applicable to patients with Marfan syndrome in view of the known issue of fibrillin fragmentation and deterioration in aortic valve leaflets and the potential for early postoperative valve failure. Evidence has, however, accumulated to suggest that valve-sparing, aortic root replacement, particularly the re-implantation method, is associated with good early and mid-term results.[15–17] These techniques have grown in popularity in recent years particularly as a result of patient demand. It should, however, be remembered that these are technically demanding operations and that, although excellent survival at 10 years has been demonstrated, there are still issues of recurrent aortic regurgitation with a number of re-operations for aortic valve failure.[14,15]

THE ROSS PROCEDURE (PULMONARY AUTOGRAFT)

Replacement of diseased aortic valve by pulmonary autograft and replacement of the pulmonary valve with a homograft, introduced by Donald Ross in 1967, has been associated with excellent haemodynamic function and with low morbidity and mortality rates.[18] Advantages identified for this operation include excellent haemodynamic profile (particularly under exercise), low risk of endocarditis, low risk of thrombo-embolism without the need for anticoagulation and a potential for growth of the aortic valve substitute in children.[18–20] These advantages are particularly relevant in the setting of children or young adults, particularly women of child-bearing age. Disadvantages include the complexity of the operation which incorporates a double valve solution to a single valve problem and the relatively unknown long-term fate of the pulmonary homograft and the aortic pulmonary autograft.[18] Evidence is steadily accumulating, however, that the procedure can be performed with acceptable mortality figures. A number of reports of low peri-operative mortality (1.8% or less) have been published with excellent long-term outcomes.[18–20] With respect to the long-term fate of the pulmonary autograft, it is now apparent that the re-operation rate for autograft failure is extremely low.[18–20] The long-term durability of the homograft with respect to the pulmonary valve is less certain, particularly in children and young adults.[19] The limited availability and durability of valved homografts for use in reconstruction of the right ventricular outflow tract including during the Ross procedure has led to the introduction of the Contegra Bovine Jugular Vein Conduit. This commercially available product incorporates a naturally integrated trileaflet valve. This conduit is available 'off-the-shelf' and has been associated with good results in 5-year follow-up.[21]

A recent development of considerable interest is the use of the tissue-engineered pulmonary valve to reconstruct the right ventricular outflow tract during the Ross procedure. Several weeks prior to the Ross procedure, the autologous vein is harvested and endothelial cells harvested and expanded in a tissue laboratory. A homograft or xenograft is next decellularised and used as a scaffold onto which the endothelial cells are seeded. The tissue-engineered heart valve is then available for implantation. In Ross procedure patients, these have shown excellent haemodynamic performance during mid-term follow-up. It is hoped that tissue degeneration will be prevented leading to improved valve durability.[22]

AORTIC ARCH SURGERY

Procedures to replace the aortic arch are associated with a significant risk of mortality and morbidity, particularly neurological deficit. There have been a number of improvements in technique which have been associated with better surgical outcome. Although a debate continues with regard to the role of deep hypothermic circulatory arrest (DHCA) at core temperatures of 15—18°C, this is still the most frequently used form of cerebral protection. Most authorities would except that the 'safe' period of deep hypothermic circulatory arrest alone is limited to 25–30 min.[23,24] Cerebral perfusion has long been considered an important adjunct in cerebral protection during DHCA for aortic arch surgery. Retrograde cerebral perfusion involves increasing the pressure within the superior vena cava. In theory, such retrograde cerebral perfusion helps to maintain intracranial hypothermia, flush out particulate matter from the aortic arch, reduce the embolic load and provide metabolic support. More recently, clinical randomised controlled trials have failed to demonstrate any benefit in terms of cerebral metabolism, neurological or neuropsychological outcomes with retrograde cerebral perfusion.[23] Selective antegrade cerebral perfusion (SACP) is now the most widely applied adjunct to DHCA in aortic arch surgery. In recent years, a variety of methods have been described in which some or all of the head and neck vessels are cannulated and perfused during the period of DHCA. One approach is to cannulate the right axillary artery as a means of perfusing the innominate artery and thus the right common carotid artery.[25] This technique may reduce the possibility of embolism from cannulation of the ascending aorta and arch vessels. However, in 15% of patients the circle of Willis is incomplete and a separate cannula is required for perfusion of the left common carotid in order to ensure adequate cerebral perfusion.[23] Excellent outcomes in terms of mortality and neurological morbidity have been demonstrated in several large series.[23]

ACUTE AORTIC DISSECTION

Acute aortic dissection is the most common aortic emergency and has a highly lethal natural history. Acute type A aortic dissection is associated with mortality of 1–3% per hour, 25% of patients are dead within 24 h, 70% by 1 week and 80% by 2 weeks. Rapid and accurate diagnosis is crucial in the management of these patients. The diagnosis is not made initially in up to 38% of patients on presentation.[26] The most useful means of confirming the diagnosis of acute aortic dissection are computerised tomography (CT), magnetic resonance imaging (MRI) and transoesophageal echocardiography (TOE). CT scanning is the most widely available initial investigation and has a reported sensitivity of 83–94% and specificity of 87–100%.[26] Potential disadvantages include the use of intravenous contrast and the relative isolation of a potentially unstable patient in the radiology department. MRI scanning, although particularly sensitive and specific for aortic dissection, is less widely available and tends not to be used in the acute setting.

TOE has a reported sensitivity of 98% and specificity of 95%; it provides valuable additional information such as:

1. The site and extent of dissection.
2. Presence of thrombus in the false lumen.
3. Location of entry and re-entry sites.
4. Involvement and patency of aortic branches, *e.g.* coronary arteries.
5. Severity and mechanism of aortic regurgitation.
6. Left ventricular function, particularly wall motion abnormalities.
7. Pleural and pericardial fluid and cardiac tamponade.[26]

It should be noted, however, that TOE is an invasive investigation and general anaesthesia or adequate sedation is of particular importance in the setting of acute aortic dissection.

The International Registry of Acute Aortic Dissection (IRAD) offers an opportunity to examine the outcomes of a large group of consecutive patients managed by 18 large referral centres world-wide. In spite of considerable advances in medical and surgical treatments, proximal aortic dissection in experienced IRAD centres is associated with a 25% mortality.[27] Attempts to improve outcomes have included an analysis of pre-operative variables and careful assessment of likely operative risk. A predictive score has been reported which aims to assist surgeons in the decision-making progress with respect to operative management in patients who present in extreme clinical conditions.[28] Further evidence has accumulated in relation to the management of specific subsets of patients with acute aortic dissection. There has been controversy with regard to the timing and sequence of interventions in patients with significant peripheral (non-coronary) malperfusion syndromes. Data now suggest that in acute type A aortic dissection, immediate aortic reconstruction should be performed as the primary procedure. Early postoperative intervention (*e.g.* percutaneous fenestration and stenting of peripheral vessels) is then recommended for persistent malperfusion.[29]

Another area of interest concerns the indications for extended aortic arch replacement in Marfan patients with acute aortic dissection. There are clear guidelines with regard to replacement of the aortic root in the elective setting for Marfan patients with aortic root aneurysms. These patients have a low risk of subsequent requirement for aortic arch replacement; in contrast, Marfan patients presenting with acute type A aortic dissection are very likely to require aortic arch replacement subsequently.[30] A number of reports of extended arch replacement at the time of acute aortic dissection repair have demonstrated acceptable outcomes.[31,32] This has encouraged a move towards more aggressive aortic arch replacement in acute type A aortic dissection in patients with Marfan syndrome.

With regard to the postoperative, long-term follow-up of patients who have undergone surgical repair of acute type A aortic dissection, recent evidence clearly supports meticulous attention to detail. Life-long follow-up is necessary with very careful blood pressure control (ideally maintaining systolic blood pressure less than 120 mmHg), β-blocker therapy regardless of blood pressure effect and life-long imaging (since as aortic enlargement may occur more than 10 years postoperatively).[33]

ENDOVASCULAR AORTIC REPAIR

The first endovascular stent graft repair of an aortic aneurysm (EVAR) was performed in Argentina by Parodi and colleagues in 1990.[34] Since then with improved technology, endovascular stent grafting is becoming the procedure of choice for descending thoracic aortic and abdominal aortic aneurysms.[35] Traditionally, these were both previously treated by open surgical repair.

The endovascular stent grafts commonly used consist of metal fixation stents which are attached to a fabric graft, thus excluding flow through the true aortic lumen over the length of the stent graft. The metal stents are usually made of Nitinol (nickel–titanium alloy) while the fabric of the graft is made of either polytetrafluoroethylene (PTFE) or a polyester fabric. The stent graft is loaded within an introducer sheath and usually introduced via formal arteriotomies of the common femoral arteries.

Stent grafts have been widely used in the treatment of thoracic aortic aneurysms of the descending thoracic aorta and in the treatment of aortic trans-sections; also, they are being used, at times, in Stanford type B aortic dissections. Further indications include the treatment of penetrating ulcers and intramural haematomas which are believed to be at risk of rupture. Treatment of aortobronchial fistulae with aortic stent grafts is also well recognised. Patients being considered for a stent graft placement will have a CT scan to assess the extent of the disease and measure the thoracic aorta to choose an appropriately sized device.

Descending thoracic aortic aneurysms (DTAs) have the same predisposing factors and occur in a similar age group to abdominal aortic aneurysms (AAAs). DTA is, however, far less common than AAA. The primary goal of aneurysm treatment is to prevent aneurysm-related deaths.

The first endovascular repair of a thoracic aneurysm (TEVAR) was performed in 1994.[36] Since then, several studies have been performed comparing TEVAR with open surgical repair.

A review of the literature on open surgical repair of DTA shows an overall operative mortality of 8.8%, renal failure in 5.3% and paraplegia in 3.7%.[37]

Technical procedural success rates with thoracic aortic stent grafting are in the region of 98%.[37] Endoleaks seen during the deployment of the stent grafts have to be characterised. Type 1 and type 3 endoleaks increase the aneurysm rupture risk. These are treated aggressively at the time of the implantation with either balloon dilatation and/or the placement of additional stent grafts being placed with sufficient overlap between individual components. Type 2 endoleaks in the presence of a growing aneurysm sac may require occlusion either via percutaneous embolisation or open surgical ligation.

The GORE TAG Phase II Trial (a multicentre, prospective non-randomised trial) compared TEVAR with open surgery controls (140 TEVAR and 94 open surgical).[37] This showed an operative mortality of 2% in the TEVAR group and 12% ($P = 0.01$) in the open surgical group. Paraplegia rates of 3% and 14% ($P = 0.01$) were seen in the two groups, while strokes occurred in 4% of both groups.

Major adverse events at 30 days were 28% for TEVAR and 70% for open surgery ($P = 0.0001$). This included major bleeding (11% versus 54%), major pulmonary complications (13% versus 38%) and major vascular complications (18% versus 6%).

Mean blood loss was 250 ml versus 1850 ml, mean hospital stay was 3 days versus 10 days and return to normal activities was 30 days versus 78 days.

TEVARs require continuous interval follow-up imaging mainly by CT scanning. This is to monitor the size of the thoracic aortic aneurysm sac, detect any endoleaks present and assess whether there has been any migration of the devices.[36] Further procedures to treat or prevent endoleaks are sometimes required. In the GORE TAG Phase II Trial, re-intervention was performed in 3.6% of cases.

The trial concluded that TEVAR significantly improved the early treatment results of DTA compared to open thoracotomy. Aneurysm-related mortality improved but no long-term survival advantage is expected. Re-intervention rates were similar between the two groups. Shorter in-hospital stay and earlier return to normal activities were seen with TEVAR.

Ancillary surgical procedures with the formation of extra-anatomical arterial bypasses of the great vessels of the aortic arch have allowed endovascular stent grafts to be placed within the ascending thoracic aorta and the aortic arch. These combined open surgical and endovascular techniques have increased the spectrum of diseases which can be treated. Similarly, extra-anatomical visceral arterial bypasses have allowed thoraco-abdominal aneurysms to be treated with a similar combined approach.

Newer endovascular stent grafts with branches have been used in specialised centres in the treatment of thoraco-abdominal aneurysms and in cases of aneurysms involving the aortic arch. With continued improvements in technology, there will undoubtedly be increased treatment of thoracic aortic disease by TEVAR with improved long-term durability.

References

1. Koullias GJ, Ravichandran P, Korkolis DP, Rimm DL, Elefteriades JA. Increased tissue microarray matrix metalloproteinase expression favors proteolysis in thoracic aortic aneurysms and dissections. *Ann Thorac Surg* 2004; **78**: 2106–2111.

Key points for clinical practice

- Thoracic aortic disease is a highly lethal condition. The natural history of aortic aneurysm and aortic dissection has been established. Clear guidelines exist with respect to indications for surgical intervention.

- The genetic aspects of aortic disease are being characterised and are likely to play a greater role in coming years.

- Valve-sparing aortic root replacement and new prostheses aim to improve the outlook for patients with aortic root disease.

- The Ross procedure (pulmonary autograft) provides an excellent aortic root substitute for children and young adults. Tissue-engineered heart valves offer the prospect of increased durability of the procedure.

- Aortic arch surgery has been refined and is now associated with excellent early outcomes.

- Acute aortic dissection remains a major problem with high morbidity and mortality. A high index of suspicion is required. Life-long follow-up with strict blood pressure control, β-blocker therapy and imaging of aorta is essential for all patients following successful surgical repair.

- Thoracic endovascular aortic repair (TEVAR) is an evolving technology which offers the prospect of less invasive means of treating thoracic aortic disease.

2. Boyum J, Fellinger EK, Schmoker JD et al. Matrix metalloproteinase activity in thoracic aortic aneurysms associated with bicuspid and tricuspid aortic valves. J Thorac Cardiovasc Surg 2004; 127: 686–691.
3. Chen L, Wang X, Carter SA et al. A single nucleotide polymorphism in the matrix metalloproteinase 9 gene (–8202A/G) is associated with thoracic aortic aneurysms and thoracic aortic dissection. J Thorac Cardiovasc Surg 2006; 131: 1045–1052.
4. Aicher D, Urbich C, Zeiher A, Dimmeler S, Schäfers H-J. Endothelial nitric oxide synthase in bicuspid aortic valve disease. Ann Thorac Surg 2007; 83: 1290–1204.
5. Williams JA, Loeys BL, Nwakanma LU et al. Early surgical experience with Loeys–Dietz: a new syndrome of aggressive thoracic aortic aneurysm disease. Ann Thorac Surg 2007; 83: s757–s763.
6. Lee RS, Fazel S, Schwarze U et al. Rapid aneurysmal degeneration of a Stanford type B aortic dissection in a patient with Loeys–Dietz syndrome. J Thorac Cardiovasc Surg 2007; 134: 242–243.
7. Davies RR, Goldstein LJ, Coady MA et al. Yearly rupture or dissection rates for thoracic aortic aneurysms: simple prediction based on size. Ann Thorac Surg 2002; 73: 17–28.
8. Davies RR, Gallo A, Coady MA et al. Novel measurement of relative aortic size predicts rupture of thoracic aortic aneurysms. Ann Thorac Surg 2006; 81: 169–177.
9. Etz CD, Homann TM, Silovitz D et al. Long-term survival after the Bentall procedure in 206 patients with bicuspid aortic valve. Ann Thorac Surg 2007; 84: 1186–1194.
10. Hagl C, Strauch JT, Spielvogel D et al. Is the Bentall procedure for ascending aorta or aortic valve replacement the best approach for long-term event-free survival. Ann Thorac Surg 2003; 76: 698–703.
11. Gott VL, Cameron DE, Alejo DE et al. Aortic root replacement in 271 Marfan patients: a 24-year experience. Ann Thorac Surg 2002; 73: 438–443.
12. Hilgenberg AD, Mora BN. Composite aortic root replacement with a bovine pericardial valve conduit. Ann Thorac Surg 2003; 75: 1338–1339.
13. Etz CD, Homann TM, Rane N et al. Aortic root reconstruction with a bioprosthetic valved conduit: a consecutive series of 275 procedures. J Thorac Cardiovasc Surg 2007; 133: 1455–1463.
14. Miller DC. Valve-sparing aortic root replacement: current state of the art and where are

we headed? *Ann Thorac Surg* 2007; **83**: s736–s739.

15. David TE, Feindel CM, Webb GD, Colman JM, Armstrong S, Maganti M. Long-term results of aortic valve-sparing operations for aortic root aneurysm. *J Thorac Cardiovasc Surg* 2006; **132**: 347–354.

16. Kallenbach K, Baraki H, Khaladj N *et al*. Aortic valve-sparing operation in Marfan syndrome: what do we know after a decade? *Ann Thorac Surg* 2007; **83**: s764–s768.

17. Settepani F, Szeto WY, Pacini D *et al*. Reimplantation valve-sparing aortic root replacement in Marfan syndrome using the Valsalva conduit: an intercontinental multicenter study. *Ann Thorac Surg* 2007; **83**: s769–s773.

18. Chiappini B, Absil B, Rubay J *et al*. The Ross procedure: clinical and echocardiographic follow-up in 219 consecutive patients. *Ann Thorac Surg* 2007; **83**: 1285–1289.

19. Böhm JO, Botha CA, Horke A *et al*. Is the Ross operation still an acceptable option in children and adolescents? *Ann Thorac Surg* 2006; **82**: 940–947.

20. Böhm JO, Botha CA, Hemmer W *et al*. Older patients fare better with the Ross operation. *Ann Thorac Surg* 2003; **75**: 796–802.

21. Sekarski N, van Meir H, Rijlaarsdam MEB *et al*. Right ventricular outflow tract reconstruction with the bovine jugular vein graft: 5 years' experience with 133 patients. *Ann Thorac Surg* 2007; **84**: 599–605.

22. Dohmen PM, Lembcke A, Holinski S *et al*. Mid-term clinical results using a tissue-engineered pulmonary valve to reconstruct the right ventricular outflow tract during the Ross procedure. *Ann Thorac Surg* 2007; **84**: 729–736.

23. Harrington DK, Fragomeni F, Bonser RS. Cerebral perfusion. *Ann Thorac Surg* 2007; **83**: s799–s804.

24. Griepp RB, Bonser R, Haverich A *et al*. Panel discussion: Session II – Aortic Arch. *Ann Thorac Surg* 2007; **83**: s824–s831.

25. Strauch JT, Spielvogel D, Lauten A *et al*. Axillary artery cannulation: routine use in ascending aorta and aortic arch replacement. *Ann Thorac Surg* 2004; **78**: 103–108.

26. Matalanis G. Acute aortic dissection: how to confirm the diagnosis? *Heart Lung Circ* 2004; **13**: 127–128.

27. Trimarchi S, Nienaber CA, Rampoldi V *et al*. Contemporary results of surgery in acute type A aortic dissection: The International Registry of Acute Aortic Dissection experience. *J Thorac Cardiovasc Surg* 2005; **129**: 112–122.

28. Rampoldi V, Trimarchi S, Eagle KA *et al*. Simple risk models to predict surgical mortality in acute type A aortic dissection: The International Registry of Acute Aortic Dissection Score. *Ann Thorac Surg* 2007; **83**: 55–61.

29. Girardi LN, Krieger KH, Lee LY, Mack CA, Tortolani AJ, Isom OW. Management strategies for type A dissection complicated by peripheral vascular malperfusion. *Ann Thorac Surg* 2004; **77**: 1309–1314.

30. Bachet J, Larrazet F, Goudot B *et al*. When should the aortic arch be replaced in Marfan patients? *Ann Thorac Surg* 2007; **83**: s774–s779.

31. Urbanski PP, Siebel A, Zacher M, Hacker RW. Is extended aortic replacement in acute type A dissection justifiable? *Ann Thorac Surg* 2003; **75**: 525–529.

32. Tan MESH, Dossche KME, Morshuis WJ, Kelder JC, Waanders FGJ, Schepens MAAM. Is extended arch replacement for acute type a aortic dissection an additional risk factor for mortality? *Ann Thorac Surg* 2003; **76**: 1209–1214.

33. Zierer A, Voeller RK, Hill KE *et al*. Aortic enlargement and late reoperation after repair of acute type A aortic dissection. *Ann Thorac Surg* 2007; **84**: 479–487.

34. Parodi JC, Palmaz JC, Barone HD. Transfemoral intraluminal graft implantation for abdominal aortic aneurysms. *Ann Thorac Surg* 1991; **5**: 491–499.

35. Greenberg RK, O'Neill S, Walker E *et al*. Endovascular repair of thoracic aortic lesions with the Zenith TX1 and TX2 thoracic grafts: intermediate-term results. *J Vasc Surg* 2005; **41**: 589–596.

36. Dake MD, Miller DC, Semba CP, Mitchell RS, Walker PJ, Liddell RP. Transluminal placement of endovascular stent-grafts for the treatment of descending thoracic aortic aneurysms. *N Engl J Med* 1994; **331**: 1729–1724.

37. Makaroun MS, Dillavou ED, Kee ST *et al*. Endovascular treatment of thoracic aortic aneurysms: Results of the phase II multicenter trial of the GORE TAG thoracic endoprosthesis. *J Vasc Surg* 2005; **41**: 1–9.

Glossary

AAC abdominal aortic calcification

ACAS Asymptomatic Carotid Atherosclerosis Study

ACC American College of Cardiology

ACE angiotensin-converting enzyme

ACHD adults with congenital heart disease

AdSPC activated, synthetic pacemaker channel

AHA American Heart Association

AICD automated implantable cardioverter–defibrillator

AP action potential

Apo apolipoprotein

ARC Academic Research Consortium

ARVC arrhythmogenic right ventricular cardiomyopathy

ARVD arrhythmogenic right ventricular dysplasia

ASI aortic size index

AVR aortic valve replacement

BARI bypass angioplasty revascularization investigation

BMS bare metal stenting

CABG coronary artery bypass grafting

CAC coronary artery calcium

CAD coronary artery disease

CAPTIM Comparison of Angioplasty and Pre-hospitalThrombolysis in acute Myocardial
    infarction

CARP coronary artery revascularization prophylaxis

CAS carotid artery stenosis

CASS Coronary Artery Surgery Study registry

CCU coronary care unit

CHD coronary heart disease

CHF congestive heart failure

CI confidence interval

CMR cardiovascular magnetic resonance

COMMIT Clopidogrel and Metoprolol in Myocardial Infarction Trial

COX cyclo-oxygenase

CREDO Clopidogrel for the reduction of events during observation

CURE Clopidogrel in Unstable angina to prevent Recurrent Events study

CVA cerebrovascular accident
CVC calcifying vascular cells
CVD cardiovascular disease
DES drug-eluting stents
DHCA deep hypothermic circulatory arrest
DSE dobutamine stress echocardiography
DTAs descending thoracic aortic aneurysms
EBCT electron beam CT
ECM extracellular matrix
EGIR European Group for the Study of Insulin Resistance
ERS early repolarisation syndrome
ERV early repolarisation variant
ESC European Society of Cardiology
ESPRIT European/Australasian Stroke Prevention In Reversible Ischaemia Trial
ESPS-2 European Stroke Prevention Study
ESRD end-stage renal disease
EVAR endovascular aortic repair
FDA Food and Drug Administration
GITS gastrointestinal therapeutic system
GRACE Global Registry of Acute Coronary Events/Syndromes
HCM hypertrophic cardiomyopathy
hESCs human embryonic stem cells
hMSCs human mesenchymal stem cells
HR hazard ratio
IART intra-atrial re-entrant tachycardia
IHT inter-hospital transfer
INSIGHT International Nifedipine once daily Study Intervention as a Goal in Hypertension
    Treatment
IRAD International Registry of Acute Aortic Dissection
IVUS intravascular ultrasonography
LACS small vessel events, the so-called lacunar strokes
LAD left anterior descending
LAS London Ambulance Service
LBBB left bundle branch block
LOS length of stay
LQTS long QT syndrome
LVADs left ventricular assist devices
LVOT left ventricular outflow tract obstruction
MACE major adverse coronary events
MATCH Management of ATherothrombosis with Clopidogrel in High-risk patients
MDCT multirow detector computed tomography
METs metabolic equivalents
MGP matrix gla protein
MI myocardial infarction
MMPs matrix metalloproteinases
MRI magnetic resonance imaging
NASCET North American Symptomatic Carotid Endarterectomy Trial
NCEP National Cholesterol Education Program
NHANES National Health and Nutrition Examination Survey
NRVM neonatal rat ventricular myocytes
OCSP Oxfordshire Community Stroke Project
OPG osteoprotegerin
OXVASC Oxford Vascular Study

PACS partial anterior circulation stroke
PAR protease-activated receptor
PCI percutaneous coronary interventions
PCT Primary Care Trust
PDU pump drive unit
PES paclitaxel-eluting stent
PGI2 prostacyclin
POCS posterior circulation stroke
POISE Perioperative Ischemia Evaluation trial
PPCI primary percutaneous coronary intervention
PRAGUE Primary Angioplasty in patients transferred from General community hospitals to
    specialized PTCA Units with or without Emergency thrombolysis
PVAD paracorporeal ventricular assist device
PVAD pneumatic ventricular assist device
RANK receptor activator of nuclear factor kappa-B
RANK-L receptor activator of nuclear factor kappa-B-ligand
RBBB right bundle branch block
RCRI Revised Cardiac Risk Index
RCTs randomised, clinical trials
REACH Reduction of Atherothrombosis for Continued Health
REMATCH Randomised Evaluation of Mechanical Assistance for the Treatment of Congestive
    Heart failure
RR relative risk
RRR relative risk reduction
SCAAR Swedish Coronary Angiography and Angioplasty Registry
SES sirolimus-eluting stent
SMCs smooth muscle cells
ST stent thrombosis
statins HMG-CoA reductase inhibitors
STEMI ST segment elevation myocardial infarction
SVG saphenous vein graft
SVT supraventricular tachycardias
TACS total anterior circulation stroke
TCPC total cavopulmonary connection
TCT transcatheter cardiovascular therapeutics
TEVAR thoracic endovascular aortic repair
TGF transforming growth factor
TGF-β transforming growth factor-beta
TIA transient ischaemic attack
TIMPs tissue inhibitor of metalloproteinases
TLR target lesion revascularisation
TOE transoesophageal echocardiography
TxA_2 thromboxane A_2
UKPDS United Kingdom Prospective Study
VAD ventricular assist device
VC vascular calcification
VCAF vascular calcification associated factor
VSMCs vascular smooth muscle cells
VT ventricular tachycardia
WHO World Health Organization

Index